The baby names almanac

2019

Emily Larson

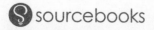

sourcebooks

Published by Sourcebooks, Inc.
P.O. Box 4410, Naperville, Illinois 60567-4410
(630) 961-3900
Fax: (630) 961-2168
sourcebooks.com

Ninth Edition

Printed and bound in the United States of America.
BVG 10 9 8 7 6 5 4 3 2 1

Contents

So, you've got a baby to name.

As if preparing for the arrival of the baby isn't enough, you're dealing with all the pressure of figuring out what, exactly, to call the little bundle of joy. It can be stressful to find a name that will do justice to the hope you have for your child.

After all, names influence first impressions. They can trigger great—or unpleasant—nicknames. They can affect your child's self-esteem. They can be a tangible, lasting link to a family legacy. But let's not forget that they can be fun. And that's what this book is all about.

Remember *The Old Farmer's Almanac*, which comes out annually as a guide to each year's trends, forecasts, and hot spots? Aimed at farmers, of course, the book provides a way to put the year into context, to navigate the shifting seasons, and to understand all the factors swirling in the atmosphere.

The 2019 Baby Names Almanac aims to be a similar lifeline for parents. With a finger on the pulse of pop culture and an ear to the ground of what's hip, new, and relevant, this book offers you an instant, idiosyncratic snapshot of how the world today is shaping what you may want to name your child tomorrow.

Jam-packed with information and ideas, plus thousands of names to browse, this book analyzes the most recent trends and fads in baby naming, offering up forecasts and predictions. You'll find our take on questions like these (and much more!):

- Which cutting-edge names are on the rise?
- Which popular names are on the decline?
- What influence do celebrities have on names?

- *Names in music:* Will your child be **Alessia** or **Hendrix**?
- *Names in entertainment:* Will **Marvel** or **Storm** be in your child's kindergarten class? Or will you see more Game of Thrones–inspired kids?
- *Names in current events*: Will royal names like **Harry** and **Meghan** inspire outside of Kensington Palace? Or will **Royalty** and **King** rule?
- How many babies get the most popular name, anyway?
- Which letter do most girls' names start with? How about boys' names?
- What are the most popular "gender-neutral" names today—and which gender uses each name more often? (If you name your daughter **Sawyer**, will she find herself playing with lots of other little girls named **Sawyer**—or little boys instead?)
- How can you take a trend and turn it into a name you love? (How about a little **Birdie** of your own?)

We understand that sometimes this information on trends and popularity is hard to digest, so we've created some easy-to-visualize graphics. Turn to page 4, for example, to see a map of the United States showing where **Emma** reigns and where little **Liam** is king.

And what baby name book would be complete without the names? Flip to page 69 to begin browsing through more than 20,000 names, including entries for the most popular names for girls and boys as reported by the most recent, complete data set from the Social Security Administration (www.ssa.gov/OACT/babynames).[1]

A little bit of a mishmash and a screenshot of the world today, *The 2019 Baby Names Almanac* is like no other book out there. Stuffed with ideas on what's hip and hot and how you can take a trend and turn it into a name you love, this book is your all-in-one guide to baby names now.

---

1 *Due to the Social Security Administration data collection cycle, the most complete dataset currently available is from the full 2017 calendar year.*

The Top 10

Let's start with the most popular names in the country. Ranked by the Social Security Administration (SSA), these names are released around Mother's Day each year. (The top 10 names get the most attention, but you may also hear about the top 100. The total number of names widely reported is 1,000.) In 2017 the top 10 names were similar to—but not identical to—the top 10 for 2016. For example, **Emma** and **Olivia** remained the top two choices for girls, but **Isabella** replaced **Sophia** for the number 4 spot beneath number 3, **Ava**. The boys' list was just as stable, though **Liam** unseated **Noah** to claim the top spot this year, and both **Logan** and **Oliver** (on the boys' side) were new additions to the top 10 list. Here's a quick comparison of 2016 and 2017:

2016 Girls	2017 Girls	2016 Boys	2017 Boys
1. Emma	1. Emma	1. Noah	1. Liam
2. Olivia	2. Olivia	2. Liam	2. Noah
3. Ava	3. Ava	3. William	3. William
4. Sophia	4. Isabella	4. Mason	4. James
5. Isabella	5. Sophia	5. James	5. Logan
6. Mia	6. Mia	6. Benjamin	6. Benjamin
7. Charlotte	7. Charlotte	7. Jacob	7. Mason
8. Abigail	8. Amelia	8. Michael	8. Elijah
9. Emily	9. Evelyn	9. Elijah	9. Oliver
10. Harper	10. Abigail	10. Ethan	10. Jacob

Just How Many Emmas Are There, Anyway?

Sure, these names are popular, but what does that mean? Well, it seems that new parents are increasingly looking for off-the-beaten-path names for their little ones, and it shows. According to the SSA, the top 1,000 names represent about 73 percent of all babies born and named in the United States in 2017—a significant drop from the 77.84 percent recorded in 2000.

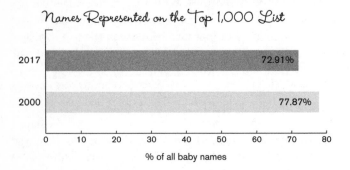

Names Represented on the Top 1,000 List

Year	% of all baby names
2017	72.91%
2000	77.87%

Although parents of either gender have always been looking beyond the top 1,000, parents of boys are more likely to pick a name in that mix—77.91 percent of boys' names are represented on the top 1,000 list, while only 67.66 percent of girls' names are.

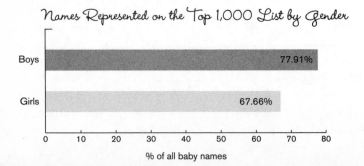

Names Represented on the Top 1,000 List by Gender

Gender	% of all baby names
Boys	77.91%
Girls	67.66%

Plus, although it may seem like you know a zillion people with daughters named **Emma** or **Olivia**, the most popular names are actually bestowed upon a relatively small number of babies each year. For example, in 2017 only 0.9539 percent of all male babies born in the United States (that's 18,728 little guys total) got the most popular name, **Liam**. There are slightly more girls (19,738) with the most popular name, **Emma**, but even that's only 1.0528 percent of all girls born. Only a fifth of the **Noah** total—3,907 babies—were given the 100th most popular name, **Jameson**.

Mary, Mary Quite Contrary

Mary has been the most popular girls' name in the last 100 years, with 3.4 million babies given the name since 1918. For boys, **James** reigns, with about 4.8 million name-sakes in the last century.

The number of babies with the number one name is dropping swiftly—back in 1999, when **Jacob** first hit number one, more than 35,000 boys got that name, which is over 16,000 more babies than got the top boys' name, **Liam**, in 2017. And back in 1970, 4.48 percent of all male babies (a staggering 85,298 tots) were named **Michael**, the most popular name of that year. So if you've got your heart set on naming your son **Noah** but you're worried that he'll be surrounded by Noahs wherever he goes, take heart!

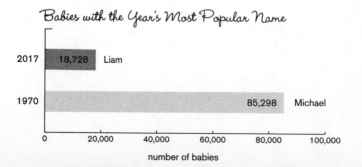

Babies with the Year's Most Popular Name

2017	18,728	Liam
1970	85,298	Michael

0   20,000   40,000   60,000   80,000   100,000

number of babies

What's Popular in My State?

It's interesting to see how some names are more popular in certain states than in others. For example, **Chloe** ranks 22nd nationally for girls, but in Hawaii, it's the fifth most popular name. Likewise, **Paisley** ranks fourth among Mississippi's baby girls, but only 45th in the nation. On the boys' side, **Santiago** was the second most popular name in New Mexico, but falls to number 93 across the country.

The following chart lists the top five names for girls and boys for each of the 50 states, and it also shows the actual number of births for each of those names in each state.

Top Five Names by State

State	Girl	Births	Boy	Births
Alabama	Ava	358	William	398
	Olivia	300	James	315
	Emma	240	Elijah	303
	Harper	192	John	297
	Amelia	190	Noah	252
Alaska	Emma	56	James	47
	Olivia	56	Liam	45
	Aurora	38	Wyatt	40
	Isabella	38	William	38
	Sophia	35	Noah	37
Arizona	Emma	446	Liam	404
	Isabella	400	Noah	380
	Olivia	394	Sebastian	344
	Mia	380	Alexander	329
	Sophia	374	Julian	298

State	Girl	Births	Boy	Births
Arkansas	Emma	176	Elijah	170
	Olivia	155	William	146
	Ava	150	Noah	142
	Harper	138	Liam	133
	Isabella	108	Mason	125
California	Emma	2,726	Noah	2,511
	Mia	2,588	Sebastian	2,264
	Olivia	2,474	Liam	2,180
	Sophia	2,430	Ethan	2,141
	Isabella	2,337	Matthew	2,120
Colorado	Emma	292	Liam	315
	Olivia	271	Oliver	297
	Charlotte	257	William	268
	Evelyn	252	Noah	267
	Isabella	246	Benjamin	253
Connecticut	Olivia	230	Noah	222
	Emma	219	Liam	208
	Ava	169	Logan	189
	Mia	162	Jacob	187
	Sophia	159	Michael	175
Delaware	Olivia	56	Logan	56
	Ava	55	Noah	55
	Charlotte	49	Liam	53
	Isabella	45	Mason	52
	Emma	44	Michael	49
District of Columbia	Ava	56	James	93
	Olivia	52	Henry	83
	Eleanor	51	William	80
	Genesis	41	Noah	76
	Elizabeth	39	Jacob	59

State	Girl	Births	Boy	Births
Florida	Isabella	1,306	Liam	1,352
	Emma	1,241	Noah	1,275
	Olivia	1,168	Lucas	1,030
	Sophia	1,057	Elijah	938
	Ava	1,019	Matthew	910
Georgia	Ava	667	William	685
	Olivia	569	Noah	609
	Emma	531	Mason	543
	Isabella	460	Elijah	522
	Charlotte	391	James	509
Hawaii	Emma	73	Liam	78
	Olivia	64	Noah	64
	Aria	51	Mason	60
	Ava	47	Elijah	56
	Chloe	46	Logan	55
Idaho	Emma	105	Oliver	115
	Olivia	96	Liam	99
	Charlotte	89	William	93
	Evelyn	88	James	83
	Harper	76	Mason	81
Illinois	Olivia	726	Noah	769
	Emma	701	Liam	662
	Ava	615	Benjamin	621
	Sophia	598	Logan	596
	Isabella	583	Alexander	583
Indiana	Emma	448	Oliver	386
	Olivia	391	Liam	384
	Amelia	352	Elijah	343
	Charlotte	342	Noah	337
	Harper	333	William	335

State	Girl	Births	Boy	Births
Iowa	Harper	173	Oliver	210
	Emma	170	Liam	180
	Olivia	166	Henry	179
	Charlotte	160	Lincoln	158
	Evelyn	155	Wyatt	153
Kansas	Emma	202	Oliver	170
	Olivia	182	William	160
	Ava	154	Liam	150
	Harper	151	Jackson	140
	Evelyn	144	Henry	139
Kentucky	Emma	290	William	302
	Ava	243	Elijah	283
	Olivia	236	Noah	275
	Harper	235	Liam	265
	Isabella	210	James	256
Louisiana	Olivia	296	Liam	253
	Ava	278	Noah	252
	Emma	228	Mason	246
	Amelia	195	Elijah	239
	Harper	187	William	228
Maine	Charlotte	89	Oliver	86
	Olivia	74	Lincoln	66
	Emma	70	Liam	62
	Harper	65	Owen	62
	Amelia	56	Wyatt	59
Maryland	Ava	341	Liam	341
	Olivia	283	Noah	297
	Emma	266	James	282
	Sophia	258	Logan	279
	Charlotte	220	Jacob	278

State	Girl	Births	Boy	Births
Massachusetts	Emma	393	Benjamin	492
	Olivia	379	William	421
	Charlotte	347	Liam	373
	Sophia	330	Lucas	373
	Isabella	294	Noah	365
Michigan	Emma	531	Liam	505
	Ava	526	Noah	476
	Olivia	505	Oliver	459
	Charlotte	421	Lucas	436
	Amelia	409	Mason	432
Minnesota	Olivia	310	Oliver	357
	Evelyn	307	William	343
	Emma	296	Henry	337
	Charlotte	259	Liam	299
	Nora	235	Theodore	264
Mississippi	Ava	211	William	180
	Emma	151	John	179
	Olivia	128	James	166
	Paisley	105	Mason	165
	Amelia	97	Elijah	157
Missouri	Olivia	367	William	345
	Ava	351	Liam	341
	Emma	341	Oliver	318
	Amelia	318	Noah	315
	Harper	296	Elijah	301
Montana	Olivia	59	James	59
	Emma	53	William	57
	Harper	45	Liam	53
	Ava	44	Oliver	50
	Charlotte	37	Wyatt	47

State	Girl	Births	Boy	Births
Nebraska	Emma	124	Oliver	147
	Olivia	115	Liam	123
	Amelia	103	William	118
	Charlotte	103	Henry	105
	Evelyn	90	Noah	96
Nevada	Emma	187	Liam	196
	Mia	181	Noah	167
	Isabella	170	Elijah	155
	Sophia	168	Michael	145
	Olivia	163	Sebastian	140
New Hampshire	Charlotte	95	Logan	78
	Evelyn	74	Henry	69
	Emma	68	Mason	67
	Olivia	67	Owen	67
	Amelia	58	Oliver	65
New Jersey	Emma	583	Liam	582
	Olivia	561	Noah	545
	Isabella	535	Matthew	521
	Mia	456	Michael	496
	Sophia	440	Jacob	474
New Mexico	Mia	107	Noah	129
	Sophia	102	Santiago	96
	Isabella	91	Elijah	94
	Olivia	88	Liam	91
	Ava	72	Daniel	89
New York	Olivia	1,227	Liam	1,427
	Emma	1,204	Noah	1,238
	Sophia	1,007	Jacob	1,141
	Mia	996	Lucas	1,047
	Ava	987	Joseph	1,014

State	Girl	Births	Boy	Births
North Carolina	Ava	649	William	629
	Emma	586	Noah	621
	Olivia	583	Liam	571
	Isabella	430	James	537
	Charlotte	417	Mason	522
North Dakota	Emma	70	Oliver	74
	Harper	61	Henry	64
	Olivia	53	Liam	61
	Amelia	51	Noah	51
	Ava	49	William	49
Ohio	Emma	669	Liam	652
	Ava	661	Carter	586
	Olivia	621	Noah	585
	Harper	559	William	556
	Charlotte	525	Lucas	539
Oklahoma	Emma	234	William	199
	Olivia	199	Liam	196
	Harper	184	Noah	189
	Ava	177	Elijah	183
	Isabella	159	James	181
Oregon	Emma	208	Oliver	229
	Olivia	207	Liam	216
	Sophia	158	Henry	193
	Charlotte	150	Benjamin	190
	Evelyn	146	William	178
Pennsylvania	Emma	778	Liam	718
	Olivia	666	Noah	683
	Ava	620	Logan	670
	Charlotte	506	Benjamin	632
	Sophia	498	Mason	616

State	Girl	Births	Boy	Births
Rhode Island	Charlotte	69	Lucas	64
	Emma	67	Liam	61
	Olivia	63	Noah	61
	Sophia	60	Julian	59
	Isabella	51	Mason	56
South Carolina	Ava	289	William	324
	Emma	255	Noah	285
	Olivia	221	Mason	267
	Charlotte	192	James	251
	Harper	187	Liam	231
South Dakota	Emma	53	Oliver	67
	Olivia	50	Owen	62
	Harper	47	Lincoln	56
	Evelyn	46	Liam	53
	Nora	45	William	50
Tennessee	Ava	435	William	526
	Olivia	394	Elijah	436
	Emma	376	James	401
	Amelia	310	Noah	367
	Harper	308	Mason	339
Texas	Emma	2,302	Noah	1,942
	Mia	1,882	Liam	1,830
	Isabella	1,828	Sebastian	1,585
	Sophia	1,814	Mateo	1,511
	Olivia	1,764	Elijah	1,469
Utah	Olivia	245	Oliver	297
	Emma	233	Liam	265
	Charlotte	211	William	247
	Evelyn	191	James	244
	Hazel	179	Benjamin	205

State	Girl	Births	Boy	Births
Vermont	Evelyn	34	Wyatt	36
	Olivia	29	William	32
	Charlotte	28	Oliver	31
	Emma	27	Liam	30
	Harper	24	Noah	29
Virginia	Olivia	474	Liam	541
	Ava	458	William	525
	Emma	437	Noah	497
	Charlotte	418	James	468
	Isabella	348	Benjamin	367
Washington	Olivia	428	Liam	421
	Emma	421	Oliver	410
	Evelyn	336	Noah	352
	Ava	309	William	347
	Isabella	308	Benjamin	341
West Virginia	Emma	111	Liam	133
	Olivia	94	Mason	98
	Harper	88	Elijah	96
	Paisley	79	Grayson	92
	Amelia	77	Carter	90
Wisconsin	Emma	312	Henry	328
	Olivia	312	Oliver	322
	Evelyn	294	Liam	283
	Charlotte	278	William	281
	Ava	273	Logan	268
Wyoming	Emma	35	Liam	30
	Harper	24	Wyatt	30
	Ava	23	Carter	28
	Avery	21	James	27
	Charlotte	21	Logan	27

What Joined—and Dropped Off—the Hot 100 in 2017?

One of the easiest ways to spot name trends is to watch what joins the Hot 100 and what drops off. For the (young) ladies, several new names joined in 2017: **Emilia**, **Everly**, **Isabelle**, **Nova**, and **Valentina**. A number of these names are following current trends, like Emilia, after *Solo: A Star Wars Story* and *Game of Thrones* starlet Emilia Clarke, and Valentina, an ode to popular television personality and contestant on the ninth season of *RuPaul's Drag Race*, which aired in 2017.

Another bunch dropped off the list: **Brianna**, number 15 in 2000, lost its Hot 100 spot, as did **Faith**, **Katherine**, **Kylie**, and **Taylor**. For the boys, a handful of newcomers joined the Hot 100. **Ezekiel**, **Jameson**, **Kayden**, **Maverick**, and **Santiago** all continued to rise, while **Bentley**, **Brandon**, **Kevin**, **Tyler**, and **Zachary** fell off.

New to the Hot 100

Emilia
Everly
Isabelle
Nova
Valentina

Off the Hot 100

Brianna
Faith
Katherine
Kylie
Taylor

New to the Top 1,000 This Year

These names are fresh faces in the top 1,000 list this year. Some of them have never set foot on the list before, but odds are they'll keep moving up.

Girls

Octavia	593	Malani	921	Sonia	983
Emberly	629	Miley	923	Sunny	984
Oaklyn	676	Melania	930	Tara	985
Amora	698	Mylah	941	Yara	987
Everlee	762	Oaklee	942	Alisa	988
Dream	828	Legacy	945	Saanvi	991
Paisleigh	840	Jurnee	950	Samira	992
Xiomara	848	Magdalena	955	Jenny	996
Lyanna	858	Kimora	960	Alora	1000
Opal	859	Ensley	965		
Raylee	881	Renee	966		
Oaklynn	886	Treasure	968		
Aminah	887	Egypt	974		
India	890	Spencer	975		
Luella	905	Emerald	979		
Meilani	911	Florence	980		
Selene	917	Marlowe	981		

Boys

Colson	736	Shepard	926	Ledger	973
Juelz	776	Kaiser	929	Simeon	974
Kairo	803	Zayd	931	Yadiel	975
Jaxxon	846	Koa	939	Kylen	980
Caspian	868	Mike	949	Rashad	981
Kace	870	Bjorn	953	Gianluca	986
Briar	880	Gatlin	957	Jovanni	987
Aaden	888	Kyng	959	Bishop	988
Frankie	898	Randall	960	Alaric	994
Ayan	907	Reign	961	Decker	995
Wells	915	Shmuel	965	Jaxx	1000
Nova	918	Zahir	966		
Dilan	920	Khari	969		

Biggest Jumper: Ensley and Wells

The rise of the girls' name **Ensley**, which shot up 1,461 slots from 2,426 in 2016 to 965 in 2017, looks to be a variation of the girls' name **Ainsley**, which sat at number 352 along with **Ansley**, 761, in 2016. This rise is most likely due to the prominent "Lee" trend taking over the charts with like names Paisley, Kinsley, Kinley, and Tinley all appearing in the top 1,000. **Wells**, on the boys' side, has raced 504 spots from 1,419 to 915, making its first appearance on the list.

What Do the Most Popular Names Start With?

You may find it surprising, but only nine of the top 1,000 girl baby names for 2017 start with an O: **Oaklee**, **Oakley**, **Oaklyn**, **Oaklynn**, **Octavia**, **Olive**, **Olivia**, **Opal**, and **Ophelia**. At the same time, you probably won't find it as surprising that the most popular letter that girls' names start with is A (169 of the top 1,000), with M as a close second with 103 names. Among the boys' names, 97 start with A, and J names comprise 95 of the total 1,000 names. However, not every letter is present and accounted for on both sides. In 2009, every single letter in the alphabet had at least one boy and girl name, as **Unique** hopped back on the chart (929) for the first time in four years. But in 2017, no U names made it on the girls' list. (The boys, however, are covered, with **Uriah**, **Uriel**, and **Ulises**). And there was only one Q (**Quinn**) and two X (**Ximena**, **Xiomara**) names for girls this year.

Gender-Neutral Options

Lots of names are popular for both boys and girls, but they're generally more popular for one gender than the other. Here's a list of names that appeared on both the boys' top 1,000 and the girls' top 1,000, plus how they ranked in 2017 for each gender. Some interesting finds here—**Charlie**, once in the top 100 for boys, is now given to nearly the same number of girls as boys. **Landry**, relatively new to the top 1,000 for both genders, is also almost equally distributed, and **Oakley** is almost exactly even, ranking at 479 for boys and 474 for girls. And **River** is seeing a huge upward swing in recent years, shooting up from 612 in 2000 to 201 for boys and 274 for girls! We'd suggest that 2019 will be a great year for **James** and **Arlo** to hit the girls' list.

Spelling Matters!

If you're going to choose…
Cameron/Camryn/Kamryn: Camryn and Kamryn are the more popular choices for girls, Cameron for boys.
Skylar/Skyler: Skylar is more popular for girls, while Skyler wins for boys.
Jordan/Jordyn: Jordyn is more popular for girls, Jordan for boys.

Nearly Equal

Name	Girl Rank	Boy Rank
Charlie	154	214
Rowan	212	140
River	274	201
Skyler	383	466
Oakley	474	479
Justice	500	563
Landry	792	848

More Popular for Girls

Name	Girl Rank	Boy Rank	Name	Girl Rank	Boy Rank
Harper	11	800	Reese	171	688
Avery	14	181	Payton	189	794
Riley	25	253	Harley	202	650
Skylar	47	808	Marley	209	948
Quinn	76	369	Kendall	225	864
Peyton	89	340	Dakota	233	344
Nova	95	918	Lyric	307	941
Taylor	112	506	Sage	309	472
Emery	115	772	Tatum	443	598
Eden	139	491	Lennon	445	667
Ariel	142	486	Leighton	467	904
Alexis	144	396	Sutton	602	809
Emerson	150	276	Jamie	615	768
London	151	819	Emory	635	807
Morgan	152	685	Jessie	657	963
Finley	159	279			

More Popular for Boys

Name	Girl Rank	Boy Rank
Logan	292	5
Carter	520	24
Jayden	933	26
Dylan	353	29
Ryan	410	43
Hunter	740	53
Cameron	535	60
Angel	350	71
Jordan	356	73
Parker	206	90
Sawyer	224	95
Micah	982	107
Kai	804	127
Blake	268	150

Name	Girl Rank	Boy Rank
Elliot	609	161
Hayden	231	174
Zion	928	199
Dallas	577	260
Phoenix	363	268
Amari	423	275
Rylan	797	287
Ellis	737	312
Rory	565	379
Ari	801	402
Lennox	665	408
Remy	605	449
Royal	694	508
Casey	916	524

Which Names Are Moving Up—and Falling Down—the Fastest?

The SSA compiles a list of names that have made the biggest moves when compared to their rank the previous year (assuming the name has made the top 1,000 at least once in the last two years). Some of these jumpers have obvious triggers, while the reasons for other jumps and declines are more open to interpretation. Take a look and see what you think.

40 Girls' Names Heating Up

Name	Number of Spots It Moved Up	Name	Number of Spots It Moved Up
Ensley	1,461	Saanvi	214
Oaklynn	1,072	Alessia	203
Dream	840	Lyra	198
Oaklyn	749	Bonnie	198
Melania	720	Mylah	196
Emberly	616	Sunny	194
Octavia	435	Everleigh	185
Paisleigh	364	Xiomara	176
Yara	352	Nalani	176
Kehlani	347	Amalia	169
Amora	317	Katalina	168
Maren	305	Ari	167
Lyanna	304	Roselyn	164
Selene	302	Ophelia	164
Luella	298	Emerald	161
Malani	271	Raylee	159
Oaklee	251	Opal	159
Everlee	250	Samara	150
Kynlee	221	Reina	142
Emmie	217	Antonella	139

40 Girls' Names Cooling Down

Name	Number of Spots It Moved Down	Name	Number of Spots It Moved Down
Julianne	263	Emilie	149
Wendy	243	Patricia	146
Milania	241	Heather	146
Montserrat	225	Ayana	146
Nathaly	225	Clare	140
Jayden	204	Breanna	140
Jessa	201	Emilee	140
Tenley	198	Kaylin	140
Aryana	184	Arden	139
Ciara	183	Hadlee	136
Amya	176	Aitana	135
Aryanna	175	Adele	133
Jaylynn	175	Tabitha	131
Ally	173	Milena	130
Maylee	170	Itzayana	127
Miah	170	Angelique	127
Arely	169	Sharon	125
Brittany	168	Chana	122
Briley	16	Courtney	122
Anabelle	151	Aislinn	121

40 Boys' Names Heating Up

Name	Number of Spots It Moved Up	Name	Number of Spots It Moved Up
Wells	504	Rowen	164
Kairo	423	Merrick	156
Caspian	328	Wilder	152
Nova	323	Ridge	149
Colson	323	Zahir	147
Kace	315	Aaden	133
Kashton	302	Yadiel	131
Koa	294	Gordon	130
Gatlin	282	Briar	128
Bjorn	276	Zaid	127
Juelz	241	Matias	126
Reign	236	Kannon	124
Jaxxon	214	Musa	123
Zayd	211	Shepard	118
Ledger	205	Kyng	112
Ayan	200	Alfonso	112
Cairo	196	Tadeo	111
Marcelo	177	Frankie	111
Khari	172	Wesson	105
Gianluca	168	Jaziel	103

40 Boys' Names Cooling Down

Name	Number of Spots It Moved Down	Name	Number of Spots It Moved Down
Riaan	421	Camdyn	105
Kylo	245	Talon	104
Kolby	195	Rolando	104
Urijah	189	Jericho	99
Kamdyn	189	Brantlee	99
Jamar	163	Camron	98
Giovani	160	Howard	98
Nickolas	155	Zackary	98
Chad	155	Vaughn	96
Jair	147	Arian	95
Gauge	144	Marc	95
Braiden	132	Bridger	94
Neymar	130	Benton	94
Karim	128	Joey	93
Konner	126	Davion	92
Maximo	119	Cain	92
Bode	119	Menachem	91
London	113	Layton	91
Hakeem	108	Xzavier	91
Coen	106	Valentin	90

What's Hot (or Not) Today
(And What Will—and Won't!—Be Tomorrow)

Now that we've seen the state of baby names today, here's a snapshot of some interesting trends we've spotted, as well as some predictions of who you may be meeting on the playground sometime soon.

You'll notice that certain names are on the rise and others are on the decline, showing how trends are morphing over time (for example, how some religious names like **Jesus** and **Rachel** are on the decline, but others like **Abel** and **Genesis** are climbing the ranks). We've also included some offbeat and unique ways to take each of these trends and find a name that really fits you and your family.

Trends Today

SHORT AND SWEET

In a world where chaos and clutter reign supreme, parents are now making an effort to tidy up—simplicity is key! In a new trend that has swept across Europe and is now making its way over to the United States, short and simple names are becoming increasingly popular, and this trend doesn't seem like it will stop anytime soon. Girls' names like **Liv**, which rose 279 spots from 2011 to 675 in 2017, and **Elle**, which currently holds the 373 spot, are looking to climb up the top 1,000. Meanwhile, boys' names like **Dax**, which jumped from 518 in 2016 to 456 in 2017, and **Finn**, a steady riser from 835 in 2000 to 167 seventeen years later, are on the move to pass their longer counterparts, **Finnegan** and **Daxton**, in the ranks.

These single syllable names are reminiscent of simpler times, and, as the trend continues, don't be surprised to see names like **Kit**, **Jude**, **Bee**, **Mac**, and **Win** appear on the list in coming years.

LITERARY INSPIRATION

Been noticing a lot of Holdens and Eloises in the sandbox lately? Names from classic children's books and novels have been heating up, perhaps because parents have such fond memories and associations with these popular characters from their own youth. On the boys' side, **Holden** (of *Catcher in the Rye*'s Holden Caulfield), **Rhett** (of *Gone with the Wind* fame), **Milo** (from *The Phantom Tollbooth*), **Sawyer** and **Finn** (the last names of popular Mark Twain heroes Tom Sawyer and Huckleberry Finn), and author inspirations like **Emerson** (Ralph Waldo Emerson) and **Beckett** (Samuel Beckett) have all been climbing the charts.

For girls, our eyes are on **Matilda** (from the Roald Dahl classic), **Frances** (the full name of *A Tree Grows in Brooklyn*'s Francie Nolan), **Eloise** (from Kay Thompson's popular series about a young girl who lives at the Plaza Hotel), **Josephine** (the full name of *Little Women*'s Jo March), **Amelia** (from the children's series *Amelia Bedelia*), and **Alice** (of Wonderland). Some beloved authors like **Maya** (Maya Angelou) and **Charlotte** (Charlotte Bronte) are sure to make a strong showing as well. Take a look at this chart to see how these literary namesakes have been trending over the past seven years.

Name	2011	2012	2013	2014	2015	2016	2017
Holden	299	296	288	292	291	271	242
Charlie	236	233	233	225	229	227	214
Rhett	564	507	425	338	274	220	180
Sawyer	172	147	120	110	94	97	95
Finn	302	291	250	234	209	175	167
Milo	358	326	311	311	288	248	224
Dorian	522	559	546	538	563	542	532
Emerson	387	363	329	323	301	296	276

Name	2011	2012	2013	2014	2015	2016	2017
Beckett	330	314	280	244	218	213	226
Matilda	769	658	645	583	535	497	521
Frances	780	763	693	602	514	446	438
Eloise	449	364	338	300	256	209	190
Josephine	182	160	160	147	131	114	107
Amelia	30	23	17	15	12	11	8
Alice	142	127	107	97	87	76	70
Charlotte	27	19	11	10	9	7	7
Maya	64	63	72	74	69	64	61
Scarlett	80	61	42	30	22	18	18

Ways to Make This Trend Your Own

Options still off the radar: Huck (Finn), Marius (Pontmercy), Abra (Bacon), Pip (Pirrup), Scout (Finch)

AN AMERICAN PRINCE(SS)

There is no monarchy on American soil, but with the royal wedding of American actress Meghan Markle and Prince Harry, Duke of Sussex captivating the world in 2018, parents will be looking toward Kensington Palace for some royal treatment in coming years—but perhaps with a more modern twist. The ruling monarchs on the boys' list: **George** (124), **Alexander** (13), and **Louis** (277) are holding strong, and we're expecting **Harry**, currently at 649, to climb the ranks as well. And for the girls, **Elizabeth** (13), **Diana** (230), and **Kate** (275) all land above the top 500, but we're waiting for **Meghan**, which fell off the list in 2012, to finally come back and claim her throne. And let's not forget about the more contemporary choices! Americans are searching for their own royal treatment, and three names are on the rise—**Royal**, **King**, and **Prince**. **Roya**l debuted at 900 in 2013 and shot up 392 spots to 508 in 2017. **King** jumped from 193 in 2013 to 147 in 2017 (its variant **Kingston** rose from 190 to 134, and **Kingsley** sits at 654 this year), and **Duke** debuted on the boys' list at 720 in 2013, and this year sits at 538. And don't forget about **Prince**! With the *Purple Rain* singer's passing in April 2016, the name has seen a steady increase to its current spot at 345. (Its counterpart **Princeton**, at number 404, has seen a bump as well.) And what about the girls? This year, **Royalty** sits at 422, jumping 729 spots since 2015. **Reign** also appeared on the ladies' list at number 830 in 2016 and now holds the 704 rank. And after sitting at 999 in 2015, **Princess** has climbed up the top 1,000 to hold the number 741 spot, and **Jewel** saw a big leap to now sit at 818.

What name will reign in 2019? We could see fairytale favorites **Knight**, **Kensington**, and **Queen** soon commanding attention on the top 1,000 in the coming years.

MAY THE FORCE BE WITH YOU

The first Star Wars film was released in 1977, but the names from the series are getting new life—perhaps due to the reboots of the popular franchise, which began premiering at the end of 2015. It seems hard to believe that many parents would want to name their little ones after Darth Vader, but the name **Anakin** had a huge rise in popularity, moving up from 1,258 in 2013 to 957 in 2014, and then to 738 in 2017. **Luke** is holding steady at 30, and **Leia**, which came back into the top 1,000 in 2006 (its other two appearances were in 1978 and 1980, no doubt due to the film), rose to 279 in 2017, its highest rank yet. And let's not forget about the new faces in the Star Wars universe! With *Star Wars: The Force Awakens* grossing over two billion in the box office and the much anticipated sequel premiering in 2017, it isn't much of a surprise to see that Kylo was the fastest rising boys' name in 2016, jumping a staggering 2,368 spots to number 901. And though it fell below the top 1,000 this year, Star Wars counterpart **Rey** has hit its peak in 2017 at 769 on the boys' list. And with **Kira**, 377, and **Emilia**, 74, (for *Solo: A Star Wars Story* actress Emilia Clarke) both peaking on the girls' list in 2017, we're expecting this trend to continue strong in the coming years. Soon enough we'll be seeing characters like **Solo**, **Lando**, **Poe**, **Jyn**, and **Cassian** storm-troopering on to our lists.

OH WELSH

For decades, American parents have been looking across the Atlantic for baby names, borrowing popular monikers like **Patrick** and **Liam** to **Erin** and **Claire** from the Irish and English. But now, parents may be looking toward the Cardiff coast for some name inspiration. Strong Welsh names are seeing a comeback, and with their rich history and traditional meanings, parents are gravitating toward these Celtic classics. For the boyos, popular names like **Owen** and **Maddox**, a contemporary spin on the more traditional **Madoc**, are thriving on our list. And the girls are seeing a rise in Welsh inspiration as well with **Gwendolyn** and **Morgan**. Here's a look at how some popular Welsh names are doing on the top 1,000:

Boys' Names	2017
Ellis	312
Owen	28
Rhys	477
Maddox	136
Vaughn	962

Ways to Make This Trend Your Own
Options still off the radar: Davies, Aeron, Cadoc, Gareth

Girls' Names	2017
Gwendolyn	674
Meredith	496
Morgan	152
Reese	171
Gwen	862

Ways to Make This Trend Your Own
Options still off the radar: Mair, Carys, Arwen, Brynna, Isolde

TO DIE FOR DIGRAPHS

Instead of one consonant ruling the schools, we're looking at the digraph *th* sound to be popular in playgrounds in the coming years. With "th" names rising in the top 1,000, we think that the digraph will be a thrilling thing in 2019. Already rising in the ranks on the girls' side are popular names like **Thalia**, at number 783, **Dorothy**, which has been rising since 2006 at 981 to 601 in 2017, and **Thea**, which has reached its highest rank since its debut in 2014, sitting at 269 today. Boys are dominating the softer "th" names as well, with **Theo** climbing from 354 to 289 in 2017, **Thiago** landing at 216, its highest rank to date, and **Thaddeus** making a steady rise since 2010 to hold the 666 spot.

Names We're Predicting to Join the Trend
Theodosia, Thayer, Matthias, Edith, Theodora, Ruth, Seth, Dorothea

IT'S A BIRD, IT'S A PLANE...

It's superhero baby! In recent years, superhero movies have taken over the silver screen, breaking box office records with classic characters that fight for justice against the wrongdoers of the world. With both Marvel and DC films drawing crowds, there is a whole batch of superhero baby names taking flight, and parents are clamoring for more innovative ways to make their child a hero on the playground. With *Wonder Woman* premiering in 2017 as the highest grossing female-directed film, it's no wonder **Diana** (Diana Prince) took a leap in 2017, rising from 269 to now hold the 230 spot. And on the boys' side, **Logan** of Wolverine fame made its biggest jump since 2010, rising 13 spots to now sit comfortably at number 5. Let's take a look at some other super names from the top 1,000:

Name	Marvel	2017	Name	DC	2017
Aurora	*X-Men*	51	Harley	*Suicide Squad* (Harley Quinn)	202
Remy	*X-Men* (Gambit)	605	Ivy	*Batman* (Poison Ivy)	108
Natasha	*Avengers* (Black Widow)	769	Diana	*Wonder Woman* (Diana Prince)	230

Ways to Make This Trend Your Own
Options still off the radar: Nakia (*Black Panther*), Storm *(X-Men)*, Lois (*Superman*)

Name	Marvel	2017	Name	DC	2017
Logan	*X-Men* (Wolverine)	5	Clark	*Superman* (Clark Kent)	380
Erik	*Black Panther* (Erik Killmonger)	367	Cain	*Batgirl* (Cassandra Cain)	840
Wade	*Deadpool* (Wade Wilson)	362	Allen	*The Flash* (Barry Allen)	230

Ways to Make This Trend Your Own
Options still off the radar: Falcon (*Captain America*), Loki (*The Avengers*), Zuri (*Black Panther*)

JUST AROUND THE RIVERBEND

As the race to find creative names heats up, parents are diving into the cool pool of water-related names, hoping to break the surface on this new trend. Spinning from celebrity siblings River and Rain Phoenix, water names have recently been cresting on our list. After musician Kelly Clarkson's daughter, River Rose, was born in 2014, **River** has risen to 201 in 2017. **Wells** is in the same boat, jumping a whopping 504 spots in 2017 to now sit at 915 as the boys' fastest rising name of the year. Riding the same wave, **Saylor** appeared on the girls' list at 909 in 2013, and has now reached its highest rank yet, floating comfortably at 430. We're predicting many more aquatic names to appear on our list in coming years like: Harbor, Aqua, Rain, Delta, Ocean, and Bay.

A-PLUS!

It's a fact, parents love names that start with A...but what about names that end with it too? In recent years we've seen an increase of little girl names that both start and end in the letter A, making for beautiful, light, airy additions to the beginning of preschool attendance sheets. Starting with names like **Ava** (3), **Amelia** (8), and **Aria** (20), these double-A names have increased to now take up a crazy fraction of the top 1,000! In 2017, 78 girl names held rank on our list, with contemporary double-A favorites like **Alexia**, **Amalia**, **Anika**, and **Ayla** leading the way. There's also the more traditional **Alma**, **Ada**, and **Alexandra** holding steady at 643, 321, and 120, respectively. Overall, we think this trend is only going to grow to include new A-plus names like Antonia, Anisha, Agatha, and Abella in the coming years.

MR. (OR MS.) PRESIDENT

With the divisive 2016 presidential election causing a major fissure along party lines, it seems America now, more than ever in recent history, has gotten political. And with an upswing in political interest comes an increase in political baby names, as parents look to their leaders to name their children. **Donald**, for current president Donald J. Trump, ranks at number 488 on the boys' side, and while **Hillary** (for Democratic nominee Hillary Clinton) hasn't been on the girls' list since 2008 (where it sat at 722), we're expecting a big rise as supporting parents declare that they're with her. Other notable 2016 election players have also appeared on the list. Senator of Massachusetts Elizabeth Warren appears both on the girls' and boys' side, with **Elizabeth** sitting steadily at 13 and **Warren** rising from 400 in 2015 to 360 in 2017. **Marco**, for Republican candidate Marco Rubio, is ranked at number 337 on the boys' end, while **Cruz** (Ted) and **Michelle** (Obama) sit at 348 and 214 on their respective lists. **Melania** (Trump) has made its first appearance in 2017, breaking onto the top 1,000 at number 930. And this trend isn't just looking at current leaders; historical presidential options are also popping up everywhere for both sexes—**Ford** entered the boys' top 1,000 in 2014 and rose to 711 in 2017, and **Hayes** (also for boys) sits comfortably at 409. **Carter** appeared on the girls' list for the first time in 2013 and shot up to now hold the 520 rank in 2017. Take a look at these other presidential name nominations over the years:

Girls' Names	2000 Rank	2017 Rank
Hillary (Clinton)	876	–
Elizabeth (Warren)	9	13
Kennedy (John F.)	139	58
Reagan (Ronald)	286	98
Taylor (Zachary)	10	112
Michelle (Obama)	52	348
McKinley (William)	–	437
Monroe (James)	–	681
Melania (Trump)	–	930

Ways to Make This Trend Your Own

Options still off the radar: Martha (Washington), Jackson (Andrew), Ivanka (Trump), Hillary (Clinton)

Boys' Names	2000 Rank	2017 Rank
Jackson (Andrew)	72	20
Carter (Jimmy)	152	24
Lincoln (Honest Abe)	711	41

Boys' Names	2000 Rank	2017 Rank
Tyler (John)	10	106
Harrison (Benjamin or William Henry)	184	113
Grant (Ulysses)	123	172
Marco (Rubio)	182	337
Warren (Elizabeth)	438	360
Hayes (Rutherford)	–	409
Donald (Trump)	217	488
Pierce (Franklin)	498	522
Wilson (Woodrow)	526	638
Ford (Gerald)	–	711
Truman (Harry S.)	–	978

Ways to Make This Trend Your Own
Options still off the radar: Madison (James), Fillmore (Millard), Garfield (James), Roosevelt (Theodore and Franklin Delano), Barack (Obama)

A LITTLE GEM

Everyone loves a little sparkle, and with parents turning toward nature for naming inspiration, we're expecting gemstone names to shine bright on our list in the coming years. **Pearl** appeared on our list in 2007 after a hiatus from the top 1,000 and now has climbed to hold the 652 spot, while **Ruby** has always been a favorite, sitting nicely at 79. And with **Opal** breaking out onto the top 1,000 on the girls' list in 2017 and **Emerald** sitting at 979, we're expecting other gemstones like Onyx, Amethyst, Garnet, and Jade to begin to shine in 2019.

KEEPING UP WITH THE KARDASHIANS

There's no question that the oldest Kardashian sister, Kourtney, bears some responsibility for the rise of **Mason** in recent years. Mason Dash Disick, Kourtney's older son, was born December 14, 2009. Since his birth, the name Mason has shot up from number 34 in 2009 to number 12 in 2010 and then all the way to number 2 in 2011. Today it sits at number 7—pretty impressive! **Dash** has also made it into the top 1,000, debuting at 948 in 2014 and then skyrocketing to hold the 743 spot in 2017. Kourtney's daughter, Penelope, was born July 8, 2012. **Penelope** climbed the name ranks from 168 in 2011 to 125 in 2012, and it rose to 24 in 2017. (Its variant **Penny** is on the climb too, entering the top 1,000 in 2013 and jumping to 772 in 2017.) In 2015, Kourtney gave birth to her third child, baby boy Reign Aston, which soon led to the debut of **Reign** on the boys' list this year at 961 (on the girls' side it sits at 704). All eyes are on **Chicago** and **Saint** as we wait for Kim Kardashian West's newest monikers to emerge on the top 1,000 in the coming years. While her first daughter's name, **North**, hasn't hit the list yet, we expect it (and the nickname **Nori**) to arrive soon. The newest additions to the family are also expected to make big waves. Khloe Kardashian and Kylie Jenner both welcomed new little ones in 2018, which means we're expecting **True** and **Stormi** to crack the list just like their cousin **Dream** (daughter of Rob Kardashian) did in 2017, hitting the 828 spot as the year's third fastest climber. And what about the Kardashian Kweens themselves? **Kimberly** (164), **Khloe** (137), **Kendall** (225), and **Kylie** (114) all sit in the top 1,000. However, **Kris** (Kardashian), **Rob** (Kardashian), and **Caitlyn** (Jenner) don't appear. In fact, four variations of Caitlyn were the four fastest dropping names of 2016, one falling 542 spots down the ranks and the others quickly following suit. There's definitely a naming hierarchy when it comes to this mega-famous clan.

POP MUSIC INSPIRING NAMES—AND NOT

Some of the fastest-rising names in popularity are thanks to pop stars...but so too are the fastest fallers. **Alessia**, as in pop songstress Alessia Cara, most definitely deserves credit for the rise of her name, which made its first appearance on the list in 2016 at a whopping 827 the same year her song "Here" hit number 1 on the Billboard charts. This year, Alessia is sitting pretty at 625 as the songstress continues to dominate the charts. Likewise, **Demi**, as in ex-Disney starlet Demi Lovato, skyrocketed 84 spots in 2017 after the release of her moving, tell-all documentary *Simply Complicated* and now sits at the 485 spot. **Camila**, as in ex-Fifth Harmony and Havana singer Camila Cabello, sits high at number 23, a 9 bump increase. And One Direction fans are probably to thank for the remarkable rise of **Zayn**, which appeared on the boys' list in 2013 at 897 and has rocketed up 556 spots to now sit at 341. Rock fans also probably helped with **Hendrix**, like Jimi, which climbed from 973 in 2011 to 349 in 2017, a peak for this boys' name. But perhaps more notable is the negative effect some pop stars have had on their names' popularity. The biggest faller of recent years was **Miley**, no doubt a nod to Miley Cyrus. But after a dramatic fall where it went from its 129 peak in 2008 to dropping off the top 1,000 in 2015, Miley has finally made her comeback, reappearing at 923 in 2017. This is most likely due to her more cleaned-up image and the success of her song "Malibu" in 2017.

THE SINGING SELENAS

We have two Selenas to thank for the continued popularity of this Latin name: Selena Quintanilla-Perez, who ruled the charts in the '80s and '90s until her sudden death in 1995 (which sparked the name's peak), and Selena Gomez, today's reigning songstress and chart topper. Here's a look at how Selena has fared over the years.

Year	Rank
1990	780
1995	91
2000	194
2005	242
2010	328
2015	321
Today	243

TOTALLY '90s

With scrunchies and chokers, tube tops and denim-everything ruling the fashion scene, it's official: the '90s have taken over, and we're expecting some of our favorite '90s names to return in a big way as well! As '90s kids have children of their own, and '90s fashion and culture continues to rise, we're expecting more Ashleys and Dylans to return to the playgrounds in 2019. Here's a look at some names from the list in 1990 and how they're doing today!

Girls' Names	1990	2017
Ashley	2	122
Courtney	17	948
Brianna	61	123
Bianca	84	375
Carly	163	455
Amber	15	401
Naomi	300	69
Lydia	204	85
Kimberly	31	164

Girls' Names	1990	2017
Sabrina	118	434
Jennifer	8	310
Stephanie	7	287

Ways to Make This Trend Your Own
Options still off the radar: Brittney, Heather, Bethany, Shannon

Boys' Names	1990	2017
Joshua	4	39
Bradley	65	230
Danny	162	504
Seth	102	322
Mitchell	93	651
Brian	27	217
Cody	31	278
Christian	60	52
Simon	374	263
Joel	95	177
Kenneth	52	218
Travis	42	300

Ways to Make This Trend Your Own
Options still off the radar: Ross, Stuart, Todd, Brock

ANYTHING YOU CAN DO, I CAN DO BETTER
We've already talked about gender-neutral names, but let's just focus on the girls for a moment. Lately, girls have been claiming typical boys' names and making them their own, and we don't see this gender-bending trend stopping anytime soon. With

celebs like Blake Lively and Ryan Reynolds naming their daughter **James**, and Rachel Bilson and Hayden Christenson and their new little girl **Arlo**, classically masculine names are about to become a huge trend for girls in 2019. **Ryan**, a typical boys' name, has risen on the girls' list from 642 in 2013 to 410 in 2017, and **Charlie** is following suit, jumping from 784 in 2007 to 154 just ten years later! Even **Sawyer**, which is at 95 on the boys' list, has jumped 22 spots in 2017 to land at 224 on the girls' side. And we're predicting even more typical boys' names like Austin, Flynn, Quincy, Ira, Lyle, Wylie, Spencer, and August to be hitting the girls' top 1,000 soon.

GAME OF THRONES REIGNS

Ever met a Daenerys, Cersei, or Tyrion? You might soon! The popular HBO series, *Game of Thrones*, based on the *Song of Ice and Fire* novels by George R. R. Martin, is a pop culture phenomenon with a legion of loyal fans—and unusual names! The TV show premiered in 2011, and in 2012, the name **Arya**—also the name of one of the series' most popular characters—shot up from number 714 to 412. In 2013, it flew another 135 slots to 278, and in 2017 it has peaked at 135. Variants of Arya are on the rise too: **Aria** rose from 91 in 2012 to 31 in 2014 and climbed all the way up to 20 in 2017, and **Ariya** debuted at 918 in 2013 and has risen to 642 in 2017. While the popular character Margaery Tyrell, with its uncommon spelling, hasn't inspired any namesakes in the top 1,000, the more common spelling, **Marjorie**, debuted in 2013 and now sits at the 946 spot in 2017. The actress who plays Daenerys Targaryen, Emilia Clarke, is another name inspiration. **Emilia** climbed from 145 in 2015 to 102 in 2016, breaking into the top 100 in 2017 (74), while **Khaleesi** (the fictional royal title given to her character) debuted on the list in 2014 and now holds the 630 rank. But plenty of names from this fantasy world are still off the radar. Try Missandei, Sansa, Ygritte, Catelyn, or Daenerys for girls, or Tyrion, Rickon, Gendry, Bran, Loras, or Theon for boys, and your little one will have a unique—but on trend!—name.

NAMES FROM THE ANCIENT GREEKS AND ROMANS

When we say these names are old, we're not kidding. They have been around for a long, long time...and may finally be making a comeback of mythic proportions. As many girls' names become more popular (with some traditional exceptions like Helen on the slide), the boys' names are making some even more surprising strides, jumping from below the top 1,000 in 2000 to sit on the list in 2017. These are the perfect names for parents looking for something that borders the line between traditional and cutting edge. Take a look at what's hot today:

Girls' Names	2000	2017
Ariadne	–	773
Athena	529	127
Chloe	38	22
Daphne	632	385
Diana	106	230
Freya	–	305
Helen	345	418
Maeve	778	360
Paris	473	303
Phoebe	441	319

Ways to Make This Trend Your Own

Options still off the radar: Artemis, Antigone, Aphrodite, Calliope, Circe, Cleopatra, Echo, Electra, Eurydice, Euterpe, Gaia, Halcyone,

Ione, Juno, Lavinia, Medea, Minerva, Persephone, Psyche, Rhea, Selene, Venus

Boys' Names	2000	2017
Alexander	20	13
Apollo	–	535
Adonis	756	390
Atlas	–	329
Cassius	–	585
Jason	39	92
Titan	–	620

Ways to Make This Trend Your Own
Options still off the radar: Achilles, Aeneas, Cadmus, Dionysus, Endymion, Hercules, Hermes, Hyperion, Icarus, Janus, Mercury, Midas, Minos, Morpheus, Odysseus, Orpheus, Pegasus, Perseus, Prometheus, Ptolemy, Theseus, Vulcan, Zeus

POSH AND PREPPY

In 2019, it's time to smooth that pencil skirt, button up your white collar, and put your best boat shoe forward, because all things preppy are taking over. People are loving the luxe life, and with country-club attire commandeering the fashion world, it's no wonder parents are also getting posh with their baby names. We've been seeing sophisticated boys' names rising across our list, with **Sebastian** being a frontrunner, sitting pretty at number 22. Loftier surnames are also gaining prestige, like **Anderson** at 295 and **Remington** at 247. And this trend isn't just for the guys in the world—waspy girls' names are taking over, like **Poppy**, which made its first appearance on the list in 2016 and now sits at 689, and **Sloane** sitting comfortably at 220. Take a look at some other names gracing our lists with some class:

Girls' Names	2013	2014	2015	2016	2017
Sloane	405	369	327	267	220
Leighton	544	543	470	429	467
Collins	958	835	702	647	608
Lennox	–	–	740	716	665
Poppy	–	–	–	747	689
Tinsley	–	–	–	963	837
Blaire	–	–	–	944	914
Ellison	948	891	950	920	970

Ways to Make This Trend Your Own
Options still off the radar: Tilly, Margaux, Palmer, Darcy, Hathaway

Boys' Names	2013	2014	2015	2016	2017
Brooks	301	246	233	231	204
Remington	–	687	623	458	247
Anderson	303	304	305	303	295
Hayes	605	545	537	433	409
Sterling	583	509	493	458	435
Briggs	910	835	743	655	615
Kingsley	827	760	748	585	654
Thatcher	991	868	901	832	847

Ways to Make This Trend Your Own
Options still off the radar: Digby, Connery, Ames, Whitaker, Montgomery

NOT YOUR GRANDMA'S NAME

Names like **Mabel**, **Walter**, **Pearl**, and **Henry** might sound like old-fashioned monikers more fit for your grandparents than your kids, but these names were once the top 20 in 1917, and some of them are still in the top 20 today! Take a look at these "old-fashioned" names (not anymore!) that were popular a century ago and are suddenly climbing again.

Girls' Names	1917	2017
Mary	1	126
Helen	2	418
Dorothy	3	601
Margaret	4	132
Ruth	5	265
Mildred	6	–
Anna	7	53
Elizabeth	8	13
Frances	9	438
Virginia	10	514
Evelyn	11	9
Marie	12	651
Alice	13	70
Florence	14	980
Lillian	15	27
Rose	16	141
Irene	17	594
Catherine	18	198
Louise	19	805
Edna	20	–

Ways to Make This Trend Your Own

Options still off the radar: Beatrice, Eleanor, Martha, Lois, Agnes, Elsie, Pauline, Marjorie

Boys' Names	1917	2017
John	1	27
William	2	3
James	3	4
Robert	4	65
Joseph	5	19
George	6	124
Charles	7	49
Edward	8	169
Frank	9	373
Thomas	10	48
Walter	11	265
Harold	12	799
Paul	13	225
Richard	14	175
Henry	15	18
Raymond	16	293
Arthur	17	244
Albert	18	430
Harry	19	649
Donald	20	488

Ways to Make This Trend Your Own

Options still off the radar: Elmer, Lawrence, Clarence, Roy, Willie, Herbert, Kenneth

FEMINIST HEROINES

With the #MeToo movement, #HeForShe, and women's marches erupting across the globe, empowered females are standing proud, speaking up, and influencing the world in a huge way. And with that, we're expecting a lot of parents to look at some of the greatest feminist heroines to inspire their daughters-to-be, and this trend is just getting started. Check out a few that have hit the top 1,000 in 2017:

Girls' Names	2017
Ruth (Bader Ginsburg)	265
Ada (Lovelace)	321
Simone (de Beauvoir)	747
Emmeline (Pankhurst)	754
Eleanor (Roosevelt)	35
Gloria (Steinem)	561
Maya (Angelou)	61
Georgia (O'Keefe)	242
Emma (Watson)	1
Margaret (Atwood)	132
Alice (Walker)	70

Ways to Make This Trend Your Own

Options still off the radar: Marlene (Dietrich), Patrisse (Cullors), Bell (hooks), Hillary (Clinton), Malala (Yousafzai), Betty (Friedan), Frida (Kahlo), Sojourner (Truth)

ANIMAL INSTINCTS

In recent years, we've seen little boys and girls racing toward the wild, and we're predicting a large leap in animal and nature inspired names in nurseries across the country. With celebrities like Liam Payne, Alicia Silverstone, and Kate Winslet naming their offspring Bear, and others following suit with names like **Koda** (866) and **Colt** (269), we're seeing this trend gaining some legs in the coming years. And let's not leave the girls out! **Oaklynn** is our second-fastest riser of the year, jumping 1,072 spots to sit at 886 in 2017, along with other nature names like **Briar** and **Wren**. Here are some more names that are already hitting our top 1,000:

Boys' Names	2017
Hunter	53
Maverick	85
Chase	94
Phoenix	268
Colt	269
Wilder	573
Talon	754
Fisher	765
Koda	866
Shepard	926

Girls' Names	2017
Wren	465
Briar	718
Hunter	740
Oaklynn	886

Ways to Make This Trend Your Own
Options still off the radar: Falcon, Lynx, Jaguar, Hawk, Wolf, Fox

FASHION FORWARD

Time to break out the baby fashionistas as the Paris, Milan, and New York shows start to inspire some chic baby names in 2019. We're predicting fashion brands and designers (along with some hot models of the moment) to spark some new trends in the baby name world. With **Valentina** finally cracking the girls' top 100 at number 94 and it's male counterpart **Valentino** holding strong at 671, we're expecting a rise out of high fashion brands like **Armani**, which sits comfortably at 509 on the boys side, and **Vivienne** (of Westwood fame), which stands at 252 for girls. And don't forget about **Stella** (McCartney) at 42 and **Ford** (Tom Ford) at 711. In 2019, we're expecting new tykes to walk the playground like it's their own runway!

Ways to Make This Trend Your Own
Options still off the radar: Donatella, Versace, Westwood, Kors, Chanel, Giorgio, Vera

VIRTUOUS NAMES

Religious names have always been popular, and even in recent years, we've seen an increase in religious classics like **Noah** and **Mary**. However, now parents are looking beyond the tried-and-true religious names toward virtuous monikers that'll inspire their baby-to-be. This is especially popular on the girls' side, with **Grace** leading the way at number 21 and **Genesis** sitting at 56 (which is also the fourth most popular girls' name in Washington, DC). **Dream** is our third fastest riser this year, jumping 782 spots to sit at 828 in 2017 (most likely due to Rob Kardashian and Blac Chyna's baby of the same name), and **Joy** is on an upswing since

2011, reaching its peak this year at 336. And let's not forget about the boys on the list! With **Justice**, **King**, and **Gabriel** all breaking the top 1,000, and **Legend** reaching its peak at 255, we're expecting more babies living up to their names in 2019.

Girls' Names	2017
Grace	21
Genesis	56
Nevaeh*	77
Faith	119
Eden	139
Trinity	160
Destiny	227
Dream	828
Legacy	945
Hope	253
Heaven	335
Joy	336
Miracle	371
Eve	436
Mercy	771

*Heaven spelled backward

Ways to Make This Trend Your Own
Options still off the radar: Charity, Amity, Constance, Temperance

Boys' Names	2017
Gabriel	31
King	147
Messiah	198

Boys' Names	2017
Zion	199
Legend	255
Royal	508
Justice	563
Dash	743
Reign	961

Ways to Make This Trend Your Own

Options still off the radar: Honor, Merritt, Noble, Regal, Swift, True

GIVE ME A LEE!

As parents try to get a more creative with their kid's names, alternative spellings for classic baby names have risen in popularity. One of the most common new spelling tricks? Adding –lee at the end of popular girls' names. Names ending in the lee sound are growing in popularity, and their spellings are becoming more and more varied as time goes on. An example of that is **Charlie**, which stands strong at number 154 on the girls' list, and its variant **Charlee** close behind it at 277. And while girls more commonly have the lee spelling, boys are jumping on the lee sound bandwagon, with names like **Brantlee** (956), **Marley** (948), and **Wesley** (111) moving up the ranks. Here's a look at how these lee-inspired name have been doing in the past five years:

Girls' Names	2013	2014	2015	2016	2017
Kaylee	41	52	61	70	84
Rylee	109	113	121	105	104
Finley	292	223	204	189	159
Brynlee	269	235	244	222	218

Girls' Names	2013	2014	2015	2016	2017
Charlee	324	313	282	296	277
Paislee	626	354	320	278	311
Kynlee	698	624	656	775	554
Haylee	339	401	482	586	576
Bailee	521	559	551	587	583
Kinslee	–	923	749	739	647
Zaylee	–	–	990	813	705
Novalee	–	–	–	949	902
Annalee	931	980	895	892	920

Ways to Make This Trend Your Own
Options still off the radar: Adalee, Blakelee, Jubilee, Hanalee, Fernley

Boys' Names	2013	2014	2015	2016	2017
Bentley	81	89	93	100	102
Wesley	139	130	126	117	111
Riley	157	174	194	225	253
Finley	292	223	204	287	279
Stanley	679	682	690	682	702
Marley	209	203	218	866	948
Brantlee	881	829	777	953	956

Ways to Make This Trend Your Own
Options still off the radar: Billie, Weslee, Henley, Radley

PAIRING SIBLING NAMES

So you've picked the perfect baby name, but now you're stuck with the question—what about the next one? Over the years, choosing sibling names that "go together" has been very on trend, and while the days of matching first consonant siblings may feel dated, there are some other surefire tricks to make sure your baby monikers match. The most important factor in creating cohesive sibling names is consistency: consistency in the style, the tradition, and sex of the names you're choosing. For example, if you're naming your child the more traditional Christopher, you may stick on the same straight and narrow for your second born Mary. On the other hand, a new baby Willow can definitely stand alongside the more unconventional Saylor. And what about the gender-neutral names? If you're looking to name a little girl the traditionally male Riley, you may want to stick with something equally gender-ambiguous for the second as well, pairing Riley with a name like Hayden, instead of going full-feminine with Isabella. Keeping the style, sex, and tradition of names consistent will make sure your kids are the perfect pair.

Predictions: Hot Names

Okay, so you've read about the trends. But what other names might be taking off in the near future? Here are some we think could be gaining ground.

GIRLS

Marvel

With superhero fever running high and celebrities like Pete Wentz christening his own daughter with this powerful name, we're expecting Marvel to finally make a comeback on our list in the coming years. Popular in the early 1900s (ranking at 522 in 1900), Marvel held steady over the years before finally falling off the top 1,000 in 1941. Coming in under our "old names making a comeback" category, Marvel is perfect for parents looking for something on trend but also cutting edge.

Saoirse

The popular Irish name meaning freedom, Saoirse (pronounced sur-sha or seer-sha) is finally coming across the pond and breaking out in a big way. Debuting on our list in 2016 at 970, Saoirse is gaining traction, moving up to 962 this year and ready to climb even higher. This increase is most likely due to popular actor Saoirse Ronan from the critically acclaimed movie *Lady Bird*, which won her a Golden Globe for Best Actress in 2017.

True

Following the popular "virtue names" trend that parents are turning to in a big way, True is likely to hit our list in 2019 and beyond due to the newest member of the Kardashian clan. Amid a media frenzy, Khloe Kardashian of the Kardashian empire and her boyfriend, Cleveland Cavaliers player Tristan Thompson, welcomed their baby girl True Thompson into the world. And with the way past Kardashian children have spurred previous naming trends, we're expecting a lot of little Trues in playgrounds and schoolyards around the country in the coming years.

Ophelia

For a name that had sailed across the top 1,000 until the late 1950's, it's amazing that Ophelia has now come back bigger and better than ever! Returning to our list for the first time since its 57-year hiatus, Ophelia broke onto the 1,000 in 2015 at the 976 spot. And it hasn't stop rising since then, jumping a whopping 562 spots to now sit at 416. What may have spurred the rising demand for this classic? It could be due to the catchy lead single "Ophelia" by American folk rock band The Lumineers, which debuted in early 2016 and earned the number 1 spot on Billboard's Alternative list in the United States. And with Ophelia's momentum, and lasting power, we think this name is going to be even bigger in 2019.

Ophelia	
Year	**Rank**
1900	268
1910	297
1920	348
1930	416
1940	570
1950	651
1958	887
2015	976
2016	580
2017	416

More 2019 Forecasts: Getting Hotter

Oakley: Outdoorsy names are all the rage, and Oakley is no exception. Debuting at 928 in 2013, this name has risen to 474 in 2017. And let's not forget any spelling variations! Oaklee, Oaklyn, and Oakley have all jumped over 100 spots in the past year, with Oaklynn being the second fastest riser of 2017, skyrocketing 1,072 spots to sit at 886 today. This name is unstoppable, and we're expecting it to climb even further in the coming years.

Maren: With country superstar Maren Morris collaborating on the hit song "The Middle" in 2017, breaking the top 10 list on the U.S. Billboard Hot 100, as well as reigning as a country queen, we're expecting Maren to continue to rise in the baby names rank as well as the Billboard charts. Currently sitting at 633 on our top 1,000, a huge leap from her previous rank (938), Maren debuted in 1979 at 733 only to fall off the list twice, both in 1982 and in

2008. Now, however, it looks like Maren is here to stay, and we're left singing her praises.

Octavia: With Octavia Spencer ruling the film industry—up for nominations in 2016 and 2017 for Best Supporting Actress in *Hidden Figures* and *The Shape of Water*—it's no surprise that Octavia has finally landed on our list once again. Falling off the list in 1998, Octavia spent 19 years below the top 1,000 before skyrocketing to hold the 593 rank in 2017, our seventh fastest riser of the year.

BOYS

Caspian

Whether for a prince in a fantastical world or the name of a beautiful sea, there's no doubt that Caspian is the perfect name for a new baby boy. Most likely inspired by C. S. Lewis's character Prince Caspian from the second installment in the fantasy series *The Chronicles of Narnia*, Caspian is a unique name for parents looking for something below the top 1,000 that has an adventurous spirit and outdoorsy vibe.

Kairo

Destination names have been increasingly popular in recent years, as have alternative spellings. Enter Kairo, the perfect blend of both! Our number 2 fastest riser on the boys' side, Kairo jumped 423 spots in 2017 to break the top 1,000 and sit at 803 on our list. Whether it's an ode to the sprawling capital of Egypt or perhaps a more celeb-focused trend (Kylie Jenner's highly publicized ex-boyfriend Tyga's child is named King Cairo, after all), we're expecting Kairo to continue to rise in popularity over the next few years.

Wells

Short for the more straight-laced Wellington, a perfect contender for our "posh and preppy" trend, Wells is our number 1 fastest riser in 2017, and is predicted to soar through the charts in the coming years. Sitting well below the top 1,000, Wells debuted on our list at number 915 this year. We're expecting Wells to stand among the future Brooks, Bennetts, Sawyers, and Grahams of the world.

Miles

Thank you, Chrissy Teigen and John Legend, for another hot name of the moment. With the pair welcoming their second child, Miles Theodore Stephens, in early 2018, we're expecting Miles to make leaps and bounds on our list. With steady growth over the years, and currently sitting at 110 on the boys' list (with Milo rising rapidly just below, at 224 in 2017), we're predicting Miles to be a hot name in 2019 and beyond. Our reasoning? Just look what the duo did for the name Luna, which has reached its highest ranking yet at number 37 on the girls' side!

More 2019 Forecasts: Getting Hotter

Ennis: With names like Dennis, Harris, and Ellis sitting comfortably in the top 1,000, we're expecting Ennis to finally make a stand in the U.S. in the coming years. A popular Irish name meaning "island," Ennis is the perfect blend of trendy and traditional, ideal for a little boy looking to break out of the mold.

Randall: Randall is back on the top 1,000, and we couldn't be happier! After falling off the list in 2015, Randall has made a comeback, arriving at 960 this year. This is most likely due to the success of *This Is Us*, the hit network show on NBC starring Sterling K. Brown as Randall Pearson, for which Brown became the first African American actor to win a Screen Actors Guild Award in the Outstanding Performance by a Male Actor in a Drama Series category.

Sutton: We can't get enough of the gender-neutral name trend, and this one might be our favorite heating up. Sutton appeared on the boys' list in 2015 at 952 and has steadily risen to now sit at 809, and it is expected to keep climbing. This is perfect for parents looking for something a bit off the radar (for now!).

Hidden Climbers

These names aren't necessarily the biggest jumpers in popularity, and we've mentioned some of them already, but we wanted to bring them to your attention, because they have steadily climbed the charts over the past few years. Look for them to gain even more ground in 2019.

Girls

Alessia	Faye	Octavia
Alma	Frankie	Paloma
Amora	Hunter	Reina
Ari	Jewel	Remy
Belle	Joelle	Royalty
Bonnie	Kalani	Sariah
Calliope	Katalina	Selene
Camilla	Khaleesi	Stevie
Collins	Kynlee	Sunny
Davina	Laney	Sutton
Demi	Lina	Tinsley
Elliott	Mabel	Veronica
Ellis	Magnollia	Winter
Emberly	Maren	Zaria
Emmie	Nalani	
Everleigh	Oakley	

Hidden Climbers

Boys

Alaric
Alfonso
Apollo
Axton
Bodhi
Briar
Briggs
Cairo
Callum
Cassius
Clyde
Colt
Dax
Ezequiel
Frankie
Gatlin
Gianni
Hassan
Hayes
Hendrix
Jaxxon

Jaziel
Jordy
Kace
Kamari
Keanu
Kyree
Leland
Lucian
Luka
Mack
Magnus
Marcelo
Matias
Merrick
Otto
Randall
Rey
Ridge
Sage
Tadeo
Wesson

Winston
Yousef
Zaid
Zayn

Predictions: The Coldest Baby Names

We think these names are over with a capital O. In some cases, they became really hot really fast, and now they're oh-so out of style. Others are surprisingly low in popularity considering their perceived "commonality." Perhaps you may want to consider some of these options if you want your baby to stand out in a crowd. See if you agree.

BOYS

Kylo: With a quick rise also comes a quick fall, and Kylo is a prime example. Debuting on the top 1,000 just last year, Kylo has dropped 245 spots in 2017, to sit well below our list today. Even though Star Wars is hot, looks like being the villain is finally cooling down.

Chad: In 2000, Chad sat at a lofty 236 on our list. Today, it has fallen to its lowest ranking, dropping a staggering 155 spots from 801 to 956. This is most likely due to the "bro" stereotype that has become synonymous with the name, creating a plummet in popularity in recent years.

Harvey: While the name hasn't fallen yet, we're expecting it to. Currently on an upswing and sitting at 382 on our list, we're predicting Harvey to take a hit after countless allegations of sexual assault and misconduct came to light against former film producer Harvey Weinstein. We wouldn't be surprised if this name has a significant drop in popularity very soon.

Neymar: Another example of the faster they rise, the faster they fall, Neymar shot to popularity in 2014, reaching its peak rank of 551, most likely due to Brazilian soccer player Neymar da Silva Santos Junior. Now, however, this name has lost some of its steam, finally falling below the top 1,000 this year.

GIRLS

Ciara: In 2004, singer Ciara (Ciara Princess Harris) debuted her studio album *Goodies*, which topped the Top R & B/Hip-Hop Albums chart and skyrocketed Ciara to fame. In 2005, the name Ciara shot up on our list to an astounding 149 rank. Since then, as Ciara's starpower has dwindled, so has the name on our list, and Ciara has fallen to its lowest spot on the top 1,000 yet, dropping 116 spots to sit at 875. We're expecting Ciara to continue to cool in the coming years.

Tenley: Not all alternative spellings are created equal—and Tenley is taking a hit. Our eighth fastest faller this year, Tenley dropped from 548 to 746, and we're expecting a continuing decline as parents hone in on some more traditional options.

Aryanna: While Ariana is still standing strong at number 66 on our list, Aryanna is not faring as well. Dropping 175 spots to 958 (with Aryana falling off the top 1,000 entirely), don't be surprised to see this spelling disappear very soon!

Milania: While we can guess our current First Lady is behind the rise of the name Melania, she may also be the reason for the decline of this variation. With more parents looking at the more traditional spelling (Melania finally broke into the top 1,000 for the first time at number 930!), Milania is now our third fastest faller of 2017, dropping to its lowest rank (944) since the name debuted on our list in 2011.

S CLUB!

The latest fashion in baby naming: the letter S. Both at the beginning and at the end, S names are hot in 2017 and are expected to become even more popular. From Sawyer to Collins, Sebastian to Brooks, these S names are the rising stars of our list!

Girls' Name	2017
Stella	42
Genesis	56
Sophie	106
Alexis	144
Sloane	220
Sawyer	224
Selena	243
Sage	309
Serena	414
Saylor	430
Frances	438
Selah	460
Sasha	517
Dallas	577

Girls' Name	2017
Shiloh	582
Sutton	602
Collins	608
Stevie	699
Ellis	737
Princess	741
Simone	747
Mavis	806
Amaris	860
Saoirse	962
Spencer	975
Sonia	983

Boys' Name	2017
James	4
Lucas	11
Sebastian	22
Thomas	48
Charles	49
Nicholas	68
Elias	78
Santiago	93
Sawyer	95
Miles	110
Luis	117
Jesus	144
Marcus	195
Maximus	200
Brooks	204
Andres	219
Tobias	273
Titus	299
Ellis	312
Sullivan	399
Hayes	409

Boys' Name	2017
Moises	416
Sterling	435
Sage	472
Saul	483
Davis	492
Sam	540
Sincere	567
Memphis	575
Santino	600
Curtis	612
Stetson	644
Samir	719
Otis	746
Stefan	750
Sonny	777
Shepherd	797
Shiloh	815
Salvatore	900
Santos	982

Celebrity-Inspired Names on the Rise

Kehlani (Ashley Parrish): Debuted in 2016 at 869, now at 522.

Milo (Ventimiglia): Debuted in 2001 at 984, now at 224.

Rhett (Thomas): Was 702 in 2007, now at 180.

Octavia (Spencer): Debuted in 2017 at 593.

Stevie (Nicks): Reappeared at 957 in 2014, now ranks 699 on the girls' side.

Zayn (Malik): Debuted in 2013 at 897, now at 341.

Alessia (Cara): Sits at 625 on the girls' side.

Kyrie (Irving): Was at 870 in 2012, now at 215.

Millie (Bobby Brown): Reappeared after 43 years off the list, now sits at 355.

Recent Celebrity Babies

Here's a quick overview of what the celebustork has dropped off.

Alayna Madaleine (Kerri Strug and Robert Fischer)

Alexandra Kalliope (Debbie Matenopoulos and Jon Falcone)

Amélie Moon (Sandra Cho Durand and Kevin Durand)

Anders Reyn (Angela and Alfonso Ribeiro)

Arlo Day (Leighton Meester and Adam Brody)

Art (Dawn O'Porter and Chris O'Dowd)

Augustus Alexis (Christina and David Arquette)

Ava Grace (Stacy Keibler and Jared Pobre)

Avri Roel (Susan and Robert Downey Jr.)

Bear (Cheryl Cole and Liam Payne)

Beau Dean (Tori Spelling and Dean McDermott)

Beckett Richard (Michael Phelps)

Bosley Jo (Bill Horn and Scout Masterson)

Bowie Ezio (Zoe Saldana and Marco Perego)

Brexton Locke (Samantha and Kyle Busch)

Briar Rose (Rachel Bilson and Hayden Christensen)

Brooklyn Elisabeth (Vanessa and Nick Lachey)
Cadence Gaëlle (Eudoxie Mbouguiengue and Ludacris)
Calder Allan William (Meghan Mikkelson and Scott Reid)
Caroline Olivia (Abby and Eli Manning)
Cash Van (Kelli Cashiola and Dave Haywood)
Chanel Nicole (Coco Austin and Ice T)
Charlie Ocean (Emilie Livingston and Jeff Goldblum)
Chicago (Kim Kardashian and Kanye West)
Chosen Sebastian (Kia Proctor and Cam Newton)
Christopher Carlton (Sophie Hunter and Benedict Cumberbatch)
Coco (Terri Seymour and Clark Mallon)
Colette Koala (Macklemore)
Conrad (Elspeth Keller and Reid Scott)
Cooper Blue (Dylan Lauren and Paul Arrouet)
Daenerys Josephine (Gina Glocksen and Joe Ruzicka)
Dashiel Edon (Milla Jovovich and Paul W. S. Anderson)
Declan (Elisa Yao and Patrick Stump)
Della Rose (Alexis and Billy Joel)
Delta Bell (Kristen Bell and Dax Shepard)
Edie (Keira Knightley and James Righton)
Edith Vivian Patricia (Cate Blanchett and Andrew Upton)
Ella and **Alexander** (Amal and George Clooney)
Elsie Otter (Zooey Deschanel and Jacob Pechenik)
Ennis Howard (Kirsten Dunst and Jesse Plemons)
Esmeralda Amada (Eva Mendes and Ryan Gosling)
Ever Belle (Gigi Yallouz and Owain Yeoman)
Florence May (Candice Accola and Joe King)
Ford Douglas Armand (Elizabeth Chambers and Armie Hammer)
Fordham Rhys (Ashley Hebert and J. P. Rosenbaum)
Forrest Bradley (Jessie James and Eric Decker)
Frances Cole (Nancy Juvonen and Jimmy Fallon)
Genesis Ali (Alicia Keys and Swizz Beatz)

Gus Monroe (Poppy Montgomery and Shawn Sanford)
Hannah Mali Rose (Sarah Drew and Peter Lanfer)
Harlow Monroe (Kimberly Caldwell and Jordan Harvey)
Henry Peet (Amanda Peet and David Benioff)
Holland Marysia Walker (Courtney Hansen and Jay Hartington)
Holt Fisher (Tiffani Thiessen and Brady Smith)
Hutton Michael (Beverly Mitchell and Michael Cameron)
Ilya Vue (Ashley Scott and Steve Hart)
Indigo (Alexandra Baretto and Rider Strong)
Ioni James (Coco Rocha and James Conran)
Isaiah Michael (Carrie Underwood and Mike Fisher)
Isley Ray (Jill Latiano and Glenn Howerton)
Jack Lion (Amy Lee and Josh Hartzler)
Jagger Snow (Ashlee Simpson and Evan Ross)
James (Blake Lively and Ryan Reynolds)
Jax Bracy (Renee Oteri and Bracy Maynard)
Jolie Rae (Jana Kramer and Michael Caussin)
Jonathan Rosebanks (Anne Hathaway and Adam Shulman)
Josey Hollis (Naya Rivera and Ryan Dorsey)
Kaya Evdokia (Hayden Panettiere and Wladimir Klitschko)
Kellen William (Kelly Stables and Kurt Patino)
Kenric Justin (Sonequa Martin-Green and Kenric Green)
Kingsley Rainbow (Dylan Lauren and Paul Arrouet)
Kinzee Cruz (Heidi and James Durbin)
Knox Blue (Sarah Shahi and Steve Howey)
Konrad (Marika Dominczyk and Scott Foley)
Lachlyn Hope (Catriona McGinn and Mark-Paul Gosselaar)
Larkin Zouey (Mireille Enos and Alan Ruck)
Lea De Seine (Irina Shayk and Bradley Cooper)
Liam James (Lauren Conrad and William Tell)
London Rose (Siri Pinter and Carson Daly)
Marvel Jane (Meagan Camper and Pete Wentz)

Matteo Oliver (Felicity Blunt and Stanley Tucci)
Miles Theodore (Chrissy Teigen and John Legend)
Montague George Hector (Geri Halliwell and Christian Horner)
Montgomery Moses Brian (Isla Fisher and Sacha Baron Cohen)
Myllena Mae (Doutzen Kroes and Sunnery James)
Nash Skan (Morgan Beck and Bode Miller)
Olive Mae (Marla Sokoloff and Alec Puro)
Ophelia Saint (Jordyn Blum and Dave Grohl)
Owen Bartlett (Heather Morris and Taylor Hubbell)
Paulina Kathleen (Kelly and Mike Myers)
Phoenix Sky (A.J. Cook and Nathan Anderson)
Poppy (Nate Berkus and Jeremiah Brent)
Qirin Love (Miranda and Terrence Howard)
Quinn Lily (Jenna Wolfe and Stephanie Gosk)
Reign Aston (Kourtney Kardashian and Scott Disick)
Remington Alexander (Kelly Clarkson and Brandon Blackstock)
Rhodes Emilio (Sara Gilbert and Linda Perry)
Ripley Dorothy (Robyn Lawley and Everest Schmidt)
Rocket Zot (Lara Bingle and Sam Worthington)
Rose Dorothy (Scarlett Johansson and Romain Dauriac)
Rumi and **Sir Carter** (Beyoncé and Jay-Z)
Ryan Carson (Ayesha and Steph Curry)
Rylen Judith (Brittany and Drew Brees)
Sailor Gene (Liv Tyler and Dave Gardner)
Saint (Kim Kardashian and Kanye West)
Saint Lazslo (Meagan Camper and Pete Wentz)
Samuel Hawke (Jennifer and Josh Turner)
Saylor James (Kristin Cavallari and Jay Cutler)
Scarlett May (Molly Sims and Scott Stuber)
Sebastian Lopeti (Agnes Bruckner and Alefaio Brewer)
Sidney Aoibheann (Vanessa Carlton and John McCauley)
Sienna Princess (Ciara and Russell Wilson)

Silas Randall (Jessica Biel and Justin Timberlake)
Sistine Sabella (Steffiana de la Cruz and Kevin James)
Stefan (Jelena and Novak Djokovic)
Stella June (Holly Williams and Chris Coleman)
Stormi (Kylie Jenner & Travis Scott)
Story Annabelle (Lauren and Aaron Paul)
Summer Rain (Christina Aguilera and Matt Rutler)
Tatum (Paulina Gretzky and Dustin Johnson)
Tennessee Hawkins (Katherine and Eric Church)
Theodore Vigo Sullivan (Rachel Leigh Cook and Daniel Gillies)
Tiana Gia (Lauren Hashian and Dwayne Johnson)
Titan Jewell (Kelly Rowland and Tim Witherspoon)
True (Khloe Kardashian and Tristan Thompson)
Vale Guthrie (Savannah Guthrie and Michael Feldman)
Vera Audrey (Emilie de Ravin and Eric Bilitch)
Victoria Isabella (Leyicet and Danny Gokey)
Viola Philomena (Megan Hilty and Brian Gallagher)
Violet Moon (Sarah Shahi and Steve Howey)
Vivienne Margaret (Ali Larter and Hayes MacArthur)
Wilder Frances (CaCee Cobb and Donald Faison)
Wolfe (Kimora Lee Simmons and Tim Leissner)
Wyatt Isabelle (Mila Kunis and Ashton Kutcher)
York (Tyra Banks and Erik Asla)
Zephyr Emerson (Alexandra and Sean Parker)
Zhuri Nova (Savannah and LeBron James)

Girls

A

Aadi (Hindi) Child of the beginning
Aadie, Aady, Aadey, Aadee, Aadea, Aadeah, Aadye

Aaliyah (Arabic) An ascender, one having the highest social standing
Aaleyah, Aaliya, Aliyah, Alliyah, Alieya, Aliyiah, Alliyia, Aleeya, Alee, Aleiya, Alia, Aleah, Alea, Aliya

Aaralyn (American) Woman with song
Aaralynn, Aaralin, Aaralinn, Aaralinne, Aralyn, Aralynn

Aba (African) Born on a Thursday
Abah, Abba, Abbah

Abarrane (Hebrew) Feminine form of Abraham; mother of a multitude; mother of nations
Abarrayne, Abarraine, Abarane, Abarayne, Abaraine, Abame, Abrahana

Abena (African) Born on a Tuesday
Abenah, Abeena, Abyna, Abina, Abeenah, Abynah, Abinah

Abiela (Hebrew) My father is Lord
Abielah, Abiella, Abiellah, Abyela, Abyelah, Abyella, Abyellah

Abigail (Hebrew) The source of a father's joy
Abagail, Abbigail, Abigael, Abigale, Abbygail, Abygail, Abygayle, Abbygayle, Abbegale, Abby, Abbagail, Abbey, Abbie, Abbi, Abigayle

Abijah (Hebrew) My father is Lord
Abija, Abisha, Abishah, Abiah, Abia, Aviah, Avia

Abila (Spanish) One who is beautiful
Abilah, Abyla, Abylah

Abilene (American / Hebrew) From a town in Texas / resembling grass
Abalene, Abalina, Abilena, Abiline, Abileene, Abileen, Abileena, Abilyn

Abir (Arabic) Having a fragrant scent
Abeer, Abyr, Abire, Abeere, Abbir, Abhir

Abira (Hebrew) A source of strength; one who is strong
Abera, Abyra, Abyrah, Abirah, Abbira, Abeerah

Abra (Hebrew / Arabic)
Feminine form of Abraham;
mother of a multitude;
mother of nations / lesson;
example
*Abri, Abrah, Abree, Abria,
Abbra, Abrah, Abbrah*

Abril (Spanish / Portuguese)
Form of April, meaning
opening buds of spring

Academia (Latin) From a com-
munity of higher learning
*Akademia, Academiah,
Akademiah*

Acantha (Greek) Thorny; in
mythology, a nymph who was
loved by Apollo
*Akantha, Ackantha, Acanthah,
Akanthah, Ackanthah*

Adah (Hebrew) Ornament;
beautiful addition to the
family
Adda, Adaya, Ada

Adanna (African) Her father's
daughter; a father's pride
*Adana, Adanah, Adannah,
Adanya, Adanyah*

Adanne (African) Her
mother's daughter; a
mother's pride
*Adane, Adayne, Adaine,
Adayn, Adain, Adaen, Adaene*

Adara (Greek / Arabic)
Beautiful girl / chaste one;
virgin
*Adair, Adare, Adaire, Adayre,
Adarah, Adarra, Adaora, Adar*

Addin (Hebrew) One who is
adorned; voluptuous
Addine, Addyn, Addyne

Addison (English) Daughter of
Adam
*Addeson, Addyson, Adison,
Adisson, Addisyn, Adyson*

Adeen (Irish) Little fire shin-
ing brightly
*Adeene, Adean, Adeane, Adein,
Adeine, Adeyn, Adeyne*

Adela (German) Of the nobil-
ity; serene; of good humor
*Adele, Adelia, Adella, Adelle,
Adelie, Adelina, Adali*

Adelaide (German) Of the
nobility; serene; of good
humor
Adelaid

Adeline (German) Form of
Adela, meaning of the nobility
*Adalyn, Adalynn, Adelyn,
Adelynn*

Adianca (Native American)
One who brings peace
Adianka, Adyanca, Adyanka

Adira (Hebrew / Arabic) Powerful, noble woman / having great strength
Adirah, Adeera, Adyra, Adeerah, Adyrah, Adeira, Adeirah, Adiera

Admina (Hebrew) Daughter of the red earth
Adminah, Admeena, Admyna, Admeenah, Admynah, Admeina

Adoración (Spanish) Having the adoration of all

Adra (Arabic) One who is chaste; a virgin

Adriana (Greek) Feminine form of Adrian; from the Adriatic Sea region; woman with dark features
Adria, Adriah, Adrea, Adreana, Adreanna, Adrienna, Adriane, Adriene, Adrie, Adrienne, Adrianna, Adrianne, Adriel

Adrina (Italian) Having great happiness
Adrinna, Adreena, Adrinah, Adryna, Adreenah, Adrynah

Aegea (Latin / Greek) From the Aegean Sea / in mythology, a daughter of the sun who was known for her beauty

Aegina (Greek) In mythology, a sea nymph
Aeginae, Aegyna, Aegynah

Aelwen (Welsh) Woman with a fair brow
Aelwenn, Aelwenne, Aelwin, Aelwinn, Aelwinne, Aelwyn, Aelwynn, Aelwynne

Afra (Hebrew / Arabic) Young doe / white; an earth color
Affra, Affrah, Afrah, Afrya, Afryah, Afria, Affery, Affrie

Afrodille (French) Daffodil; showy and vivid
Afrodill, Afrodil, Afrodile, Afrodilla, Afrodila

Afton (English) From the Afton river

Agave (Greek) In mythology, a queen of Thebes

Agnes (Greek) One who is pure; chaste
Agneis, Agnese, Agness, Agnies, Agnus, Agna, Agne, Agnesa, Nessa, Oona

Agraciana (Spanish) One who forgives
Agracianna, Agracyanna, Agracyana, Agraciann, Agraciane, Agracyann, Agracyane, Agracianne

Agrona (Celtic) In mythology, the goddess of war and death
Agronna, Agronia, Agrone

Ahelia (Hebrew) Breath; a source of life
Ahelie, Ahelya, Aheli, Ahelee, Aheleigh, Ahelea, Aheleah, Ahely

Ahellona (Greek) Woman who has masculine qualities
Ahelona, Ahellonna, Ahelonna

Ahinoam (Hebrew) In the Bible, one of David's wives

Ahuva (Hebrew) One who is dearly loved
Ahuvah, Ahuda, Ahudah

Aida (English / French / Arabic) One who is wealthy; prosperous / one who is helpful / a returning visitor
Ayda, Aydah, Aidah, Aidee, Aidia, Aieeda, Aaida

Aidan (Gaelic) One who is fiery; little fire
Aiden, Adeen, Aden, Aideen, Adan, Aithne, Aithnea, Ajthne

Aiko (Japanese) Little one who is dearly loved

Ailbhe (Irish) Of noble character; one who is bright

Aileen (Irish / Scottish) Light bearer / from the green meadow
Ailean, Ailein, Ailene, Ailin, Aillen, Ailyn, Alean, Aleane

Ailis (Irish) One who is noble and kind
Ailish, Ailyse, Ailesh, Ailisa, Ailise

Ailna (German) One who is sweet and pleasant; of the nobility
Ailne

Ain (Irish / Arabic) In mythology, a woman who wrote laws to protect the rights of women / precious eye

Aine (Celtic) One who brings brightness and joy

Aingeal (Irish) Heaven's messenger; angel
Aingealag

Ainsley (Scottish) One's own meadow
Ainslie, Ainslee, Ainsly, Ainslei, Aynslie, Aynslee, Aynslie, Ansley

Aionia (Greek) Everlasting life
Aioniah, Aionea, Aioneah, Ayonia, Ayoniah, Ayonea, Ayoneah

Airic (Celtic) One who is pleasant and agreeable
Airick, Airik, Aeric, Aerick, Aerik

Aisha (Arabic / African) lively / womanly
Aiesha, Ayisha, Myisha

Aisling (Irish) A dream or
vision; an inspiration
*Aislin, Ayslin, Ayslinn, Ayslyn,
Ayslynn, Aislyn, Aisylnn,
Aislinn, Isleen*

Aitheria (Greek) Of the wind
*Aitheriah, Aitherea, Aithereah,
Aytheria, Aytheriah, Aytherea,
Aythereah*

Ajaya (Hindi) One who is
invincible; having the power
of a god
Ajay

Aka (Maori / Turkish)
Affectionate one / in mythol-
ogy, a mother goddess
Akah, Akka, Akkah

Akili (Tanzanian) Having great
wisdom
*Akilea, Akilee, Akilie, Akylee,
Akylie, Akyli, Akileah*

Akilina (Latin) Resembling an
eagle
*Akilinah, Akileena, Akilyna,
Akilinna, Ackilina, Acilina,
Akylina, Akylyna*

Akira (Scottish) One who acts
as an anchor
*Akera, Akerra, Akiera, Akirah,
Akiria, Akyra, Akirrah, Akeri,
Akeira, Akeara*

Aksana (Russian) Form of
Oksana, meaning "hospitality"
Aksanna, Aksanah, Aksannah

Alaia (Arabic / Basque) One
who is majestic, of high
worth joy
Alaya, Alayah, Alaiah

Alaina (French) Beautiful and
fair woman; dear child
*Alayna, Alaine, Alayne,
Alainah, Alana, Alanah,
Alanna, Alannah, Alanis, Alyn,
Alani, Alanni, Alaney; Alanney;
Alanie*

Alair (French) One who has a
cheerful disposition
*Alaire, Allaire, Allair, Aulaire,
Alayr, Alayre, Alaer*

Alanza (Spanish) Feminine
form of Alonzo; noble and
ready for battle

Alarice (German) Feminine
form of Alaric; ruler of all
*Alarise, Allaryce, Alarica,
Alarisa, Alaricia, Alrica*

Alcina (Greek) One who is
strong-willed and opinionated
*Alceena, Alcyna, Alsina,
Alsyna, Alzina, Alcine, Alcinia,
Alcyne*

Alda (German / Spanish) Long-lived, old / wise; an elder
Aldah, Aldine, Aldina, Aldinah, Aldene, Aldona

Aldis (English) From the ancient house
Aldys, Aldiss, Aldisse, Aldyss, Aldysse

Aldonsa (Spanish) One who is kind and gracious
Aldonza, Aldonsia, Aldonzia

Aleah (Arabic) Exalted
Alea, Alia, Aliah, Aliana, Aleana

Aleen (Celtic) Form of Helen, meaning "the shining light"
Aleena, Aleenia, Alene, Alyne, Alena, Alenka, Alynah, Aleine

Alegria (Spanish) One who is cheerful and brings happiness to others
Alegra, Aleggra, Allegra, Alleffra, Allecra

Alera (Latin) Resembling an eagle
Alerra, Aleria, Alerya, Alerah, Alerrah

Alethea (Greek) One who is truthful
Altheia, Lathea, Lathey, Olethea

Alexa (Greek) Form of Alexandra, meaning "helper and defender of mankind"
Aleka, Alexia

Alexandra (Greek) Feminine form of Alexander; a helper and defender of mankind
Alexandria, Alexandrea, Alixandra, Alessandra, Alexis, Alondra, Aleksandra, Alejandra, Sandra, Sandrine, Sasha

Alexis (Greek) Form of Alexandra, meaning "helper and defender of mankind"
Alexus, Alexys, Alexia

Ali (English) Form of Allison or Alice, meaning "woman of the nobility"
Allie, Alie, Alli, Ally

Aliana (English) Form of Eliana, meaning "the Lord answers our prayers"
Alianna

Alice (German) Woman of the nobility; truthful; having high moral character
Ally, Allie, Alyce, Alesia, Aleece

Alicia (Spanish) Form of Alice, meaning "woman of the nobility"
Alecia, Aleecia, Aliza, Aleesha, Alesha, Alisha, Alisa

Alika (Hawaiian) One who is honest
Alicka, Alicca, Alyka, Alycka, Alycca

Alina (Arabic / Polish) One who is noble / one who is beautiful and bright
Aline, Aleena, Alena, Alyna

Alivia (Spanish) Form of Olivia, meaning of the olive tree

Allison (English) Form of Alice, meaning "woman of the nobility, truthful; having high moral character"
Alisanne, Alison, Alicen, Alisen, Alisyn, Allyson, Alyson, Allisson

Alma (Latin / Italian) One who is nurturing and kind / refers to the soul
Almah

Almira (English) A princess; daughter born to royalty
Almeera, Almeira, Almiera, Almyra, Almirah, Almeerah, Almeirah

Aloma (Spanish) Form of Paloma, meaning "dove-like"
Alomah, Alomma, Alommah

Alondra (Spanish) Form of Alexandra, meaning "helper and defender of mankind"

Alpha (Greek) The firstborn child; the first letter of the Greek alphabet

Alphonsine (French) Feminine form of Alphonse; one who is ready for battle
Alphonsina, Alphonsyne, Alphonsyna, Alphonseene, Alphonseena, Alphonseane, Alphonseana, Alphonsiene

Alura (English) A divine counselor
Allura, Alurea, Alhraed

Alvera (Spanish) Feminine of Alvaro; guardian of all; speaker of the truth
Alveria, Alvara, Alverna, Alvernia, Alvira, Alvyra, Alvarita, Alverra

Alyssa (German) Form of Alice, meaning "woman of the nobility, truthful; having high moral character"
Alisa, Alissya, Alyssaya, Alishya, Alisia, Alissa, Allisa, Allyssa, Alysa, Alysse, Alyssia

Amada (Spanish) One who is loved by all
Amadia, Amadea, Amadita, Amadah

Amadea (Latin) Feminine form of Amedeo; loved by God
Amadya, Amadia, Amadine, Amadina, Amadika, Amadis

Amadi (African) One who rejoices
Amadie, Amady, Amadey, Amadye, Amadee, Amadea, Amadeah

Amalia (German) One who is industrious and hardworking
Amelia, Amalya, Amalie, Amalea, Amylia, Amyleah, Amilia, Neneca

Amalthea (Greek) One who soothes; in mythology, the foster mother of Zeus
Amaltheah, Amalthia, Amalthya

Amanda (Latin) One who is much loved
Amandi, Amandah, Amandea, Amandee, Amandey, Amande, Amandie, Amandy, Mandy

Amani (African / Arabic) One who is peaceful / one with wishes and dreams
Amanie, Amany, Amaney, Amanee, Amanye, Amanea, Amaneah

Amara (Greek) One who will be forever beautiful
Amarah, Amarya, Amaira, Amaria, Amar

Amari (African) Having great strength, a builder
Amaree, Amarie

Amaya (Japanese) Of the night rain
Amayah, Amaia, Amaiah

Amber (French) Resembling the jewel; a warm honey color
Ambur, Ambar, Amberly, Amberlyn, Amberli, Amberlee, Ambyr, Ambyre

Ambrosia (Greek) Immortal; in mythology, the food of the gods
Ambrosa, Ambrosiah, Ambrosyna, Ambrosina, Ambrosyn, Ambrosine, Ambrozin, Ambrozyn, Ambrozyna, Ambrozyne, Ambrozine, Ambrose, Ambrotosa, Ambruslne, Amhrosine

Amelia (German) Form of Amalia or (Latin) form of Emily, meaning "one who is industrious and hardworking"
Amelie, Amelita, Amylia, Amely

America (Latin) A powerful ruler
Americus, Amerika, Amerikus

Amina (Arabic) A princess, one who commands; truthful, trustworthy
Amirah, Ameera, Amyra, Ameerah, Amyrah, Ameira, Ameirah, Amiera

Amissa (Hebrew) One who is honest; a friend
Amisa, Amise, Amisia, Amiza, Amysa, Amysia, Amysya, Amyza

Amiyah (American) Form of Amy, meaning "beloved"
Amiah, Amiya, Amya

Amrita (Hindi) Having immortality; full of ambrosia
Amritah, Amritta, Amryta, Amrytta, Amrytte, Amritte, Amryte, Amreeta

Amser (Welsh) A period of time

Amy (Latin) Dearly loved
Aimee, Aimie, Aimi, Aimy, Aimya, Aimey, Amice, Amicia

Anaba (Native American) A woman returning from battle
Anabah, Annaba, Annabah

Anabal (Gaelic) One who is joyful
Anaball, Annabal, Annaball

Anahi (Latin) Immortal

Analia (Spanish) Combination of Ana and Lea or Lucia
Annalee, Annali, Annalie, Annaleigh, Annalea, Analeigh, Anali, Analie, Annalina, Anneli, Annaleah, Annaliese, Annalise, Annalisa, Analise, Analiese, Analisa

Anarosa (Spanish) A graceful rose
Annarosa, Anarose, Annarose

Anastasia (Greek) One who shall rise again
Anastase, Anastascia, Anastasha, Anastasie, Stacia, Stasia, Stacy, Stacey

Ancina (Latin) Form of Ann, meaning "a woman graced with God's favor"
Ancyna, Anncina, Anncyna, Anceina, Annceina, Anciena, Annciena, Anceena

Andrea (Greek / Latin) Courageous and strong / feminine form of Andrew; womanly
Andria, Andrianna, Andreia, Andreina, Andreya, Andriana, Andreana, Andera

Angel (Greek) A heavenly messenger

Angela (Greek) A heavenly messenger; an angel
Angelica, Angelina, Angelique, Anjela, Anjelika, Angella, Angelita, Angeline, Angie, Angy

Angelina (Greek) Form of Angela, meaning "a heavenly messenger, an angel"
Angeline, Angelyn, Angelene, Angelin

Ani (Hawaiian) One who is very beautiful
Aneesa, Aney, Anie, Any, Aany, Aanye, Anea, Aneah

Aniceta (French) One who is unconquerable
Anicetta, Anniceta, Annicetta

Aniya (American) Form of Anna, meaning "a woman graced with God's favor"
Aniyah, Anaya

Anna (Latin) A woman graced with God's favor
Annah, Ana, Ann, Anne, Anya, Ane, Annika, Anouche, Annchen, Ancina, Annie, Anika

Annabel (Italian) Graceful and beautiful woman
Annabelle, Annabell, Annabella, Annabele, Anabel, Anabell, Anabelle, Anabella

Annabeth (English) Graced with God's bounty
Anabeth, Annabethe, Annebeth, Anebeth, Anabethe

Annalynn (English) From the graceful lake
Analynn, Annalyn, Annaline, Annalin, Annalinn, Analyn, Analine, Analin

Annmarie (English) Filled with bitter grace
Annemarie, Annmaria, Annemaria, Annamarie, Annamaria, Anamarie, Anamaria, Anamari

Annora (Latin) Having great honor
Anora, Annorah, Anorah, Anoria, Annore, Annorya, Anorya, Annoria

Anouhea (Hawaiian) Having a soft, cool fragrance

Ansley (English) From the noble's pastureland
Ansly, Anslie, Ansli, Anslee, Ansleigh, Anslea, Ansleah, Anslye, Ainsley

Antalya (Russian) Born with the morning's first light
Antaliya, Antalyah, Antaliyah, Antalia, Antaliah

Antea (Greek) In mythology, a woman who was scorned and committed suicide
Anteia, Anteah

Antoinette (French) Praiseworthy
Toinette

Anwen (Welsh) A famed beauty
Anwin, Anwenne, Anwinne, Anwyn, Anwynn, Anwynne, Anwenn, Anwinn

Anya (Russian) Form of Anna, meaning "a woman graced with God's favor"

Aphrah (Hebrew) From the house of dust
Aphra

Aphrodite (Greek) Love; in mythology, the goddess of love and beauty
Afrodite, Afrodita, Aphrodita, Aphrodyte, Aphhrodyta, Aphrodytah

Aponi (Native American) Resembling a butterfly
Aponni, Apponni, Apponi

Apphia (Hebrew) One who is productive
Apphiah

Apple (American) Sweet fruit; one who is cherished
Appel, Aple, Apel

April (English) Opening buds of spring, born in the month of April
Avril, Averel, Averill, Avrill, Apryl, Apryle, Aprylle, Aprel, Aprele, Aprila, Aprile, Aprili, Aprilla, Aprille, Aprielle, Aprial, Abrielle, Avrielle, Avrial, Abrienda, Avriel, Averyl, Averil, Avryl, Apryll

Aquene (Native American) One who is peaceful
Aqueena, Aqueene, Aqueen

Arabella (Latin) An answered prayer; beautiful altar
Arabela, Arabel, Arabell

Araceli (Spanish) From the altar of heaven
Aracely, Aracelie, Areli, Arely

Aranka (Hungarian) The golden child

Ararinda (German) One who is tenacious
Ararindah, Ararynda, Araryndah

Arava (Hebrew) Resembling a willow; of an arid land
Aravah, Aravva, Aravvah

Arcadia (Greek / Spanish) Feminine form of Arkadios; woman from Arcadia / one who is adventurous
Arcadiah, Arkadia, Arcadya, Arkadya, Arckadia, Arckadya

Ardara (Gaelic) From the stronghold on the hill
Ardarah, Ardarra, Ardaria, Ardarrah, Ardariah

Ardel (Latin) Feminine form of Ardos; industrious and eager
Ardelle, Ardella, Ardele, Ardelia, Ardelis, Ardela, Ardell

Arden (Latin / English) One who is passionate and enthusiastic / from the valley of the eagles
Ardin, Ardeen, Ardena, Ardene, Ardan, Ardean, Ardine, Ardun

Ardra (Celtic / Hindi) One who is noble / the goddess of bad luck and misfortune

Argea (Greek) In mythology, the wife of Polynices
Argeia

Aria (English) A beautiful melody
Ariah

Ariana (Welsh / Greek) Resembling silver / one who is holy
Ariane, Arian, Arianna, Arianne, Aerian, Aerion, Arianie, Arieon, Aryana, Aryanna

Ariel (Hebrew) A lionness of God
Arielle, Ariele, Airial, Ariela, Ariella, Aryela, Arial, Ari, Ariely, Arely, Arieli, Areli

Arietta (Italian) A short but beautiful melody
Arieta, Ariete, Ariet, Ariett, Aryet, Aryeta, Aryetta, Aryette

Arin (English) Form of Erin, meaning "woman of Ireland"
Aryn

Arisje (Danish) One who is superior

Arissa (Greek) One who is superior
Arisa, Aris, Aryssa, Arysa, Arys

Arizona (Native American) From the little spring / from the state of Arizona

Armani (Persian) One who is desired
Armanee, Armahni, Armaney, Armanie, Armaney

Arnette (English) A little eagle
Arnett, Arnetta, Arnete, Arneta, Arnet

Aroha (Maori) One who loves and is loved

Arona (Maori) One who is colorful and vivacious
Aronah, Aronnah, Aronna

Arrosa (Basque) Sprinkled with dew from heaven; resembling a rose
Arrose

Artis (Irish / English / Icelandic) Lofy hill; noble / rock / follower of Thor
Artisa, Artise, Artys, Artysa, Artyse, Artiss, Arti, Artina

Arusi (African) A girl born during the time of a wedding
Arusie, Arusy, Arusey, Arusee, Arusea, Aruseah, Arusye

Arwa (Arabic) A female mountain goat

Arya (Indian) One who is noble and honored
Aryah, Aryana, Aryanna, Aryia

Ascención (Spanish) Refers to the Ascension

Ashby (English) Home of the ash tree
Ashbea, Ashbie, Ashbeah, Ashbey, Ashbi, Ashbee

Asherat (Syrian) In mythology, goddess of the sea

Ashima (Hebrew) In the Bible, a deity worshipped at Hamath
Ashimah, Ashyma, Asheema, Ashimia, Ashymah, Asheemah, Asheima, Asheimah

Ashira (Hebrew) One who is wealthy; prosperous
Ashyra, Ashyrah, Ashirah, Asheera, Asheerah, Ashiera, Ashierah, Asheira

Ashley (English) From the meadow of ash trees
Ashlie, Ashlee, Ashleigh, Ashly, Ashleye, Ashlya, Ashala, Ashleay

Ashlyn (American) Combination of Ashley and Lynn
Ashlynn, Ashlynne

Asia (Greek / English) Resurrection / the rising sun; in the Koran, the woman who raised Moses; a woman from the east
Aysia, Asya, Asyah, Azia, Asianne

Asis (African) Of the sun
Asiss, Assis, Assiss

Asli (Turkish) One who is genuine and original
Aslie, Asly, Asley, Aslee, Asleigh, Aslea, Asleah, Alsye

Aspen (English) From the aspen tree
Aspin, Aspine, Aspina, Aspyn, Aspyna, Aspyne

Assana (Irish) From the waterfall
Assane, Assania, Assanna, Asanna, Asana

Astra (Latin) Of the stars; as bright as a star
Astera, Astrea, Asteria, Astrey, Astara, Astraea, Astrah, Astree

Astrid (Scandinavian / German) One with divine strength
Astryd, Estrid

Asunción (Spanish) Refers to the Virgin Mary's assumption into heaven

Athena (Greek) One who is wise; in mythology, the goddess of war and wisdom
Athina, Atheena, Athene

Aubrey (English) One who rules with elf-wisdom
Aubree, Aubrie, Aubry, Aubri, Aubriana

Audrey (English) Woman with noble strength
Audree, Audry, Audra, Audrea, Adrey, Audre, Audray, Audrin, Audrina

Augusta (Latin) Feminine form of Augustus; venerable, majestic
Augustina, Agustina, Augustine, Agostina, Agostine, Augusteen, Augustyna, Agusta

Aurora (Latin) Morning's first light; in mythology, the goddess of the dawn
Aurore, Aurea, Aurorette

Autumn (English) Born in the fall
Autum

Ava (German / Iranian) A bird-like woman / from the water
Avah, Avalee, Avaleigh, Avali, Avalie, Avaley, Avelaine, Avelina, Ayva, Avalynn

Avasa (Indian) One who is independent
Avasah, Avassa, Avasia, Avassah, Avasiah, Avasea, Avaseah

Avena (English) From the oat field
Avenah, Aviena, Avyna, Avina, Avinah, Avynah, Avienah, Aveinah

Avera (Hebrew) One who transgresses
Averah, Avyra, Avira

Avery (English) One who is a wise ruler; of the nobility
Avrie, Averey, Averie, Averi, Averee, Averea, Avereah

Aviana (Latin) Blessed with a gracious life
Avianah, Avianna, Aviannah, Aviane, Avianne, Avyana, Avyanna, Avyane

Aviva (Hebrew) One who is innocent and joyful; resembling springtime
Avivi, Avivah, Aviv, Avivie, Avivice, Avni, Avri, Avyva

Awel (Welsh) One who is as refreshing as a breeze
Awell, Awele, Awela, Awella

Awen (Welsh) A fluid essence; a muse; a flowing spirit
Awenn, Awenne, Awin, Awinn, Awinne, Awyn, Awynn, Awynne

Axelle (German / Latin / Hebrew) Source of life; small oak / ax / peace
Axella, Axell, Axele, Axl, Axela, Axelia, Axellia

Ayala (Hebrew) Resembling a gazelle
Ayalah, Ayalla, Ayallah, Aylin, Ayleen, Ayline, Aileen

Ayanna (Hindi / African) One who is innocent / resembling a beautiful flower
Ayana, Ayania, Ahyana, Ayna, Anyaniah, Ayannah, Aiyanna, Aiyana

Ayla (Hebrew) From the oak tree
Aylah, Aylana, Aylanna, Aylee, Aylea, Aylene, Ayleena, Aylena, Aylin, Ayleen, Ayline, Aileen

Aza (Arabic / African) One who provides comfort / powerful
Azia, Aiza, Aizia, Aizha

Azana (African) One who is superior
Azanah, Azanna, Azannah

Azar (Persian) One who is fiery; scarlet
Azara, Azaria, Azarah, Azarra, Azarrah, Azarr

Aznii (Chechen) A famed beauty
Azni, Aznie, Azny, Azney, Aznee, Aznea, Azneah

Azriel (Hebrew) God is my helper
Azrael, Azriell, Azrielle, Azriela, Azriella, Azraela

Azul (Spanish) Blue

Badia (Arabic) An elegant lady; one who is unique
Badiah, Badi'a, Badiya, Badea, Badya, Badeah

Bahija (Arabic) A cheerful woman
Bahijah, Bahiga, Bahigah, Bahyja, Bahyjah, Bahyga, Bahygah

Bailey (English) From the courtyard within castle walls; a public official
Bailee, Bayley, Baylee, Baylie, Baili, Bailie, Baileigh, Bayleigh

Baligha (Arabic) One who is forever eloquent
Balighah, Baleegha, Balygha, Baliegha, Baleagha, Baleigha

Banba (Irish) In mythology, a patron goddess of Ireland

Bansuri (Indian) One who is musical
Bansurie, Bansari, Banseri, Bansurri, Bansury, Bansurey, Bansuree

Bara (Hebrew) One who is chosen
Barah, Barra, Barrah

Barbara (Latin) A traveler from a foreign land; a stranger
Barbra, Barbarella, Barbarita, Baibin, Babette, Bairbre, Barbary, Barb

Barika (African) A flourishing woman; one who is successful
Barikah, Baryka, Barikka, Barykka, Baricka, Barycka, Baricca, Barycca

Barras (English) From among the trees

Beatrice (Latin) One who blesses others
Beatrix, Beatriz, Beatriss, Beatrisse, Bea, Beatrize, Beatricia, Beatrisa

Becky (English) Form of Rebecca, meaning "one who is bound to God"
Beckey, Becki, Beckie, Becca, Becka, Bekka, Beckee, Beckea

Bel (Indian) From the sacred wood

Belen (Spanish) Woman from Bethlehem

Belinda (English) A beautiful and tender woman
Belindah, Belynda, Balynda, Belienda, Bleiendah, Balyndah, Belyndah

Belisama (Celtic) In mythology, a goddess of rivers and lakes
Belisamah, Belisamma, Belysama, Belisma, Belysma, Belesama

Bella (Italian) A woman famed for her beauty
Belle, Bela, Bell, Belita, Bellissa, Belia, Bellanca, Bellany

Bena (Native American) Resembling a pheasant
Benah, Benna, Bennah

Benigna (Spanish) Feminine form of Benigno; one who is kind; friendly

Bernice (Greek) One who brings victory
Berenisa, Berenise, Berenice, Bernicia, Bernisha, Berniss, Bernyce, Bernys

Bertha (German) One who is famously bright and beautiful
Berta, Berthe, Berth, Bertina, Bertyna, Bertine, Bertyne, Birte

Beryl (English) Resembling the pale-green precious stone
Beryll, Berylle, Beril, Berill, Berille

Bess (English) Form of Elizabeth, meaning "my God is bountiful; God's promise"
Besse, Bessi, Bessie, Bessy, Bessey, Bessee, Bessea

Beth (English) Form of Elizabeth, meaning "my God is bountiful; God's promise"
Bethe

Bethany (Hebrew) From the house of figs
Bethan, Bethani, Bethanie, Bethanee, Bethaney, Bethane, Bethann, Bethanne

Beyonce (American) One who surpasses others
Beyoncay, Beyonsay, Beyonsai, Beyonsae, Beyonci, Beyoncie, Beyoncee, Beyoncea

Bianca (Italian) A shining, fair-skinned woman
Bianka, Byanca, Byanka

Bibiana (Italian) Form of Vivian, meaning "lively woman"
Bibiane, Bibianna

Bijou (French) As precious as a jewel

Billie (English) Feminine form of William; having a desire to protect
Billi, Billy, Billey, Billee, Billeigh, Billea, Billeah

Blaine (Scottish / Irish) A saint's servant / a thin woman
Blayne, Blane, Blain, Blayn, Blaen, Blaene

Blair (Scottish) From the field of battle
Blaire, Blare, Blayre, Blaer, Blaere, Blayr

Blake (English) A dark beauty
Blayk, Blayke, Blaik, Blaike, Blaek, Blaeke

Blue (English) A color, lighter than purple-indigo but darker than green

Blythe (English) Filled with happiness
Blyth, Blithe, Blith

Bonamy (French) A very good friend
Bonamey, Bonami, Bonamie, Bonamee, Bonamei, Bonamea, Bonameah

Bonnie (English) Pretty face
Boni, Bona, Bonea, Boneah, Bonee

Brady (Irish) A large-chested woman
Bradey, Bradee, Bradi, Bradie, Bradea, Bradeah

Braelyn (American) Combination of Braden and Lynn
Braylin, Braelin, Braylyn, Braelen, Braylen

Braima (African) Mother of multitudes
Braimah, Brayma, Braema, Braymah, Braemah

Brandy (English) A woman wielding a sword; an alcoholic drink
Brandey, Brandi, Brandie, Brandee, Branda, Brande, Brandelyn, Brandilyn

Brazil (Spanish) Of the ancient tree
Brasil, Brazile, Brazille, Brasille, Bresil, Brezil, Bresille, Brezille

Brenda (Irish) Feminine form of Brendan; a princess; wielding a sword
Brynda, Brinda, Breandan, Brendalynn, Brendolyn, Brend, Brienda

Brenna (Welsh) A raven-like woman
Brinna, Brenn, Bren, Brennah, Brina, Brena, Brenah

Brianna (Irish) Feminine form of Brian; from the high hill; one who ascends
Breanna, Breanne, Breana, Breann, Breeana, Breeanna, Breona, Breonna, Bryana, Bryanna, Briana

Brice (Welsh) One who is alert; ambitious
Bryce

Bridget (Irish) A strong and protective woman; in mythology, goddess of fire, wisdom, and poetry
Bridgett, Bridgette, Briget, Brigette, Bridgit, Bridgitte, Birgit, Birgitte

Brie (French) Type of cheese
Bree, Breeyah, Bria, Briya, Briah, Briyah, Brya

Briella (Italian / Spanish) Form of Gabriella, meaning "heroine of God"

Brielle (French) Form of Brie, meaning "type of cheese"

Brilliant (American) A dazzling and sparkling woman

Brisa (Spanish) Beloved
Brisia, Brisha, Brissa, Briza, Bryssa, Brysa

Bristol (English) From the city in England
Brystol, Bristow, Brystow

Brittany (English) A woman from Great Britain
Britany, Brittanie, Brittaney, Brittani, Brittanee, Britney, Britnee, Britny

Brook (English) From the running stream
Brooke, Brookie

Brooklyn (American) Borough of New York City
Brooklin, Brooklynn, Brooklynne

Brylee (American) Variation of Riley
Brilee, Brylie, Briley, Bryli

Brynley (English) From the burnt meadow
Brynlee, Brynly, Brinley, Brinli, Brynlie

Brynn (Welsh) Hill
Brin, Brinn, Bryn, Brynlee, Brynly, Brinley, Brinli, Brynlie

Bryony (English) Of the healing place
Briony, Brionee

Cabrina (American) Form of Sabrina, meaning "a legendary princess"
Cabrinah, Cabrinna

Cabriole (French) An adorable girl
Cabriolle, Cabrioll, Cabriol, Cabryole, Cabryolle, Cabryoll, Cabryol, Cabriola

Cacalia (Latin) Resembling the flowering plant
Cacaliah, Cacalea, Cacaleah

Caden (English) A battle maiden
Cadan, Cadin, Cadon

Cadence (Latin) Rhythmic and melodious; a musical woman
Cadena, Cadenza, Cadian, Cadienne, Cadianne, Cadiene, Caydence, Cadencia, Kadence, Kaydence

Caia (Latin) One who rejoices
Cai, Cais

Cailyn (Gaelic) A young woman
Cailin

Cainwen (Welsh) A beautiful treasure
Cainwenn, Cainwenne, Cainwin, Cainwinn, Cainwinne, Cainwyn, Cainwynn, Cainwynne

Cairo (African) From the city in Egypt

Caitlin (English) Form of Catherine, meaning one who is pure, virginal
Caitlyn, Catlin, Catline, Catlyn, Caitlan, Caitlinn, Caitlynn

Calais (French) From the city in France

Cale (Latin) A respected woman
Cayl, Cayle, Cael, Caele, Cail, Caile

Caledonia (Latin) Woman of Scotland
Caledoniah, Caledoniya, Caledona, Caledonya, Calydona

California (Spanish) From paradise; from the state of California
Califia

Calise (Greek) A gorgeous woman
Calyse, Calice, Calyce

Calista (Greek) Most beautiful; in mythology, a nymph who changed into a bear and then into the Great Bear constellation
Calissa, Calisto, Callista, Calyssa, Calysta, Calixte, Colista, Collista

Calla (Greek) Resembling a lily; a beautiful woman
Callah

Callie (Greek) A beautiful girl
Cali, Callee, Kali, Kallie

Calypso (Greek) A woman with secrets; in mythology, a nymph who captivated Odysseus for seven years

Cambay (English) From the town in India
Cambaye, Cambai, Cambae

Cambria (Latin) A woman of Wales
Cambriah, Cambrea, Cambree, Cambre, Cambry, Cambrey, Cambri, Cambrie, Cambreah

Camdyn (English) Of the enclosed valley
Camden, Camdan, Camdon, Camdin

Cameron (Scottish) Having a crooked nose
Cameryn, Camryn, Camerin, Camren, Camrin, Camron

Camila (Italian) Feminine form of Camillus; a ceremonial attendant; a noble virgin
Camile, Camille, Camilla, Camillia, Caimile, Camillei, Cam, Camelai

Campbell (Scottish) Having a crooked mouth
Campbel, Campbelle, Campbele

Candace (Ethiopian / Greek) A queen / one who is white and glowing
Candice, Candiss, Candyce, Candance, Candys, Candyss, Candy

Candra (Latin) One who is glowing

Candy (English) A sweet girl; form of Candida, meaning "white-skinned"; form of Candace, meaning "a queen / one who is white and glowing"
Candey, Candi, Candie, Candee, Candea, Candeah

Caneadea (Native American) From the horizon
Caneadeah, Caneadia, Caneadiah

Canika (American) A woman shining with grace
Canikah, Caneeka, Canicka, Canyka, Canycka, Caneekah, Canickah, Canykah

Canisa (Greek) One who is very much loved
Canisah, Canissa, Canysa, Caneesa, Canyssa

Cannes (French) A woman from Cannes

Cantabria (Latin) From the mountains
Cantabriah, Cantebria, Cantabrea, Cantebrea

Caprina (Italian) Woman of the island Capri
Caprinah, Caprinna, Capryna, Capreena, Caprena, Capreenah, Caprynah, Capriena

Cara (Italian / Gaelic) One who is dearly loved / a good friend
Carah, Caralee, Caralie, Caralyn, Caralynn, Carrah, Carra, Chara

Carina (Latin) Little darling
Carinna, Cariana, Carine, Cariena, Caryna, Carinna, Carynna

Carissa (Greek) A woman of grace
Carisa, Carrisa, Carrissa, Carissima

Carla (Latin) Feminine form of Carl; a free woman
Carlah, Carlana, Carleen, Carlena, Carlene, Carletta

Carlessa (American) One who is restless
Carlessah, Carlesa, Carlesah

Carly (American) Form of Carla, meaning "a free woman"
Carlee, Carleigh, Carli, Carlie, Carley

Carmel (Hebrew) Of the fruitful orchid
Carmela, Carmella, Karmel

Carmen (Latin) A beautiful song
Carma, Carmelita, Carmencita, Carmia, Carmie, Carmina, Carmine, Carmita

Carna (Latin) In mythology, a goddess who ruled the heart

Carni (Latin) One who is vocal
Carnie, Carny, Carney, Carnee, Carnea, Carneah, Carnia, Carniah

Carol (English) Form of Caroline, meaning "joyous song"; feminine form of Charles; a small, strong woman
Carola, Carole, Carolle, Carolla, Caroly, Caroli, Carolie, Carolee

Caroline (Latin) Joyous song; feminine form of Charles; a small, strong woman
Carol, Carolina, Carolyn, Carolann, Carolanne, Carolena, Carolene, Carolena, Caroliana

Carrington (English) A beautiful woman; a woman of Carrington
Carington, Carryngton, Caryngton

Carson (Scottish) Son of the marshland
Carsan, Carsen, Carsin, Carsyn

Carys (Welsh) One who loves and is loved
Caryss, Carysse, Caris, Cariss, Carisse, Cerys, Ceryss, Cerysse

Casey (Greek / Irish) A vigilant woman
Casie, Casy, Caysie, Kasey

Cason (Greek) A seer
Cayson, Caison, Caeson

Cassandra (Greek) An unheeded prophetess; in mythology, King Priam's daughter who foretold the fall of Troy
Casandra, Cassandrea, Cassaundra, Cassondra, Cass, Cassy, Cassey, Cassi, Cassie

Cassidy (Irish) Curly-haired girl
Cassady, Cassidey, Cassidi, Cassidie, Cassidee, Cassadi, Cassadie, Cassadee, Casidhe, Cassidea, Cassadea

Casta (Spanish) One who is pure; chaste
Castah, Castalina, Castaleena, Castaleina, Castaliena, Castaleana, Castalyna, Castara

Catherine (English) One who is pure; virginal
Catharine, Cathrine, Cathryn, Catherin, Catheryn, Catheryna, Cathi, Cathy, Katherine, Catalina

Catrice (Greek) A wholesome woman
Catrise, Catryce, Catryse, Catreece, Catreese, Catriece

Cayenne (French) Resembling the hot and spicy pepper

Cayla (American) Form of Kaila, meaning "crowned with laurel"
Caila, Caylah, Cailah

Caylee (American) Form of Kayla, meaning "crowned with laurel"
Caleigh, Caley, Cayley, Cailey, Caili, Cayli

Cecilia (Latin) Feminine form of Cecil; one who is blind; patron saint of music
Cecelia, Cecile, Cecilee, Cicely, Cecily, Cecille, Cecilie, Cicilia, Sheila, Silka, Sissy, Celia

Celand (Latin) One who is meant for heaven
Celanda, Celande, Celandia, Celandea

Celandine (English) Resembling a swallow
Celandyne, Celandina, Celandyna, Celandeena, Celandena, Celandia

Celeste (Latin) A heavenly daughter
Celesta, Celestia, Celisse, Celestina, Celestyna, Celestine

Celia (Latin) Form of Cecelia, meaning patron saint of music

Celina (Latin) In mythology, one of the daughters of Atlas who was turned into a star of the Pleiades constellation; of the heavens; form of Selena, meaning "of the moon"
Celena, Celinna, Celene, Celenia, Celenne, Celicia

Celosia (Greek) A fiery
woman; burning; aflame
Celosiah, Celosea, Celoseah

Cera (French) A colorful woman
Cerah, Cerrah, Cerra

Cerina (Latin) Form of Serena,
meaning "having a peaceful
disposition"
*Cerinah, Ceryna, Cerynah,
Cerena, Cerenah, Ceriena*

Cerise (French) Resembling
the cherry
Cerisa

Chai (Hebrew) One who gives
life
*Chae, Chaili, Chailie, Chailee,
Chaileigh, Chaily, Chailey,
Chailea*

Chailyn (American)
Resembling a waterfall
*Chailynn, Chailynne, Chaelyn,
Chaelynn, Chaelynne, Chaylyn*

Chakra (Arabic) A center of
spiritual energy

Chalette (American) Having
good taste
*Chalett, Chalet, Chalete,
Chaletta, Chaleta*

Chalina (Spanish) Form
of Rosalina, meaning
"resembling a gentle horse /
resembling the beautiful and
meaningful flower"
*Chalinah, Chalyna, Chaleena,
Chalena, Charo, Chaliena,
Chaleina, Chaleana*

Chameli (Hindi) Resembling
jasmine
*Chamelie, Chamely, Chameley,
Chamelee*

Chan (Sanskrit) A shining
woman

Chana (Hebrew) Form of
Hannah, meaning "having
favor and grace"
*Chanah, Channa, Chaanach,
Chaanah, Chanach, Channah*

Chance (American) One who
takes risks
*Chanci, Chancie, Chancee,
Chancea, Chanceah, Chancy,
Chancey*

Chanda (Sanskrit) An enemy
of evil
*Chandy, Chaand, Chand,
Chandey, Chandee, Chandi,
Chandie, Chandea*

Chandra (Hindi) Of the moon; another name for the goddess Devi
Chandara, Chandria, Chaundra, Chandrea, Chandreah

Chanel (French) From the canal; a channel
Chanell, Chanelle, Channelle, Chenelle, Chenel, Chenell

Channary (Cambodian) Of the full moon
Channarie, Channari, Channarey, Channaree, Chantrea, Chantria

Chantrice (French) A singer
Chantryce, Chantrise, Chantryse

Charisma (Greek) Blessed with charm
Charismah, Charizma, Charysma, Karisma

Charity (Latin) A woman of generous love
Charitey, Chariti, Charitie, Charitee

Charlesia (American) Feminine form of Charles; small, strong woman
Charlesiah, Charlesea, Charleseah, Charlsie, Charlsi

Charlie (English) Form of Charles, meaning "one who is strong"
Charlee, Charli, Charley, Charlize, Charlene, Charlyn, Charlaine, Charlisa, Charlena

Charlotte (French) Form of Charles, meaning "a small, strong woman"
Charlize, Charlot, Charlotta

Charlshea (American) Filled with happiness
Charlsheah, Charlshia, Charlshiah

Charnee (American) Filled with joy
Charny, Charney, Charnea, Charneah, Charni, Charnie

Charnesa (American) One who gets attention
Charnessa, Charnessah

Charsetta (American) An emotional woman
Charsett, Charsette, Charset, Charsete, Charseta

Chartra (American) A classy lady
Chartrah

Charu (Hindi) One who is gorgeous
Charoo, Charou

Chasia (Hebrew) One who is protected; sheltered
Chasiah, Chasea, Chaseah, Chasya, Chasyah

Chasidah (Hebrew) A religious woman; pious
Chasida, Chasyda, Chasydah

Chavi (Egyptian) A precious daughter
Chavie, Chavy, Chavey, Chavee, Chavea, Chaveah

Chaya (Hebrew) Life
Chaia

Chedra (Hebrew) Filled with happiness
Chedrah

Cheer (American) Filled with joy
Cheere

Chekia (American) A saucy woman
Cheekie, Checki, Checkie, Checky, Checkey, Checkee, Checkea, Checkeah

Chelone (English) Resembling a flowering plant

Chelsea (English) From the landing place for chalk
Chelcie, Chelsa, Chelsee, Chelseigh, Chelsey, Chelsi, Chelsie, Chelsy

Chemarin (French) A dark beauty
Chemarine, Chemaryn, Chemareen, Chemarein, Chemarien

Chemda (Hebrew) A charismatic woman
Chemdah

Chenille (American) A soft-skinned woman
Chenill, Chenil, Chenile, Chenilla, Chenila

Cherika (French) One who is dear
Chericka, Cheryka, Cherycka, Cherieka, Cheriecka, Chereika, Chereicka, Cheryka

Cherish (English) To be held dear, valued

Cherry (English) Resembling a fruit-bearing tree
Cherrie, Cherri, Cherrey, Cherree, Cherrea, Cherreah

Chesney (English) One who promotes peace
Chesny, Chesni, Chesnie, Chesnea, Chesneah, Chesnee

Cheyenne (Native American) Unintelligible speaker
Chayanne, Cheyane, Cheyene, Shayan, Shyann

Chiante (Italian) Resembling the wine
Chianti, Chiantie, Chiantee, Chianty, Chiantey, Chiantea

Chiara (Italian) Daughter of the light
Chiarah, Chiarra, Chiarrah

Chiba (Hebrew) One who loves and is loved
Chibah, Cheeba, Cheebah, Cheiba, Cheibah, Chieba, Chiebah, Cheaba

Chidi (Spanish) One who is cheerful
Chidie, Chidy, Chidey, Chidee, Chidea, Chideah

Chidori (Japanese) Resembling a shorebird
Chidorie, Chidory, Chidorey, Chidorea, Chidoreah, Chidoree

Chikira (Spanish) A talented dancer
Chikirah, Chikiera, Chikierah, Chikeira, Chikeirah, Chikeera, Chikeerah, Chikyra

Chiku (African) A talkative girl

Chinara (African) God receives
Chinarah, Chinarra, Chinarrah

Chinue (African) God's own blessing
Chinoo, Chynue, Chynoo

Chiriga (African) One who is triumphant
Chyriga, Chyryga, Chiryga

Chislaine (French) A faithful woman
Chislain, Chislayn, Chislayne, Chislaen, Chislaene, Chyslaine, Chyslain, Chyslayn

Chitsa (Native American) One who is fair
Chitsah, Chytsa, Chytsah

Chizoba (African) One who is well-protected
Chizobah, Chyzoba, Chyzobah

Chloe (Greek) A flourishing woman; blooming
Clo, Cloe, Cloey, Chloë

Christina (English) Follower of Christ
Christinah, Cairistiona, Christine, Christin, Christian, Christiana, Christiane, Christianna, Kristina, Cristine, Christal, Crystal, Chrystal, Cristal

Chula (Native American) Resembling a colorful flower
Chulah, Chulla, Chullah

Chulda (Hebrew) One who can tell fortunes
Chuldah

Chun (Chinese) Born during the spring

Chyou (Chinese) Born during autumn

Ciara (Irish) A dark beauty
Ceara, Ciaran, Ciarra, Ciera, Cierra, Ciere, Ciar, Ciarda

Cidrah (American) One who is unlike others
Cidra, Cydrah, Cydra

Cinnamon (American) Resembling the reddish-brown spice
Cinnia, Cinnie

Ciona (American) One who is steadfast
Cionah, Cyona, Cyonah

Claennis (Anglo-Saxon) One who is pure
Claenis, Claennys, Claenys, Claynnis, Claynnys, Claynys, Claynyss

Claire (French) Form of Clara, meaning "famously bright"
Clare, Clair

Clancey (American) A light-hearted woman
Clancy, Clanci, Clancie, Clancee, Clancea, Clanceah

Clara (Latin) One who is famously bright
Clarie, Clarinda, Clarine, Clarita, Claritza, Clarrie, Clarry, Clarabelle, Claire, Clarice

Clarice (French) A famous woman; also a form of Clara, meaning "one who is famously bright"
Claressa, Claris, Clarisa, Clarise, Clarisse, Claryce, Clerissa, Clerisse, Clarissa

Claudia (Latin / German / Italian) One who is lame
Claudelle, Gladys

Clelia (Latin) A glorious woman
Cloelia, Cleliah, Clelea, Cleleah, Cloeliah, Cloelea, Cloeleah

Clementine (French) Feminine form of Clement; one who is merciful
Clem, Clemence, Clemency, Clementia, Clementina, Clementya, Clementyna, Clementyn

Cleodal (Latin) A glorious woman
Cleodall, Cleodale, Cleodel, Cleodell, Cleodelle

Cleopatra (Greek) A father's glory; of the royal family
Clea, Cleo, Cleona, Cleone, Cleonie, Cleora, Cleta, Cleoni

Clever (American) One who is quick-witted and smart

Cloris (Greek) A flourishing woman; in mythology, the goddess of flowers
Clores, Clorys, Cloriss, Clorisse, Cloryss, Clorysse

Cloud (American) A light-hearted woman
Cloude, Cloudy, Cloudey, Cloudee, Cloudea, Cloudeah, Cloudi, Cloudie

Clydette (American) Feminine form of Clyde, meaning "from the river"
Clydett, Clydet, Clydete, Clydetta, Clydeta

Clymene (Greek) In mythology, the mother of Atlas and Prometheus
Clymena, Clymyne, Clymyn, Clymyna, Clymeena, Clymeina, Clymiena, Clymeana

Clytie (Greek) The lovely one; in mythology, a nymph who was changed into a sunflower
Clyti, Clytee, Clyty, Clytey, Clyte, Clytea, Clyteah

Coby (Hebrew) Feminine form of Jacob; the supplanter
Cobey, Cobi, Cobie, Cobee, Cobea, Cobeah

Coffey (American) A lovely woman
Coffy, Coffe, Coffee, Coffea, Coffeah, Coffi, Coffie

Coira (Scottish) Of the churning waters
Coirah, Coyra, Coyrah

Colanda (American) Form of Yolanda, meaning "resembling the violet flower; modest"
Colande, Coland, Colana, Colain, Colaine, Colane, Colanna, Corlanda, Calanda, Calando, Calonda, Colantha, Colanthe, Culanda, Culonda, Coulanda, Colonda

Cole (English) A swarthy woman; having coal-black hair
Col, Coal, Coale, Coli, Colie, Coly, Coley, Colee

Colette (French) Victory of the people
Collette, Kolette

Coligny (French) Woman from Cologne
Coligney, Colignie, Coligni, Colignee, Colignea, Coligneah

Colisa (English) A delightful young woman
Colisah, Colissa, Colissah, Colysa, Colysah, Colyssa, Colyssah

Colola (American) A victorious woman
Colo, Cola

Comfort (English) One who strengthens or soothes others
Comforte, Comfortyne, Comfortyna, Comforteene, Comforteena, Comfortene, Comfortena, Comfortiene

Conary (Gaelic) A wise woman
Conarey, Conarie, Conari, Conaree, Conarea, Conareah

Concordia (Latin) Peace and harmony; in mythology, goddess of peace
Concordiah, Concordea, Concord, Concorde, Concordeah

Constanza (American) One who is strong-willed
Constanzia, Constanzea

Consuela (Spanish) One who provides consolation
Consuelia, Consolata, Consolacion, Chela, Conswela, Conswelia, Conswelea, Consuella

Contessa (Italian) A titled woman; a countess
Countess, Contesse, Countessa, Countesa, Contesa

Cooper (English) One who makes barrels
Couper

Copper (American) A red-headed woman
Coper, Coppar, Copar

Cora (English) A young maiden
Corah, Coraline, Corra

Coral (English) Resembling the semiprecious sea growth; from the reef
Coralee, Coralena, Coralie, Coraline, Corallina, Coralline, Coraly, Coralyn

Corazon (Spanish) Of the heart
Corazana, Corazone, Corazona

Cordelia (Latin) A good-hearted woman; a woman of honesty
Cordella, Cordelea, Cordilia, Cordilea, Cordy, Cordie, Cordi, Cordee

Corey (Irish) From the hollow; of the churning waters
Cory, Cori, Coriann, Corianne, Corie, Corri, Corrianna, Corrie

Corgie (American) A humorous woman
Corgy, Corgey, Corgi, Corgee, Corgea, Corgeah

Coriander (Greek) A romantic woman; resembling the spice
Coryander, Coriender, Coryender

Corina (Latin) A spear-wielding woman
Corinne, Corine, Corinna, Corrinne, Corryn, Corienne, Coryn, Corynna

Corinthia (Greek) A woman of Corinth
Corinthiah, Corinthe, Corinthea, Corintheah, Corynthia, Corynthea, Corynthe

Cornelia (Latin) Feminine form of Cornelius; referring to a horn
Cornalia, Corneelija, Cornela, Cornelija, Cornelya, Cornella, Cornelle, Cornie

Cota (Spanish) A lively woman
Cotah, Cotta, Cottah

Coty (French) From the riverbank
Cotey, Coti, Cotie, Cotee, Cotea, Coteah

Courtney (English) A courteous woman; courtly
Cordney, Cordni, Cortenay, Corteney, Cortland, Cortnee, Cortneigh, Cortney, Courteney

Covin (American) An unpredictable woman
Covan, Coven, Covyn, Covon

Coy (English) From the woods, the quiet place
Coye, Coi

Cree (Native American) A tribal name
Crei, Crey, Crea, Creigh

Cressida (Greek) The golden girl; in mythology, a woman of Troy
Cressa, Criseyde, Cressyda, Crissyda

Cristos (Greek) A dedicated and faithful woman
Crystos, Christos, Chrystos

Cwen (English) A royal woman; queenly
Cwene, Cwenn, Cwenne, Cwyn, Cwynn, Cwynne, Cwin, Cwinn

Cylee (American) A darling daughter
Cyleigh, Cyli, Cylie, Cylea, Cyleah, Cyly, Cyley

Cynthia (Greek) Moon goddess
Cinda, Cindy, Cinthia, Cindia
Cinthea

Cyrene (Greek) In mythology, a maiden-huntress loved by Apollo
Cyrina, Cyrena, Cyrine,
Cyreane, Cyreana, Cyreene,
Cyreena

Czigany (Hungarian) A gypsy girl; one who moves from place to place
Cziganey, Czigani, Cziganie,
Cziganee

D

Dacey (Irish) Woman from the south
Daicey, Dacee, Dacia, Dacie,
Dacy, Daicee, Daicy, Daci

Daffodil (French) Resembling the yellow flower
Daffodill, Daffodille, Dafodil,
Dafodill, Dafodille, Daff,
Daffodyl, Dafodyl

Dahlia (Swedish) From the valley; resembling the flower
Dahlea, Dahl, Dahiana,
Dayha, Daleia, Dalia

Daira (Greek) One who is well-informed
Daeira, Danira, Dayeera

Daisy (English) Of the day's eye; resembling a flower
Daisee, Daisey, Daisi, Daisie,
Dasie, Daizy, Daysi, Deysi

Dakota (Native American) A friend to all
Dakotah, Dakotta, Dakoda,
Dakodah

Damali (Arabic) A beautiful vision
Damalie, Damaly, Damaley,
Damalee, Damaleigh, Damalea

Damani (American) Of a bright tomorrow
Damanie, Damany, Damaney,
Damanee, Damanea,
Damaneah

Damaris (Latin) A gentle woman
Damara, Damaress, Damariss,
Damariz, Dameris, Damerys,
Dameryss, Damiris

Dana (English) Woman from Denmark
Danna, Daena, Daina,
Danaca, Danah, Dane, Danet,
Daney, Dania

Danica (Slavic) Of the morning star
Danika

Daniela (Spanish) Form of Danielle, meaning "God is my judge"
Daniella

Danielle (Hebrew) Feminine form of Daniel; God is my judge
Daanelle, Danee, Danele, Danella, Danelle, Danelley, Danette, Daney

Danna (American) Variation of Dana, meaning woman from Denmark
Dannah

Daphne (Greek) Of the laurel tree; in mythology, a virtuous woman transformed into a laurel tree to protect her from Apollo
Daphna, Daphney, Daphni, Daphnie, Daffi, Daffie, Daffy, Dafna

Darby (English) Of the deer park
Darb, Darbee, Darbey, Darbie, Darrbey, Darrbie, Darrby, Derby, Larby

Daria (Greek) Feminine form of Darius; possessing good fortune; wealthy
Dari, Darian, Dariane, Darianna, Dariele, Darielle, Darien, Darienne

Daring (American) One who takes risks; a bold woman
Daryng, Derring, Dering, Deryng

Darlene (English) Our little darling
Dareen, Darla, Darleane, Darleen, Darleena, Darlena, Darlenny, Darlina

Daryn (Greek) Feminine form of Darin; a gift of God
Darynn, Darynne, Darinne, Daren, Darenn, Darene

Dawn (English) Born at daybreak; of the day's first light
Dawna, Dawne, Dawnelle, Dawnetta, Dawnette, Dawnielle, Dawnika, Dawnita

Day (American) A father's hope for tomorrow
Daye, Dai, Dae

Daya (Hebrew) Resembling a bird of prey
Dayah, Dayana, Dayanara, Dayania, Dayaniah, Dayanea, Dayaneah

Dayton (English) From the sunny town
Dayten, Daytan

Dea (Greek) Resembling a goddess
Deah, Diya, Diyah

Deborah (Hebrew)
Resembling a bee; in the
Bible, a prophetess
*Debbera, Debbey, Debbi,
Debbie, Debbra, Debby*

Deidre (Gaelic) A broken-
hearted or raging woman
*Deadra, Dede, Dedra, Deedra,
Deedre, Deidra, Deirdre,
Deidrie*

Deiondre (American) From
the lush valley
*Deiondra, Deiondria,
Deiondrea, Deiondriya*

Deja (French) One of remem-
brance
*Dayja, Dejah, Daejah, Daijia,
Daija, Daijah, Deijah, Deija*

Dekla (Latvian) In mythology,
a trinity goddess
*Decla, Deckla, Deklah,
Decklah, Declah*

Delaney (Irish / French) The
dark challenger / from the
elder-tree grove
*Delaina, Delaine, Delainey,
Delainy, Delane, Delanie,
Delany, Delayna*

Delaware (English) From the
state of Delaware
*Delawair, Delaweir, Delwayr,
Delawayre, Delawaire,
Delawaer, Delawaere*

Delilah (Hebrew) A seductive
woman
Delila, Delyla, Delylah

Delta (Greek) From the mouth
of the river; the fourth letter
of the Greek alphabet
Dellta, Deltah, Delltah

Delyth (Welsh) A pretty young
woman
Delythe, Delith, Delithe

Demeter (Greek) In mythology,
the goddess of the harvest
*Demetra, Demitra, Demitras,
Dimetria, Demetre, Demetria,
Dimitra, Dimitre*

Demi (Greek) A petite woman
*Demie, Demee, Demy, Demiana,
Demianne, Demianna, Demea*

Denali (Indian) A superior
woman
*Denalie, Denaly, Denally,
Denalli, Denaley, Denalee,
Denallee, Denallie*

Dendara (Egyptian) From the
town on the river
*Dendera, Dendaria, Denderia,
Dendarra*

Denise (French) Feminine
form of Dennis; a follower of
Dionysus
*Denese, Denyse, Denice,
Deniece, Denisa, Denissa,
Denize, Denyce, Denys*

Denver (English) From the green valley

Derora (Hebrew) As free as a bird
Derorah, Derorra, Derorit, Drora, Drorah, Drorit, Drorlya, Derorice

Derry (Irish) From the oak grove
Derrey, Derri, Derrie, Derree, Derrea, Derreah

Deryn (Welsh) A birdlike woman
Derran, Deren, Derhyn, Deron, Derrin, Derrine, Derron, Derrynne

Desiree (French) One who is desired
Desaree, Desirae, Desarae, Desire, Desyre, Dezirae, Deziree, Desirat

Destiny (English) Recognizing one's certain fortune; fate
Destanee, Destinee, Destiney, Destini, Destinie, Destine, Destina, Destyni

Deva (Hindi) A divine being
Devi, Daeva

Devera (Latin) In mythology, goddess of brooms
Deverah

Devon (English) From the beautiful farmland; of the divine
Devan, Deven, Devenne, Devin, Devona, Devondra, Devonna, Devonne, Devyn

Dextra (Latin) Feminine form of Dexter; one who is skillful
Dex

Dharma (Hindi) The universal law of order
Darma

Dhyana (Hindi) One who meditates

Diamond (French) Woman of high value
Diamanta, Diamonique, Diamante

Diana (Latin) Of the divine; in mythology, goddess of the moon and the hunt
Dianna, Dayanna, Dayana, Deanna

Diane (Latin) Form of Diana, meaning "of the divine"
Dayann, Dayanne, Deana, Deane, Deandra, Deann

Dido (Latin) In mythology, the queen of Carthage who committed suicide
Dydo

Dielle (Latin) One who worships God
Diele, Diell, Diella, Diela, Diel

Dimity (English) Resembling a sheer cotton fabric
Dimitee, Dimitey, Dimitie, Dimitea, Dimiteah, Dimiti

Dimona (Hebrew) Woman from the south
Dimonah, Dymona, Demona, Demonah, Dymonah

Disa (English) Resembling an orchid

Discordia (Latin) In mythology, goddess of strife
Dyscordia, Diskordia, Dyskordia

Diti (Hindi) In Hinduism, an earth goddess
Dyti, Ditie, Dytie, Dity, Dyty, Ditey, Dytey, Ditee

Dixie (English) Woman from the South
Dixi, Dixy, Dixey, Dixee

Dolores (Spanish) Woman of sorrow; refers to the Virgin Mary
Dalores, Delora, Delores, Deloria, Deloris, Dolorcita, Dolorcitas, Dolorita

Domina (Latin) An elegant lady
Dominah, Domyna, Domynah

Dominique (French) Feminine form of Dominic; born on the Lord's day
Domaneke, Domanique, Domenica, Domeniga, Domenique, Dominee, Domineek, Domineke

Doreen (French / Gaelic) The golden one / a brooding woman
Dorene, Doreyn, Dorine, Dorreen, Doryne, Doreena, Dore, Doirean, Doireann, Doireanne, Doireana, Doireanna

Dorothy (Greek) A gift of God
Dasha, Dasya, Dodie, Dody, Doe, Doll, Dolley, Dolli

Dove (American) Resembling a bird of peace
Duv

Drisana (Indian) Daughter of the sun
Dhrisana, Drisanna, Drysana, Drysanna, Dhrysana, Dhrisanna, Dhrysanna

Drury (French) One who is greatly loved
Drurey, Druri, Drurie, Druree, Drurea, Drureah

Duana (Irish) Feminine form of Dwayne; little, dark one
Duane, Duayna, Duna, Dwana, Dwayna, Dubhain, Dubheasa

Dulce (Latin) A very sweet woman
Dulcina, Dulcee, Dulcie

Dumia (Hebrew) One who is silent
Dumiya, Dumiah, Dumiyah, Dumea, Dumeah

Duvessa (Irish) A dark beauty
Duvessah, Duvesa, Dubheasa, Duvesah

Dylan (Welsh) Daughter of the waves
Dylana, Dylane, Dyllan, Dyllana, Dillon, Dillan, Dillen, Dillian

Dyre (Scandinavian) One who is dear to the heart

Dysis (Greek) Born at sunset
Dysiss, Dysisse, Dysys, Dysyss, Dysysse

E

Eadlin (Anglo-Saxon) Born into royalty
Eadlinn, Eadlinne, Eadline, Eadlyn, Eadlynn, Eadlynne, Eadlina, Eadlyna

Eara (Scottish) Woman from the east
Earah, Earra, Earrah, Earia, Earea, Earie, Eari, Earee

Earla (English) A great leader
Earlah

Earna (English) Resembling an eagle
Earnah, Earnia, Earnea, Earniah, Earneah

Easter (American) Born during the religious holiday
Eastere, Eastre, Eastir, Eastar, Eastor, Eastera, Easteria, Easterea

Easton (American) A wholesome woman
Eastan, Easten, Eastun, Eastyn

Eathelin (English) Noble woman of the waterfall
Eathelyn, Eathelinn, Eathelynn, Eathelina, Eathelyna, Ethelin, Ethelyn, Eathelen

Eber (Hebrew) One who moves beyond

Ebere (African) One who shows mercy
Eberre, Ebera, Eberia, Eberea, Eberria, Eberrea, Ebiere, Ebierre

Ebony (Egyptian) A dark beauty
Eboni, Ebonee, Ebonie, Ebonique, Eboney, Ebonea, Eboneah

Ebrill (Welsh) Born in April
Ebrille, Ebril, Evril, Evrill, Evrille

Edana (Irish) Feminine form of Aidan; a fiery woman
Edanah, Edanna, Ena, Eideann, Eidana

Eden (Hebrew) Place of pleasure
Edan, Edin, Edon

Edith (English) The spoils of war; one who is joyous; a treasure
Edyth, Eda, Edee, Edie, Edita, Edelina, Edeline, Edelyne, Edelynn, Edalyn, Edalynn, Edita, Edyta, Eydie

Edna (Hebrew) One who brings pleasure; a delight
Ednah, Edena, Edenah

Edra (English) A powerful and mighty woman
Edrah, Edrea, Edreah, Edria, Edriah

Eduarda (Portugese) Feminine form of Edward; a wealthy protector
Eduardia, Eduardea, Edwarda, Edwardia, Edwardea, Eduardina, Eduardyna, Edwardina

Egan (American) A wholesome woman
Egann, Egen, Egun, Egon

Egeria (Latin) A wise counselor; in mythology, a water nymph
Egeriah, Egerea, Egereah, Egeriya, Egeriyah

Eileen (Gaelic) Form of Evelyn, meaning "a birdlike woman"
Eila, Eileene, Eilena, Eilene, Eilin, Eilleen, Eily, Eilean

Eilwen (Welsh) One with a fair brow
Eilwenne, Eilwin, Eilwinne, Eilwyn, Eilwynne

Eirene (Greek) Form of Irene, meaning "a peaceful woman"
Eireen, Eireene, Eiren, Eir, Eireine, Eirein, Eirien, Eiriene

Eires (Greek) A peaceful woman
Eiress, Eiris, Eiriss, Eirys, Eiryss

Eirian (Welsh) One who is bright and beautiful
Eiriann, Eiriane, Eiriana, Eirianne, Eirianna

Ekron (Hebrew) One who is firmly rooted
Eckron, Ecron

Elaine (French) Form of Helen, meaning "the shining light"
Ellaine, Ellayne, Elaina, Elayna, Elayne, Elaene, Elaena, Ellaina

Elana (Hebrew) From the oak tree
Elanna, Elanah, Elanie, Elani, Elany, Elaney, Elanee, Elan

Elata (Latin) A high-spirited woman
Elatah, Elatta, Elattah, Elatia, Elatea, Elatiah, Elateah

Elath (Hebrew) From the grove of trees
Elathe, Elatha, Elathia, Elathea

Eldora (Greek) A gift of the sun
Eleadora, Eldorah, Eldorra, Eldoria, Eldorea

Eldoris (Greek) Woman of the sea
Eldorise, Eldoriss, Eldorisse, Eldorys, Eldoryss, Eldorysse

Eleanor (Greek) Form of Helen, meaning "the shining light"
Eleanora, Eleni, Eleonora, Eleonore, Elinor, Elnora, Eleanore, Elinora, Nora

Elena (Spanish) Form of Helen, meaning "the shining light"
Elenah, Eleena, Eleenah, Elyna, Elynah, Elina, Elinah, Eleni, Eliana

Eliana (Hebrew) The Lord answers our prayers
Eleana, Elia, Eliane, Elianna, Elianne, Eliann, Elyana, Elyanna, Elyann, Elyan, Elyanne

Elica (German) One who is noble
Elicah, Elicka, Elika, Elyca, Elycka, Elyka, Elsha, Elsje

Elida (English) Resembling a winged creature
Elidah, Elyda, Eleeda, Eleda, Elieda, Eleida, Eleada

Elika (Hebrew) God will judge
Elikah, Elyka, Elicka, Elycka, Elica, Elyca

Elisa (English) Form of Elizabeth, meaning "my God is bountiful"
Elisha, Elishia, Elissa, Elisia, Elysa, Elysha, Elysia, Elyssa

Elise (English) Form of Elizabeth, meaning "my God is bountiful"
Elle, Elice, Elisse, Elyse, Elysse, Ilyse

Elita (Latin) The chosen one
Elitah, Elyta, Elytah, Eleta, Eletah, Elitia, Elitea, Electa

Elizabeth (Hebrew) My God is bountiful; God's promise
Liz, Elisabet, Elisabeth, Elisabetta, Elissa, Eliza, Elizabel, Elizabet, Elsa, Beth, Babette, Libby, Lisa, Itzel, Ilsabeth, Ilsabet

Ella (German) From a foreign land
Elle, Ellee, Ellesse, Elli, Ellia, Ellie, Elly, Ela

Ellen (English) Form of Helen, meaning "the shining light"
Elin, Elleen, Ellena, Ellene, Ellyn, Elynn, Elen, Ellin

Ellery (English) Form of Hilary, meaning "a cheerful woman"
Ellerey, Elleri, Ellerie, Elleree, Ellerea, Ellereah

Elliana (Hebrew) The Lord answers our prayers
Eliana

Ellie (English) Form of Eleanor, meaning "the shining light"
Elli, Elly, Elley, Elleigh

Ellyanne (American) A shining and gracious woman
Ellianne, Ellyanna, Ellianna, Ellyann, Elliann, Ellyan, Ellian

Elma (German) Having God's protection
Elmah

Eloisa (Latin) Form of Louise, meaning "a famous warrior"
Eloise, Eloiza, Eloisee, Eloize, Eloizee, Aloisa, Aloise

Elrica (German) A great ruler
Elricah, Elrika, Elrikah, Elryca, Elrycah, Elryka, Elrykah, Elrick

Elsie (English) Form of Elizabeth, meaning "my god is bountiful"

Elvia (Irish) A friend of the elves
Elva, Elvie, Elvina, Elvinia, Elviah, Elvea, Elveah, Elvyna

Elvira (Latin) A truthful woman; one who can be trusted
Elvera, Elvita, Elvyra

Ema (Polynesian / German) One who is greatly loved / a serious woman

Ember (English) A low-burning fire
Embar, Embir, Embyr

Emerson (German) Offspring of Emery
Emmerson, Emyrson

Emery (German) Industrious
Emeri, Emerie, Emori, Emorie, Emory

Emily (Latin) An industrious and hardworking woman
Emilee, Emilie, Emilia, Emelia, Emileigh, Emeleigh, Emeli, Emelie, Emely, Emmalee

Emma (German) One who is complete; a universal woman
Emmy, Emmajean, Emmalee, Emmi, Emmie, Emmaline, Emelina, Emeline

Emmylou (American) A universal ruler
Emmilou, Emmielou, Emylou, Emilou, Emielou

Ena (Irish) A fiery and passionate woman
Enah, Enat, Eny, Enya

Encarnación (Spanish) Refers to the Incarnation festival

Engracia (Spanish) A graceful woman
Engraciah, Engracea, Engraceah

Enslie (American) An emotional woman
Ensli, Ensley, Ensly, Enslee, Enslea, Ensleigh

Eranthe (Greek) As delicate as a spring flower
Erantha, Eranth, Eranthia, Eranthea

Erasta (African) A peaceful woman

Ercilia (American) One who is frank
Erciliah, Ercilea, Ercileah, Ercilya, Ercilyah, Erciliya, Erciliyah

Erendira (Spanish) Daughter born into royalty
Erendirah, Erendiria, Erendirea, Erendyra, Erendyria, Erendyrea, Erendeera, Erendiera

Erica (Scandinavian / Latin) Feminine form of Eric; ever the ruler / resembling heather
Erika, Ericka, Erikka, Eryka, Erike, Ericca, Erics, Eiric, Rica

Erimentha (Greek) A devoted
protector
*Erimenthe, Erimenthia,
Erimenthea*

Erin (Gaelic) Woman from
Ireland
*Erienne, Erina, Erinn, Erinna,
Erinne, Eryn, Eryna, Erynn,
Arin*

Ernestina (German) Feminine
form of Ernest; one who is
determined; serious
Ernesta, Ernestine, Ernesha

Eshah (African) An exuberant
woman
Esha

Eshe (African) Giver of life
Eshey, Eshay, Esh, Eshae, Eshai

Esme (French) An esteemed
woman
*Esmai, Esmae, Esmay, Esmaye,
Esmee*

Esmeralda (Spanish) Resembling
a prized emerald
*Esmerald, Emerald, Emeralda,
Emelda, Esma*

Esne (English) Filled with
happiness
*Esnee, Esney, Esnea, Esni,
Esnie, Esny*

Essence (American) A
perfumed woman
*Essince, Esense, Esince, Essynce,
Esynce*

Esthelia (Spanish) A shining
woman
*Estheliah, Esthelea, Estheleah,
Esthelya, Esthelyah, Estheliya,
Estheliyah*

Esther (Persian) Resembling
the myrtle leaf
Ester, Eszter, Eistir, Eszti

Estrella (Spanish) Star
Estrela

Estrid (Norse) Form of Astrid,
meaning "one with divine
strength"
*Estread, Estreed, Estrad, Estri,
Estrod, Estrud, Estryd, Estrida*

Etana (Hebrew) A strong and
dedicated woman
*Etanah, Etanna, Etannah,
Etania, Etanea, Ethana,
Ethanah, Ethania*

Etaney (Hebrew) One who is
focused
*Etany, Etanie, Etani, Etanee,
Etanea*

Eternity (American) Lasting
forever
*Eternitie, Eterniti, Eternitey,
Eternitee, Eternyty, Eternyti,
Eternytie, Eternytee*

Ethna (Irish) A graceful
woman
*Ethnah, Eithne, Ethne, Eithna,
Eithnah*

Eudlina (Slavic) A generous
woman
Eudlinah, Eudleena, Eudleenah

Eugenia (Greek) A well-born
woman
Eugenie, Gina, Zenechka

Eulanda (American) A fair
woman
*Eulande, Euland, Eulandia,
Eulandea*

Eunice (Greek) One who con-
quers
*Eunise, Eunyce, Eunis, Euniss,
Eunyss, Eunysse*

Eurybia (Greek) In mythology,
a sea goddess and mother of
Pallas, Perses, and Astraios
Eurybiah, Eurybea, Eurybeah

Eurynome (Greek) In mythology, the mother of the Graces
Eurynomie, Eurynomi

Euvenia (American) A
hardworking woman

Eva (Hebrew) Giver of life; a
lively woman
*Eve, Evetta, Evette, Evia,
Eviana, Evie, Evita, Eeva*

Evangeline (Greek) A bringer
of good news
Evangelina, Evangelyn

Evelyn (German) A birdlike
woman
*Evaleen, Evalina, Evaline,
Evalyn, Evelin, Evelina, Eveline,
Evelyne, Eileen, Evelynn*

Evline (French) One who loves
nature
*Evleen, Evleene, Evlean,
Evleane, Evlene, Evlyn, Evlyne*

Everly (English) Boar in a wild
field
*Everleigh, Everley, Everlie,
Everlee*

F

Fairly (English) From the far
meadow
*Fairley, Fairlee, Fairleigh,
Fairli, Fairlie, Faerly, Faerli,
Faerlie*

Faith (English) Having a belief
and trust in God
*Faythe, Faithe, Faithful,
Fayana, Fayanna, Fayanne,
Fayane, Fayth*

Fakhira (Arabic) A magnificent woman
Fakhirah, Fakhyra, Fakhyrah, Fakheera, Fakira, Fakirah, Fakeera, Fakyra

Fala (Native American) Resembling a crow
Falah, Falla, Fallah

Fallon (Irish) A commanding woman
Fallyn, Faline, Falinne, Faleen, Faleene, Falynne, Falyn, Falina

Fantasia (Latin) From the fantasy land
Fantasiah, Fantasea, Fantasiya, Fantazia, Fantazea, Fantaziya

Farley (English) From the fern clearing
Farly, Farli, Farlie, Farlee, Farleigh, Farlea, Farleah

Fate (Greek) One's destiny
Fayte, Faite, Faete, Faet, Fait, Fayt

Fatima (Arabic) The perfect woman
Fatimah, Fahima, Fahimah

Fatinah (Arabic) A captivating woman
Fatina, Fateena, Fateenah, Fatyna, Fatynah, Fatin, Fatine, Faatinah, Fateana, Fateanah, Fatiena, Fatienah, Fateina, Fateinah

Favor (English) One who grants her approval
Faver, Favar, Favorre

Fay (English) From the fairy kingdom; a fairy or an elf
Faye, Fai, Faie, Fae, Fayette, Faylinn, Faylyn, Faylynn

Fayina (Russian) An independent woman
Fayinah, Fayena, Fayeena, Fayeana, Fayiena, Fayeina

February (American) Born in the month of February
Februari, Februarie, Februarey, Februaree, Februarea

Felicity (Latin) Form of Felicia, meaning "happy"
Felicy, Felicie, Felisa

Femi (African) God loves me
Femmi, Femie, Femy, Femey, Femee, Femea, Femeah

Fenia (Scandinavian) A gold worker
Feniah, Fenea, Feneah, Feniya, Feniyah, Fenya, Fenyah, Fenja

Fernanda (Spanish) Feminine form of Fernando; an adventurous woman

Fernilia (American) A successful woman
Ferniliah, Fernilea, Fernileah, Fernilya, Fernilyah

Fia (Portuguese / Italian / Scottish) A weaver / from the flickering fire / arising from the dark of peace
Fiah, Fea, Feah, Fya, Fiya, Fyah, Fiyah

Fianna (Irish) A warrior huntress
Fiannah, Fiana, Fianne, Fiane, Fiann, Fian

Fielda (English) From the field
Fieldah, Felda, Feldah

Fife (American) Having dancing eyes
Fyfe, Fifer, Fify, Fifey, Fifee, Fifea, Fifi, Fifie

Fifia (African) Born on a Friday
Fifiah, Fifea, Fifeah, Fifeea, Fifeeah

Filipa (Spanish) Feminine form of Phillip; a friend of horses
Filipah, Filipina, Filipeena, Filipyna, Filippa, Fillipa, Fillippa

Fina (English) Feminine form of Joseph; God will add
Finah, Feena, Fyna, Fifine, Fifna, Fifne, Fini, Feana

Finley (Gaelic) A fair-haired hero
Finlay, Finly, Finlee, Finli, Finlie, Finnley, Finnlee, Finnli, Finn, Fin

Finnea (Gaelic) From the stream of the wood
Finneah, Finnia, Fynnea, Finniah, Fynnia

Fiona (Gaelic) One who is fair; a white-shouldered woman
Fionna, Fione, Fionn, Finna, Fionavar, Fionnghuala, Fionnuala, Fynballa

Firdaus (Arabic) From the garden in paradise

Flair (English) An elegant woman of natural talent
Flaire, Flare, Flayr, Flayre, Flaer, Flaere

Flame (American) A passionate and fiery woman
Flaym, Flayme, Flaime, Flaim, Flaem, Flaeme

Flannery (Gaelic) From the flatlands
Flanery, Flanneri, Flannerie, Flannerey, Flannaree, Flannerea

Fleta (English) One who is swift
Fletah, Flete, Fleda, Flita, Flyta

Florence (Latin) A flourishing woman; a blooming flower
Florencia, Florentina, Florenza, Florentine, Florentyna, Florenteena, Florenteene, Florentyne

Florizel (English) A young woman in bloom
Florizell, Florizelle, Florizele, Florizel, Florizella, Florizela, Florazel, Florazell

Fola (African) Woman of honor
Folah, Folla, Follah

Forest (English) A woodland dweller
Forrest

Forever (American) Everlasting

Francesca (Italian) Form of Frances, meaning "one who is free"
Francia, Francina, Francisca, Franchesca, Francie, Frances

Frederica (German) Peaceful ruler
Freda, Freida, Freddie, Rica

Freira (Spanish) A sister
Freirah, Freyira, Freyirah

Freya (Norse) A lady
Freyah, Freyja, Freja

Freydis (Norse) Woman born into the nobility
Freydiss, Freydisse, Freydys, Fredyss, Fraidis, Fradis, Fraydis, Fraedis

Frida (German) Peaceful
Frieda, Fryda

Fuchsia (Latin) Resembling the flower
Fusha, Fushia, Fushea, Fewsha, Fewshia, Fewshea

Fury (Greek) An enraged woman; in mythology, a winged goddess who punished wrongdoers
Furey, Furi, Furie, Furee

G

Gabriella (Italian / Spanish) Feminine form of Gabriel; heroine of God
Gabriela, Gabriellia, Gabrila, Gabryela, Gabryella

Gabrielle (Hebrew) Feminine form of Gabriel; heroine of God
Gabriel, Gabriela, Gabriele, Gabriell, Gabriellen, Gabriellia, Gabrila

Galena (Greek) Feminine form of Galen; one who is calm and peaceful
Galene, Galenah, Galenia, Galenea

Galiana (Arabic) The name of a Moorish princess
Galianah, Galianna, Galianne, Galiane, Galian, Galyana, Galyanna, Galyann

Galila (Hebrew) From the rolling hills
Galilah, Gelila, Gelilah, Gelilia, Gelilya, Glila, Glilah, Galyla

Galilee (Hebrew) From the sacred sea
Galileigh, Galilea, Galiley, Galily, Galili, Galilie

Galina (Russian) Form of Helen, meaning "the shining light"
Galinah, Galyna, Galynah, Galeena, Galeenah, Galine, Galyne, Galeene

Gardenia (English) Resembling the sweet-smelling flower
Gardeniah, Gardenea, Gardyna

Garima (Indian) A woman of importance
Garimah, Garyma, Gareema

Garnet (English) Resembling the dark-red gem
Garnette, Granata, Grenata, Grenatta

Gasha (Russian) One who is well-behaved
Gashah, Gashia, Gashea, Gashiah, Gasheah

Gavina (Latin) Feminine form of Gavin; resembling the white falcon; woman from Gabio

Gaza (Hebrew) Having great strength
Gazah, Gazza, Gazzah

Geila (Hebrew) One who brings joy to others
Geela, Geelah, Geelan, Geilah, Geiliya, Geiliyah, Gelisa, Gellah

Gemma (Latin) As precious as a jewel
Gemmalyn, Gemmalynn, Gem, Gema, Gemmaline, Jemma

Genesis (Hebrew) Of the beginning; the first book of the Bible
Genesies, Genesiss, Genessa, Genisis

Genevieve (French) White wave; fair-skinned
Genavieve, Geneve, Genevie, Genivee, Genivieve, Genoveva, Gennie, Genny

Georgia (Greek) Feminine form of George; one who works the earth; a farmer; from the state of Georgia
Georgeann, Georgeanne, Georgina, Georgena, Georgene, Georgetta, Georgette, Georgiana, Jeorjia

Gerardine (English) Feminine form of Gerard; one who is mighty with a spear
Gerarda, Gerardina, Gerardyne, Gererdina, Gerardyna, Gerrardene, Gerhardina, Gerhardine

Gertrude (German) Adored warrior
Geertruide, Geltruda, Geltrudis, Gert, Gerta, Gerte, Gertie, Gertina, Trudy

Gia (Italian) Form of Gianna, meaning "God is Gracious"
Giah

Giada (Italian) Jade
Giadda

Gianna (Italian) Feminine form of John, meaning "God is gracious"
Gia, Giana, Giovana

Gillian (Latin) One who is youthful
Gilian, Giliana, Gillianne, Ghilian

Gina (Japanese / English) A silvery woman / form of Eugenia, meaning "a well-born woman"; form of Jean, meaning "God is gracious"
Geana, Geanndra, Geena, Geina, Gena, Genalyn, Geneene, Genelle

Ginger (English) A lively woman; resembling the spice
Gingee, Gingie, Ginjer, Gingea, Gingy, Gingey, Gingi

Ginny (English) Form of Virginia, meaning "one who is chaste; virginal"
Ginnee, Ginnelle, Ginnette, Ginnie, Ginnilee, Ginna, Ginney, Ginni

Giona (Italian) Resembling the bird of peace
Gionah, Gionna, Gyona, Gyonna, Gionnah, Gyonah, Gyonnah

Giovanna (Italian) Feminine form of Giovanni; God is gracious
Geovana, Geovanna, Giavanna, Giovana, Giovani, Giovanni, Giovanie, Giovanee

Giselle (French) One who offers her pledge
Gisel, Gisela, Gisella, Jiselle

Gita (Hindi / Hebrew) A beautiful song / a good woman
Gitah, Geeta, Geetah, Gitika, Gatha, Gayatri, Gitel, Gittel

Gitana (Spanish) A gypsy woman
Gitanah, Gitanna, Gitannah, Gitane

Githa (Anglo-Saxon) A gift from God
Githah, Gytha

Giulia (Italian) Form of Julia, meaning "one who is youthful, daughter of the sky"
Giuliana, Giulie, Giulietta, Giuliette

Gladys (Welsh) Form of Claudia, meaning "one who is lame"
Gladdis, Gladdys, Gladi, Gladis, Gladyss, Gwladys, Gwyladyss, Gleda

Glenna (Gaelic) From the valley between the hills
Gleana, Gleneen, Glenene, Glenine, Glen, Glenn, Glenne, Glennene

Glenys (Welsh) A holy woman
Glenice, Glenis, Glennice, Glennis, Glennys, Glynis

Gloria (Latin) A renowned and highly praised woman
Gloriana, Glorianna, Glorya, Glorie, Gloree, Gloriane

Golda (English) Resembling the precious metal
Goldarina, Goldarine, Goldee, Goldi, Goldie, Goldina, Goldy, Goldia

Gordana (Serbian / Scottish) A proud woman / one who is heroic
Gordanah, Gordanna, Gordania, Gordaniya, Gordanea, Gordannah, Gordaniah, Gordaniyah

Grace (Latin) Having God's favor; in mythology, the Graces were the personification of beauty, charm, and grace
Gracee, Gracella, Gracelynn, Gracelynne, Gracey, Gracia, Graciana, Gracie, Gracelyn

Gracie (Latin) Form of Grace, meaning "having God's favor"
Gracee, Gracey, Graci

Granada (Spanish) From the Moorish kingdom
Granadda, Grenada, Grenadda

Greer (Scottish) Feminine form of Gregory; one who is alert and watchful
Grear, Grier, Gryer

Gregoria (Latin) Feminine form of Gregory; one who is alert and watchful
Gregoriana, Gregorijana, Gregorina, Gregorine, Gregorya, Gregoryna, Gregorea, Gregoriya

Greta (German) Resembling a pearl
Greeta, Gretal, Grete, Gretel, Gretha, Grethe, Grethel, Gretna, Gretchen

Guadalupe (Spanish) From the valley of wolves
Guadelupe, Lupe, Lupita

Guinevere (Welsh) One who is fair; of the white wave; in mythology, King Arthur's queen
Guenever, Guenevere, Gueniver, Guenna, Guennola, Guinever, Guinna, Gwen

Guiseppina (Italian) Feminine form of Guiseppe; the Lord will add
Giuseppyna, Giuseppa, Giuseppia, Giuseppea, Guiseppie, Guiseppia, Guiseppa, Giuseppina

Gulielma (German) Feminine form of Wilhelm; determined protector
Guglielma, Guillelmina, Guillielma, Gulielmina, Guillermina

Gulinar (Arabic) Resembling the pomegranate
Gulinare, Gulinear, Gulineir, Gulinara, Gulinaria, Gulinarea

Gwendolyn (Welsh) One who is fair; of the white ring
Guendolen, Guendolin, Guendolinn, Guendolynn, Guenna, Gwen, Gwenda, Gwendaline, Wendy

Gwyneth (Welsh) One who is blessed with happiness
Gweneth, Gwenith, Gwenyth, Gwineth, Gwinneth, Gwinyth, Gwynith, Gwynna

Gytha (English) One who is treasured
Gythah

Habbai (Arabic) One who is much loved
Habbae, Habbay, Habbaye

Habiba (Arabic) Feminine form of Habib; one who is dearly loved; sweetheart
Habibah, Habeeba, Habyba

Hachi (Native American / Japanese) From the river / having good fortune
Hachie, Hachee, Hachiko, Hachiyo, Hachy, Hachey, Hachikka

Hadara (Hebrew) A spectacular ornament; adorned with beauty
Hadarah, Hadarit, Haduraq, Hadarra, Hadarrah

Hadassah (Hebrew) From the myrtle tree
Hadassa, Hadasah, Hadasa

Hadiya (Arabic) A gift from God; a righteous woman
Hadiyah, Hadiyyah, Haadiyah, Haadiya, Hadeeya, Hadeeyah, Hadieya, Hadieyah

Hadlai (Hebrew) In a resting state; one who hinders
Hadlae, Hadlay, Hadlaye

Hadley (English) From the field of heather
Hadlea, Hadleigh, Hadly, Hedlea, Hedleigh, Hedley, Hedlie, Hadlee

Hadria (Latin) From the town in northern Italy
Hadrea, Hadriana, Hadriane, Hadrianna, Hadrien, Hadrienne, Hadriah, Hadreah

Hafthah (Arabic) One who is protected by God
Haftha

Hagab (Hebrew) Resembling a grasshopper
Hagabah, Hagaba, Hagabe

Hagai (Hebrew) One who has been abandoned
Hagae, Hagay, Hagaye, Haggai, Haggae, Hagie, Haggie, Hagi

Hagen (Irish) A youthful woman
Hagan, Haggen, Haggan

Haidee (Greek) A modest woman; one who is well-behaved
Hadee, Haydee, Haydy, Haidi, Haidie, Haydi, Haydie, Haidy

Hailey (English) from the field of hay
Haley, Hayle, Hailee, Haylee, Haylie, Haleigh, Hayley, Haeleigh

Haimati (Indian) A queen of the snow-covered mountains
Haimatie, Haimaty, Haimatey, Haimatee, Haymati, Haymatie, Haymatee, Haimatea

Haimi (Hawaiian) One who searches for the truth
Haimie, Haimy, Haimey, Haimee, Haymi, Haymie, Haymee, Haimea

Hakana (Turkish) Feminine form of Hakan; ruler of the people; an empress
Hakanah, Hakanna, Hakane, Hakann, Hakanne

Hakkoz (Hebrew) One who has the qualities of a thorn
Hakoz, Hakkoze, Hakoze, Hakkoza, Hakoza

Halak (Hebrew) One who is bald; smooth

Haleigha (Hawaiian) Born with the rising sun
Haleea, Haleya, Halya

Hall (American) One who is distinguished
Haul

Hallie (Scandinavian / Greek / English) From the hall / woman of the sea / from the field of hay
Halley, Hallie, Halle, Hallee, Hally, Halleigh, Hallea, Halleah

Halo (Latin) Having a blessed aura
Haylo, Haelo, Hailo

Halsey (American) A playful woman
Halsy, Halsee, Halsea, Halsi, Halsie, Halcie, Halcy, Halcey

Halyn (American) A unique young woman
Halynn, Halynne, Halin, Halinn, Halinne

Hammon (Hebrew) Of the warm springs

Hamula (Hebrew) Feminine form of Hamul; spared by God
Hamulah, Hamulla, Hamullah

Hana (Japanese / Arabic) Resembling a flower blossom / a blissful woman
Hanah, Hanako

Hanan (Arabic) One who shows mercy and compassion

Hang (Vietnamese) Of the moon

Hanika (Hebrew) A graceful woman
Hanikah, Haneeka, Haneekah, Hanyka, Hanykah, Haneika, Haneikah, Hanieka

Hanita (Indian) Favored with divine grace
Hanitah, Hanyta, Haneeta, Hanytah, Haneetah, Haneita, Haneitah, Hanieta

Haniyah (Arabic) One who is pleased; happy
Haniya, Haniyyah, Haniyya, Hani, Hanie, Hanee, Hany, Haney

Hannah (Hebrew) Having favor and grace; in the Bible, mother of Samuel
Hanalee, Hanalise, Hanna, Hanne, Hannele, Hannelore, Hannie, Hanny, Chana

Hanya (Aboriginal) As solid as a stone

Hara (Hebrew) From the mountainous land
Harah, Harra, Harrah

Haradah (Hebrew) One who is filled with fear
Harada

Harika (Turkish) A superior woman
Harikah, Haryka, Hareeka, Harykah, Hareekah, Hareaka, Hareakah

Hariti (Indian) In mythology, the goddess for the protection of children
Haritie, Haryti, Harytie, Haritee, Harytee, Haritea, Harytea

Harley (English) From the meadow of the hares
Harlea, Harlee, Harleen, Harleigh, Harlene, Harlie, Harli, Harly

Harlow (American) An impetuous woman

Harmony (English / Latin) Unity / musically in tune
Harmonie, Harmoni, Harmonee

Harper (English) One who plays or makes harps

Harriet (German) Feminine form of Henry; ruler of the house
Harriett, Hanriette, Hanrietta, Harriette, Harrietta, Harrette

Harva (English) A warrior of the army

Hasibah (Arabic) Feminine form of Hasib; one who is noble and respected
Hasiba, Hasyba, Hasybah, Haseeba, Haseebah

Hasina (African) One who is good and beautiful
Hasinah, Hasyna, Hasynah

Haurana (Hebrew) Feminine form of Hauran; woman from the caves
Hauranna, Hauranah, Haurann, Hauranne

Haven (English) One who provides a safe haven
Hayven, Havan, Hayvan, Havon, Hayvon, Havin, Hayvin, Havyn, Hayvyn, Haeven, Haevin, Haevan

Havva (Turkish) A giver of the breath of life
Havvah, Havvia, Havviah

Hayden (English) From the hedged valley
Haden, Haydan, Haydn, Haydon, Haeden, Haedyn, Hadyn

Hayud (Arabic) From the mountain
Hayuda, Hayudah, Hayood, Hayooda

Hazel (English) From the hazel tree
Hazell, Hazelle, Haesel, Hazle, Hazal, Hayzel, Haezel, Haizel

Heather (English) Resembling the evergreen flowering plant
Hether, Heatha, Heath, Heathe

Heaven (American) From paradise; from the sky
Heavely, Heavenly, Hevean, Hevan, Heavynne, Heavenli, Heavenlie, Heavenleigh, Heavenlee, Heavenley, Heavenlea, Heavyn

Hecate (Greek) In mythology, a goddess of fertility and witchcraft
Hekate

Heidi (German) Of the nobility, serene
Heidy, Heide, Hydie

Heirnine (Greek) Form of Helen, meaning "the shining light"
Heirnyne, Heirneine, Heirniene, Heirneene, Heirneane

Helen (Greek) The shining light; in mythology, Helen was the most beautiful woman in the world
Helene, Halina, Helaine, Helana, Heleena, Helena, Helenna, Hellen, Aleen, Elaine, Eleanor, Elena, Ellen, Galina, Heirnine, Helice, Leanna, Yalena

Helia (Greek) Daughter of the sun
Heliah, Helea, Heleah, Heliya, Heliyah, Heller, Hellar

Helice (Greek) Form of Helen, meaning "the shining light"
Helyce, Heleece, Heliece, Heleace

Helike (Greek) In mythology, a willow nymph who nurtured Zeus
Helica, Helyke, Helika, Helyka, Helyca

Helle (Greek) In mythology, the daughter of Athamas who escaped sacrifice on the back of a golden ram

Helma (German) Form of Wilhelmina, meaning "determined protector"
Helmah, Helmia, Helmea, Helmina, Helmyna, Helmeena, Helmine, Helmyne

Heloise (French) One who is famous in battle
Helois, Heloisa, Helewidis

Henrietta (German) Feminine form of Henry; ruler of the house
Henretta, Henrieta, Henriette, Henrika, Henryetta, Hetta, Hette, Hettie

Herdis (Scandinavian) A battle maiden
Herdiss, Herdisse, Herdys

Hermelinda (Spanish) Bearing a powerful shield
Hermelynda, Hermalinda, Hermalynda, Hermelenda

Hermia (Greek) Feminine form of Hermes; a messenger of the gods
Hermiah, Hermea, Hermila

Hermona (Hebrew) From the mountain peak
Hermonah, Hermonna

Hernanda (Spanish) One who is daring
Hernandia, Hernandea, Hernandiya

Herra (Greek) Daughter of the earth
Herrah

Hersala (Spanish) A lovely woman
Hersalah, Hersalla, Hersallah, Hersalia, Hersaliah, Hersalea, Hersaleah

Hesiena (African) The first-born of twins
Hesienna, Hesienah, Heseina

Hesione (Greek) In mythology, a Trojan princess saved by Hercules from a sea monster

Hester (Greek) A starlike woman
Hestere, Hesther, Hesta, Hestar

Heven (American) A pretty young woman
Hevin, Hevon, Hevun, Hevven, Hevvin, Hevvon, Hevvun

Hezer (Hebrew) A woman of great strength
Hezir, Hezyr, Hezire, Hezyre, Hezere

Hiah (Korean) A bright woman
Heija, Heijah, Hia

Hibiscus (Latin) Resembling the showy flower
Hibiskus, Hibyscus, Hibyskus, Hybiscus, Hybiskus, Hybyscus, Hybyskus

Hikmah (Arabic) Having great wisdom
Hikmat, Hikma

Hilan (Greek) Filled with happines
Hylan, Hilane, Hilann, Hilanne, Hylane, Hylann, Hylanne

Hilary (Latin) A cheerful woman
Hillary, Hillery, Ellery

Hina (Polynesian) In mythology, a dual goddess symbolizing day and night
Hinna, Henna, Hinaa, Hinah, Heena, Hena

Hind (Arabic) Owning a group of camels; a wife of Muhammed
Hynd, Hinde, Hynde

Hinda (Hebrew) Resembling a doe
Hindah, Hindy, Hindey, Hindee, Hindi, Hindie, Hynda, Hyndy

Hitomi (Japanese) One who has beautiful eyes
Hitomie, Hitomee, Hitomea, Hitomy, Hitomey

Holda (German) A secretive woman; one who is hidden
Holde

Hollander (Dutch) A woman from Holland
Hollynder, Hollender, Holander, Holynder, Holender, Hollande, Hollanda

Holly (English) Of the holly tree
Holli, Hollie, Hollee, Holley, Hollye, Hollyanne, Holle, Hollea

Holton (American) One who is whimsical
Holten, Holtan, Holtin, Holtyn, Holtun

Holy (American) One who is pious or sacred
Holey, Holee, Holeigh, Holi, Holie, Holye, Holea, Holeah

Hope (English) One who has high expectations through faith

Hortensia (Latin) Woman of
the garden
*Hartencia, Hartinsia,
Hortencia, Hortense,
Hortenspa, Hortenxia,
Hortinzia, Hortendana*

Hova (African) Born into the
middle class

Hoyden (American) A spirited
woman
*Hoiden, Hoydan, Hoidan,
Hoydyn, Hoidyn, Hoidin,
Hoidin*

Hudson (English) One who is
adventurous; an explorer
*Hudsen, Hudsan, Hudsun,
Hudsyn, Hudsin*

Hueline (German) An intelli-
gent woman
*Huelene, Huelyne, Hueleine,
Hueliene, Hueleene, Huleane*

Huhana (Maori) Form of
Susannah, meaning "white lily"
*Huhanah, Huhanna,
Huhanne, Huhann, Huhane*

Humita (Native American)
One who shells corn
*Humitah, Humyta, Humeeta,
Humieta, Humeita, Humeata,
Humytah, Humeetah*

Hutena (Hurrian) In mythol-
ogy, the goddess of fate
*Hutenah, Hutenna, Hutyna,
Hutina*

Huwaidah (Arabic) One who
is gentle
Huwaydah, Huwaida

Huyen (Vietnamese) A woman
with jet-black hair

Hypatia (Greek) An intellectu-
ally superior woman
Hypasia, Hypacia, Hypate

I

Ianthe (Greek) Resembling the
violet flower; in mythology,
a sea nymph, a daughter of
Oceanus
Iantha, Ianthia, Ianthina

Ibtesam (Arabic) One who
smiles often
Ibtisam, Ibtysam

Ibtihaj (Arabic) A delight;
bringer of joy
Ibtehaj, Ibtyhaj

Ida (Greek) One who is
diligent; hardworking; in
mythology, the nymph who
cared for Zeus on Mount Ida
*Idania, Idaea, Idalee, Idaia,
Idania, Idalia, Idalie, Idana*

Idil (Latin) A pleasant woman
Idyl, Idill, Idyll

Idoia (Spanish) Refers to the Virgin Mary
Idoea, Idurre, Iratze, Izazkun

Idona (Scandinavian) A fresh-faced woman
Idonah, Idonna, Idonnah

Ife (African) One who loves and is loved
Ifeh, Iffe

Ikeida (American) A spontaneous woman
Ikeidah, Ikeyda, Ikeydah

Ilamay (French) From the island
Ilamaye, Ilamai, Ilamae

Ilia (Greek) From the ancient city
Iliah, Ilea, Ileah, Iliya, Iliyah, Ilya, Ilyah

Iliana (English) Form of Aileen, meaning, "the light-bearer"
Ilianna, Ilyana, Ilyanna, Ilene, Iline, Ilyne

Ilithyia (Greek) In mythology, goddess of childbirth
Ilithya, Ilithiya, Ilithyiah

Ilma (German) Form of Wilhelmina, meaning "determined protector"
Ilmah, Illma, Illmah

Ilori (African) A special child; one who is treasured
Illori, Ilorie, Illorie, Ilory, Illory, Ilorey, Illorey, Iloree

Ilta (Finnish) Born at night
Iltah, Illta

Ilyse (German / Greek) Born into the nobility / form of Elyse, meaning "blissful"
Ilysea, Ilysia, Ilysse, Ilysea

Imala (Native American) One who disciplines others
Imalah, Imalla, Imallah, Immala, Immalla

Iman (Arabic) Having great faith
Imani, Imanie, Imania, Imaan, Imany, Imaney, Imanee, Imanea, Imain, Imaine, Imayn

Imanuela (Spanish) A faithful woman
Imanuella, Imanuel, Imanuele, Imanuell

Imari (Japanese) Daughter of today
Imarie, Imaree, Imarea, Imary, Imarey

Imelda (Italian) Warrior in the universal battle
Imeldah, Imalda, Imaldah

Imperia (Latin) A majestic woman
Imperiah, Imperea, Impereah, Imperial, Imperiel, Imperielle, Imperialle

Ina (Polynesian) In mythology, a moon goddess
Inah, Inna, Innah

Inaki (Asian) Having a generous nature
Inakie, Inaky, Inakey, Inakea, Inakee

Inanna (Sumerian) A lady of the sky; in mythology, goddess of love, fertility, war, and the earth
Inannah, Inana, Inanah, Inann, Inanne, Inane

Inara (Arabic) A heaven-sent daughter; one who shines with light
Inarah, Innara, Inarra, Innarra

Inari (Finnish / Japanese) Woman from the lake / one who is successful
Inarie, Inaree, Inary, Inarey, Inarea, Inareah

Inaya (Arabic) One who cares for the well-being of others
Inayah, Inayat

Inca (Indian) An adventurer
Incah, Inka, Inkah, Incka, Inckah

India (English) From the river; woman from India
Indea, Indiah, Indeah, Indya, Indiya, Indee, Inda, Indy

Indiana (English) From the land of the Indians; from the state of Indiana
Indianna, Indyana, Indyanna

Indigo (English) Resembling the plant; a purplish-blue dye
Indygo, Indeego

Ineesha (American) A sparkling woman
Ineeshah, Ineisha, Ineishah, Iniesha, Inieshah, Ineasha, Ineashah, Ineysha

Ingalls (American) A peaceful woman

Ingelise (Danish) Having the grace of the god Ing
Ingelisse, Ingeliss, Ingelyse, Ingelisa, Ingelissa, Ingelysa, Ingelyssa

Ingrid (Scandinavian) Having the beauty of the God Ing
Ingred, Ingrad, Inga, Inge, Inger, Ingmar, Ingrida, Ingria, Ingrit, Inkeri

Inis (Irish) Woman from Ennis
Iniss, Inisse, Innis, Inys, Innys, Inyss, Inysse

Intisar (Arabic) One who is victorious; triumphant
Intisara, Intisarah, Intizar, Intizara, Intizarah, Intisarr, Intysarr, Intysar

Iolanthe (Greek) Resembling a violet flower
Iolanda, Iolanta, Iolantha, Iolante, Iolande, Iolanthia, Iolanthea

Iona (Greek) Woman from the island
Ionna, Ioane, Ioann, Ioanne

Ionanna (Hebrew) Filled with grace
Ionannah, Ionana, Ionann, Ionane, Ionanne

Ionia (Greek) Of the sea and islands
Ionya, Ionija, Ioniah, Ionea, Ionessa, Ioneah, Ioniya

Iosepine (Hawaiian) Form of Josephine, meaning "God will add"
Iosephine, Iosefa, Iosefena, Iosefene, Iosefina, Iosefine, Iosepha, Iosephe

Iowa (Native American) Of the Iowa tribe; from the state of Iowa

Iphedeiah (Hebrew) One who is saved by the Lord

Iphigenia (Greek) One who is born strong; in mythology, daughter of Agamemnon
Iphigeneia, Iphigenie

Ipsa (Indian) One who is desired
Ipsita, Ipsyta, Ipseeta, Ipseata, Ipsah

Iratze (Basque) Refers to the Virgin Mary
Iratza, Iratzia, Iratzea, Iratzi, Iratzie, Iratzy, Iratzey, Iratzee

Ireland (Celtic) The country of the Irish
Irelan, Irelann

Irem (Turkish) From the heavenly gardens
Irema, Ireme, Iremia, Iremea

Irene (Greek) A peaceful woman; in mythology, the goddess of peace
Ira, Irayna, Ireen, Iren, Irena, Irenea, Irenee, Irenka, Eirene

Ireta (Greek) One who is serene
Iretah, Iretta, Irettah, Irete, Iret, Irett, Ireta

Iris (Greek) Of the rainbow; a flower; a messenger goddess
Irida, Iridiana, Iridianny, Irisa, Irisha, Irita, Iria, Irea, Iridian, Iriss, Irys, Iryss

Irma (German) A universal woman

Irta (Greek) Resembling a pearl
Irtah

Irune (Basque) Refers to the Holy Trinity
Iroon, Iroone, Iroun, Iroune

Isabel (Spanish) Form of Elizabeth, meaning "my God is bountiful; God's promise"
Isabeau, Isabela, Isabele, Isabelita, Isabell, Isabelle, Ishbel, Ysabel

Isabella (Italian / Spanish) Form of Isabel, meaning consecrated to God
Isabela, Isabelita, Isobella, Izabella, Isibella, Isibela

Isadore (Greek) A gift from the goddess Isis
Isadora, Isador, Isadoria, Isidor, Isidoro, Isidorus, Isidro, Isidora

Isana (German) A strong-willed woman
Isanah, Isanna, Isane, Isann

Isela (American) A giving woman
Iselah, Isella, Isellah

Isis (Egyptian) In mythology, the most powerful of all goddesses

Isla (Gaelic) From the island
Islae, Islai, Isleta

Isleen (Gaelic) Form of Aisling, meaning "a dream or vision; an inspiration"
Isleene, Islyne, Islyn, Isline, Isleine, Isliene, Islene, Isleyne

Isolde (Celtic) A woman known for her beauty; in mythology, the lover of Tristan
Iseult, Iseut, Isold, Isolda, Isolt, Isolte, Isota, Isotta

Isra (Arabic) One who travels in the evening
Israh, Isria, Isrea, Israt

Itiah (Hebrew) One who is comforted by God
Itia, Iteah, Itea, Itiyah, Itiya, Ityah, Itya

Itidal (Arabic) One who is cautious
Itidalle, Itidall, Itidale

Itsaso (Basque) Woman of the ocean
Itasasso, Itassaso, Itassasso

Iudita (Hawaiian) An affectionate woman
Iuditah, Iudyta, Iudytah, Iudeta, Iudetah

Iuginia (Hawaiian) A high-born woman
Iuginiah, Iuginea, Iugineah, Iugynia

Ivana (Slavic) Feminine form of Ivan; God is gracious
Iva, Ivah, Ivania, Ivanka, Ivanna, Ivanya, Ivanea, Ivane, Ivanne

Ivory (English) Having a creamy-white complexion; as precious as elephant tusks
Ivorie, Ivorine, Ivoreen, Ivorey, Ivoree, Ivori, Ivoryne, Ivorea

Ivy (English) Resembling the evergreen vining plant
Ivie, Ivi, Ivea

Ixchel (Mayan) The rainbow lady; in mythology, the goddess of the earth, moon, and healing
Ixchell, Ixchelle, Ixchela, Ixchella, Ixchal, Ixchall, Ixchalle, Ixchala

Iyabo (African) The mother is home

Izanne (American) One who calms others
Izann, Izane, Izana, Izan, Izanna

Izolde (Greek) One who is philosophical
Izold, Izolda

J

Jacey (American) Form of Jacinda, meaning "resembling the hyacinth"
Jacee, Jacelyn, Jaci, Jacine, Jacy, Jaicee, Jaycee, Jacie

Jacinda (Spanish) Resembling the hyacinth
Jacenda, Jacenia, Jacenta, Jacindia, Jacinna, Jacinta, Jacinth, Jacintha, Jacinthe, Jacinthia, Jacynth, Jacyntha, Jacynthe, Jacynthia, Jakinda, Jakinta, Jaikinda, Jaekinda

Jacqueline (French) Feminine form of Jacques; the supplanter
Jackie, Xaquelina, Jacalin, Jacalyn, Jacalynn, Jackalin, Jackalinne, Jackelyn, Jacquelyn

Jade (Spanish) Resembling the green gemstone
Jadeana, Jadee, Jadine, Jadira, Jadrian, Jadrienne, Jady

Jaden (Hebrew / English) One who is thankful to God / form of Jade, meaning "resembling the green gemstone"
Jadine, Jadyn, Jadon, Jayden, Jadyne, Jaydyn, Jaydon, Jaidyn

Jadzia (Polish) A princess; born into royalty
Jadziah, Jadzea, Jadzeah

Jae (English) Feminine form of Jay; resembling a jaybird
Jai, Jaelana, Jaeleah, Jaelyn, Jaenelle, Jaya

Jael (Hebrew) Resembling a mountain goat
Jaella, Jaelle, Jayel, Jaele, Jayil

Jaffa (Hebrew) A beautiful woman
Jaffah, Jafit, Jafita

Jalila (Arabic) An important woman; one who is exalted
Jalilah, Jalyla, Jalylah, Jaleela

Jamaica (American) From the island of springs
Jamaeca, Jamaika, Jemaica, Jamika, Jamieka

Jamie (Hebrew) Feminine form of James; she who supplants
Jaima, Jaime, Jaimee, Jaimelynn, Jaimey, Jaimi, Jaimie, Jaimy

Janan (Arabic) Of the heart and soul

Jane (Hebrew) Feminine form of John; God is gracious
Jaina, Jaine, Jainee, Janey, Jana, Janae, Janaye, Jandy, Sine, Janel, Janelle

Janet (Scottish) Feminine form of John, meaning "God is gracious"
Janetta, Jenetta, Janeta, Janette, Janit

Janis (English) Feminine form of John; God is gracious
Janice, Janeece, Janess, Janessa, Janesse, Janessia, Janicia, Janiece

Janiyah (American) Form of Jana, meaning gracious, merciful
Janiya, Janiah

Jarah (Hebrew) A sweet and kind woman

Jasher (Hebrew) One who is righteous; upright
Jashiere, Jasheria, Jasherea

Jaslene (American) Form of Jocelyn, meaning joy
Jaslin, Jaslyn, Jazlyn, Jazlynn

Jasmine (Persian) Resembling the climbing plant with fragrant flowers
Jaslyn, Jaslynn, Jasmin, Jasmyn, Jazmin, Jazmine, Jazmyn

Javiera (Spanish) Feminine form of Xavier; one who is bright; the owner of a new home
Javierah, Javyera, Javyerah, Javeira, Javeirah

Jayda (English) Resembling the green gemstone
Jada, Jaydah, Jaida, Jaidah

Jayla (Arabic) One who is charitable
Jaela, Jaila, Jaylah, Jaylee, Jaylen, Jaylene, Jayleen, Jaylin, Jaylyn, Jaylynn

Jean (Hebrew) Feminine form of John; God is gracious
Jeanae, Jeanay, Jeane, Jeanee, Jeanelle, Jeanetta, Jeanette, Jeanice, Gina

Jemma (English) Form of Gemma, meaning "as precious as a jewel"
Jemmah, Jema, Jemah, Jemmalyn, Jemalyn

Jena (Arabic) Our little bird
Jenna, Jenah

Jendayi (Egyptian) One who is thankful
Jendayie, Jendayey, Jendayee

Jennifer (Welsh) One who is fair; a beautiful girl
Jenefer, Jeni, Jenifer, Jeniffer, Jenn, Jennee, Jenni, Jen, Jenna, Jenny

Jereni (Slavic) One who is peaceful
Jerenie, Jereny, Jereney, Jerenee

Jermaine (French) Woman from Germany
Jermainaa, Jermane, Jermayne, Jermina, Jermana, Jermayna

Jessica (Hebrew) The Lord sees all
Jess, Jessa, Jessaca, Jessaka, Jessalin, Jessalyn, Jesse, Jesseca, Yessica, Jessie

Jetta (Danish) Resembling the jet-black lustrous gemstone
Jette, Jett, Jeta, Jete, Jettie, Jetty, Jetti, Jettey

Jewel (French) One who is playful; resembling a precious gem
Jewell, Jewelle, Jewelyn, Jewelene, Jewelisa, Jule, Jewella, Juelline

Jezebel (Hebrew) One who is not exalted; in the Bible, the queen of Israel punished by God
Jessabell, Jetzabel, Jezabel, Jezabella, Jezebelle, Jezibel, Jezibelle, Jezybell

Jie (Chinese) One who is pure; chaste

Jiera (Lithuanian) A lively woman
Jierah, Jyera, Jyerah, Jierra, Jyerra

Jillian (English) Form of Gillian, meaning "one who is youthful"
Jilian, Jiliana, Jillaine, Jillan, Jillana, Jillane, Jillanne, Jillayne, Jillene, Jillesa, Jilliana, Jilliane, Jilliann, Jillianna, Jill

Jimena (Spanish) One who is heard

Jinelle (Welsh) Form of Genevieve, meaning "white wave; fair-skinned"
Jinell, Jinele, Jinel, Jynelle, Jynell, Jynele, Jynel

Jiselle (American) Form of Giselle, meaning "one who offers her pledge"
Jisell, Jisele, Jisela, Jizelle, Joselle, Jisella, Jizella, Jozelle

Jo (English) Feminine form of Joseph; God will add
Jobelle, Jobeth, Jodean, Jodelle, Joetta, Joette, Jolinda, Jolisa

Joanna (French) Feminine form of John, meaning "God is Gracious"
Joana

Jocelyn (German / Latin) From the tribe of Gauts / one who is cheerful, happy
Jocelin, Jocelina, Jocelinda, Joceline, Jocelyne, Jocelynn, Jocelynne, Josalind, Joslyn, Joslynn, Joselyn

Joda (Hebrew) An ancestor of Christ

Jolan (Greek) Resembling a violet flower
Jola, Jolaine, Jolande, Jolanne, Jolanta, Jolantha, Jolandi, Jolanka

Jolene (English) Feminine form of Joseph; God will add
Joeline, Joeleen, Joeline, Jolaine, Jolean, Joleen, Jolena, Jolina

Jolie (French) A pretty young woman
Joly, Joely, Jolee, Joleigh, Joley, Joli

Jonina (Israeli) Resembling a little dove
Joninah, Jonyna, Jonynah, Joneena, Joneenah, Jonine, Jonyne, Joneene

Jorah (Hebrew) Resembling an autumn rose
Jora

Jord (Norse) In mythology, goddess of the earth
Jorde

Jordan (Hebrew) Of the down-flowing river; in the Bible, the river where Jesus was baptized
Jardena, Johrdan, Jordain, Jordaine, Jordana, Jordane, Jordanka, Jordyn, Jordin

Josephine (French) Feminine form of Joseph; God will add
Josefina, Josephene, Jo, Josie, Iosepine

Journey (American) One who likes to travel
Journy, Journi, Journie, Journee

Jovana (Spanish) Feminine form of Jovian; daughter of the sky
Jeovana, Jeovanna, Jovanna, Jovena, Jovianne, Jovina, Jovita, Joviana

Joy (Latin) A delight; one who brings pleasure to others
Jioia, Jioya, Joi, Joia, Joie, Joya, Joyann, Joyanna

Joyce (English) One who brings joy to others
Joice, Joyceanne, Joycelyn, Joycelynn, Joyse, Joyceta

Judith (Hebrew) Woman from Judea
Judithe, Juditha, Judeena, Judeana, Judyth, Judit, Judytha, Judita, Hudes

Julia (Latin) One who is youthful; daughter of the sky
Jiulia, Joleta, Joletta, Jolette, Julaine, Julayna, Julee, Juleen, Julie, Julianne, Julieta

Juliana (Spanish) Form of Julia, meaning "one who is youthful"
Julianna

Juliet (French) Form of Julia, meaning one who is youthful
Juliette, Julitta, Julissa

July (Latin) Form of Julia, meaning "one who is youthful; daughter of the sky"; born during the month of July
Julye

June (Latin) One who is youthful; born during the month of June
Junae, Junel, Junelle, Junette, Junita, Junia

Justice (English) One who upholds moral rightness and fairness
Justyce, Justiss, Justyss, Justis, Justus, Justise

Kachina (Native American) A spiritual dancer
Kachine, Kachinah, Kachineh, Kachyna, Kacheena, Kachynah, Kacheenah, Kacheana

Kadin (Arabic) A beloved companion
Kadyn, Kadan, Kaden, Kadon, Kadun, Kaedin, Kaeden, Kaydin

Kaelyn (English) A beautiful girl from the meadow
Kaelynn, Kaelynne, Kaelin, Kailyn, Kaylyn, Kaelinn, Kaelinne

Kagami (Japanese) Displaying one's true image
Kagamie, Kagamy, Kagamey, Kagamee, Kagamea

Kailasa (Indian) From the silver mountain
Kailasah, Kailassa, Kaylasa, Kaelasa, Kailas, Kailase

Kaitlyn (Greek) Form of Katherine, meaning "one who is pure, virginal"
Kaitlin, Kaitlan, Kaitleen, Kaitlynn, Katalin, Katalina, Katalyn, Katelin, Kateline, Katelinn, Katelyn, Katelynn, Katilyn, Katlin

Kala (Arabic / Hawaiian) A moment in time / form of Sarah, meaning "a princess; lady"
Kalah, Kalla, Kallah

Kalifa (Somali) A chaste and holy woman
Kalifah, Kalyfa, Kalyfah, Kaleefa, Kaleefah, Kalipha, Kalypha, Kaleepha, Kaleafa, Kaleafah, Kaleapha

Kalinda (Indian) Of the sun
Kalindah, Kalynda, Kalinde, Kalindeh, Kalindi, Kalindie, Kalyndi, Kalyndie

Kallie (English) Form of Callie, meaning "a beautiful girl"
Kalli, Kallita, Kally, Kalley, Kallee, Kalleigh, Kallea, Kalleah

Kalma (Finnish) In mythology, goddess of the dead

Kalyan (Indian) A beautiful and auspicious woman
Kalyane, Kalyanne, Kalyann, Kaylana, Kaylanna, Kalliyan, Kaliyan, Kaliyane

Kama (Indian) One who loves and is loved
Kamah, Kamma, Kammah

Kamala (Arabic) A woman of perfection
Kamalah, Kammala, Kamalla

Kamaria (African) Of the moon
Kamariah, Kamarea, Kamareah, Kamariya, Kamariyah

Kambiri (African) Newest addition to the family
Kambirie, Kambiry, Kambyry

Kamea (Hawaiian) The one and only; precious one
Kameo

Kamila (Spanish) Form of Camilla, meaning ceremonial attendant
Kamilah

Kamyra (American) Surrounded by light
Kamira, Kamera, Kamiera, Kameira, Kameera, Kameara

Kanda (Native American) A magical woman
Kandah

Kanika (African) A dark, beautiful woman
Kanikah, Kanyka, Kanicka

Kantha (Indian) A delicate woman
Kanthah, Kanthe, Kantheh

Kanya (Thai) A young girl; a virgin

Kaoru (Japanese) A fragrant girl
Kaori

Kara (Greek / Italian / Gaelic) One who is pure / dearly loved / a good friend
Karah, Karalee, Karalie, Karalyn, Karalynn, Karrah, Karra, Khara

Karcsi (French) A joyful singer
Karcsie, Karcsy, Karcsey, Karcsee, Karcsea

Karen (Greek) Form of Katherine, meaning "one who is pure; virginal"
Karan, Karena, Kariana, Kariann, Karianna, Karianne, Karin, Karina

Karina (Scandinavian / Russian) One who is dear and pure
Karinah, Kareena, Karyna

Karisma (English) Form of Charisma, meaning "blessed with charm"
Kharisma, Karizma, Kharizma

Karissa (Greek) Filled with grace and kindness; very dear
Karisa, Karyssa, Karysa, Karessa, Karesa, Karis, Karise

Karla (German) Feminine form of Karl; a small strong, woman
Karly, Karli, Karlie, Karleigh, Karlee, Karley, Karlin, Karlyn, Karlina, Karleen

Karmel (Latin) Form of Carmel, meaning "of the fruitful orchard"
Karmelle, Karmell, Karmele, Karmela, Karmella

Karoline (English) A small and strong woman
Karolina, Karolinah, Karolyne, Karrie, Karie, Karri, Kari, Karry

Karsen (American) Variation of the Scottish Carson, meaning "from the swamp"
Karsyn, Karsin

Karsten (Greek) The anointed one
Karstin, Karstine, Karstyn, Karston, Karstan, Kiersten, Keirsten

Kasey (Irish) Form of Casey, meaning "a vigilant woman"
Kacie, Kaci, Kacy, KC, Kacee, Kacey, Kasie, Kasi

Kasi (Indian) From the holy city; shining

Kasmira (Slavic) A peacemaker
Kasmirah, Kasmeera

Kate (English) Form of Katherine, meaning "one who is pure, virginal"
Katie, Katey, Kati

Katherine (Greek) Form of Catherine, meaning "one who is pure; virginal"
Katharine, Katharyn, Kathy, Kathleen, Katheryn, Kathie, Kathrine, Kathryn, Karen, Kay

Katriel (Hebrew) Crowned by God
Katriele, Katrielle, Katriell

Kaveri (Indian) From the sacred river
Kaverie, Kauveri, Kauverie, Kavery, Kaverey, Kaveree, Kaverea, Kauvery

Kay (English / Greek) The keeper of the keys / form of Katherine, meaning "one who is pure; virginal"
Kaye, Kae, Kai, Kaie, Kaya, Kayana, Kayane, Kayanna

Kayden (American) Form of Kaden, meaning "a beloved companion"

Kayla (Arabic / Hebrew) Crowned with laurel
Kaylah, Kalan, Kalen, Kalin, Kalyn, Kalynn, Kaylan, Kaylana, Kaylin, Kaylen, Kaylynn, Kaylyn, Kayle

Kaylee (American) Form of Kayla, meaning "crowned with laurel"
Kaleigh, Kaley, Kaelee, Kaeley, Kaeli, Kailee, Kailey, Kalee, Kayleigh, Kayley, Kayli, Kaylie

Kearney (Irish) The winner
Kearny, Kearni, Kearnie, Kearnee, Kearnea

Keaton (English) From a shed town
Keatan, Keatyn, Keatin, Keatun

Keavy (Irish) A lovely and graceful girl
Keavey, Keavi, Keavie, Keavee, Keavea

Keeya (African) Resembling a flower
Keeyah, Kieya, Keiya, Keyya

Kefira (Hebrew) Resembling a young lioness
Kefirah, Kefiera, Kefeira

Keira (Irish) Form of Kiera, meaning "little dark-haired one"
Kierra, Kyera, Kyerra, Keiranne, Kyra, Kyrie, Kira, Kiran

Keisha (American) The favorite child; form of Kezia, meaning "of the spice tree"
Keishla, Keishah, Kecia, Kesha, Keysha, Keesha, Kiesha, Keshia

Kelly (Irish) A lively and bright-headed woman
Kelley, Kelli, Kellie, Kellee, Kelliegh, Kellye, Keely, Keelie, Keeley, Keelyn

Kelsey (English) From the island of ships
Kelsie, Kelcey, Kelcie, Kelcy, Kellsie, Kelsa, Kelsea, Kelsee, Kelsi, Kelsy, Kellsey

Kendall (Welsh) From the royal valley
Kendal, Kendyl, Kendahl, Kindall, Kyndal, Kenley

Kendra (English) Feminine form of Kendrick; having royal power; from the high hill
Kendrah, Kendria, Kendrea, Kindra, Kindria

Kenley (American) Variation of Kinley and McKinley

Kennedy (Gaelic) A helmeted chief
Kennedi, Kennedie, Kennedey, Kennedee, Kenadia, Kenadie, Kenadi, Kenady, Kenadey

Kensington (English) A brash lady
Kensyngton, Kensingtyn, Kinsington, Kinsyngton, Kinsingtyn

Kenzie (American) Diminutive of McKenzie

Kerensa (Cornish) One who loves and is loved
Kerinsa, Keransa, Kerensia, Kerensea, Kerensya, Kerenz, Kerenza, Keranz

Kerr (Scottish) From the marshland

Kevina (Gaelic) Feminine form of Kevin; a beautiful and beloved child
Kevinah, Keva, Kevia, Kevinne, Kevyn, Kevynn

Keyla (English) A wise daughter

Kezia (Hebrew) Of the spice tree
Keziah, Kesia, Kesiah, Kesi, Kessie, Ketzia, Keisha

Khai (American) Unlike the others; unusual
Khae, Khay, Khaye

Khalida (Arabic) Feminine form of Khalid; an immortal woman
Khalidah, Khaleeda, Khalyda

Khaliqa (Arabic) Feminine form of Khaliq; a creator; one who is well-behaved
Khaliqah, Khalyqa, Khaleeqa

Khepri (Egyptian) Born of the morning sun
Kheprie, Kepri, Keprie, Khepry, Kepry, Khepree, Kepree, Kheprea

Khiana (American) One who is different
Khianna, Khiane, Khianne, Khian, Khyana, Khyanna, Kheana, Kheanna

Khloe (Greek) Form of Chloe, meaning "a flourishing woman, blooming"

Kiara (American) Form of Chiara, meaning "daughter of the light"

Kichi (Japanese) The fortunate one

Kidre (American) A loyal woman
Kidrea, Kidreah, Kidria, Kidriah, Kidri, Kidrie, Kidry, Kidrey

Kiele (Hawaiian) Resembling the gardenia
Kielle, Kiel, Kiell, Kiela, Kiella

Kikka (German) The mistress of all
Kika, Kykka, Kyka

Kiley (American) Form of Kylie, meaning "a boomerang"
Kylie

Kimana (American) Girl from the meadow
Kimanah, Kimanna

Kimball (English) Chief of the warriors; possessing royal boldness
Kimbal, Kimbell, Kimbel, Kymball, Kymbal

Kimberly (English) Of the royal fortress
Kimberley, Kimberli, Kimberlee, Kimberleigh, Kimberlin, Kimberlyn, Kymberlie, Kymberly

Kimeo (American) Filled with happiness
Kimeyo

Kimetha (American) Filled with joy
Kimethah, Kymetha

Kimiko (Japanese) A noble child; without equal

Kimora (American) Form of Kimberly, meaning "royal"

Kina (Hawaiian) Woman of China

Kinley (American) Variation of McKinley, Scottish, meaning offspring of the fair hero

Kinsey (English) The king's victory
Kinnsee, Kinnsey, Kinnsie, Kinsee, Kinsie, Kinzee, Kinzie, Kinzey

Kinsley (English) From the king's meadow
Kinsly, Kinslee, Kinsleigh, Kinsli, Kinslie, Kingsley, Kingslee, Kingslie

Kioko (Japanese) A daughter born with happiness

Kirima (Eskimo) From the hill
Kirimah, Kiryma, Kirymah, Kirema, Kiremah, Kireema, Kireemah, Kireama

Kismet (English) One's destiny; fate

Kiss (American) A caring and compassionate woman
Kyss, Kissi, Kyssi, Kissie, Kyssie, Kissy, Kyssy, Kissey

Kobi (American) Woman from California
Kobie, Koby, Kobee, Kobey, Kobea

Kolette (English) Form of Colette, meaning "victory of the people"
Kolete, Kolett, Koleta, Koletta, Kolet

Komala (Indian) A delicate and tender woman
Komalah, Komalla, Komal, Komali, Komalie, Komalee

Kona (Hawaiian) A girly woman
Konah, Konia, Koniah, Konea, Koneah, Koni, Konie, Koney

Konane (Hawaiian) Daughter of the moonlight

Kreeli (American) A charming and kind girl
Kreelie, Krieli, Krielie, Kryli, Krylie, Kreely, Kriely, Kryly

Kristina (English) Form of Christina, meaning "follower of Christ"
Kristena, Kristine, Kristyne, Kristyna, Krystina, Krystine

Kumi (Japanese) An everlasting beauty
Kumie, Kumy, Kumey, Kumee

Kyla (English) Feminine form of Kyle; from the narrow channel
Kylah, Kylar, Kyle

Kylie (Australian) A boomerang
Kylee, Kyleigh, Kyley, Kyli, Kyleen, Kyleen, Kyler, Kily,Kileigh, Kilee, Kilie, Kili, Kilea, Kylea

Kyra (Greek) Form of Cyrus, meaning "noble"
Kyrah, Kyria, Kyriah, Kyrra, Kyrrah

L

Lacey (French) Woman from Normandy; as delicate as lace
Lace, Lacee, Lacene, Laci, Laciann, Lacie, Lacina, Lacy

Lael (Hebrew) One who belongs to God
Laele, Laelle

Laila (Arabic) A beauty of the night, born at nightfall
Layla, Laylah

Lainil (American) A softhearted woman
Lainill, Lainyl, Lainyll, Laenil, Laenill, Laenyl, Laenyll, Laynil

Lais (Greek) A legendary courtesan
Laise, Lays, Layse, Laisa, Laes, Laese

Lajita (Indian) A truthful woman
Lajyta, Lajeeta, Lajeata

Lake (American) From the still waters
Laken, Laiken, Layken, Layk, Layke, Laik, Laike, Laeken

Lala (Slavic) Resembling a tulip
Lalah, Lalla, Lallah, Laleh

Lalaine (American) A hardworking woman
Lalain, Lalaina, Lalayn, Lalayne, Lalayna, Lalaen, Lalaene, Lalaena

Lalia (Greek) One who is well-spoken
Lali, Lallia, Lalya, Lalea, Lalie, Lalee, Laly, Laley

Lalita (Indian) A playful and charming woman
Lalitah, Laleeta, Laleetah, Lalyta, Lalytah, Laleita, Laleitah, Lalieta

Lamia (Greek) In mythology, a female vampire
Lamiah, Lamiya, Lamiyah, Lamea, Lameah

Lamya (Arabic) Having lovely dark lips
Lamyah, Lamyia, Lama

Lanassa (Russian) A lighthearted woman; cheerful
Lanasa, Lanassia, Lanasia, Lanassiya, Lanasiya

Landon (English) From the long hill
Landyn, Landen

Lang (Scandinavian) Woman of great height

Lani (Hawaiian) From the sky; one who is heavenly
Lanikai

Lanza (Italian) One who is noble and willing
Lanzah, Lanzia, Lanziah, Lanzea, Lanzeah

Lapis (Egyptian) Resembling the dark-blue gemstone
Lapiss, Lapisse, Lapys, Lapyss, Lapysse

Laquinta (American) The fifth-born child

Laramie (French) Shedding tears of love
Larami, Laramy, Laramey, Laramee, Laramea

Larby (American) Form of Darby, meaning "of the deer park"
Larbey, Larbi, Larbie, Larbee, Larbea

Lark (English) Resembling the songbird
Larke

Larue (American) Form of Rue, meaning "a medicinal herb"
LaRue, Laroo, Larou

Lashawna (American) Filled with happiness
Lashauna, Laseana, Lashona, Lashawn, Lasean, Lashone, Lashaun

Lata (Indian) Of the lovely vine
Latah

Latanya (American) Daughter of the fairy queen
Latanyah, Latonya, Latania, Latanja, Latonia, Latanea

Latona (Latin) In mythology, the Roman equivalent of Leto, the mother of Artemis and Apollo
Latonah, Latonia, Latonea, Lantoniah, Latoneah

Latrelle (American) One who laughs a lot
Latrell, Latrel, Latrele, Latrella, Latrela

Laudonia (Italian) Praises the house
Laudonea, Laudoniya, Laudomia, Laudomea, Laudomiya

Laura (Latin) Crowned with laurel; from the laurel tree
Lauraine, Lauralee, Laralyn, Laranca, Larea, Lari, Lauralee, Lauren, Loretta

Lauren (French) Form of Laura, meaning "crowned with laurel; from the laurel tree"
Laren, Larentia, Larentina, Larenzina, Larren, Laryn, Larryn, Larrynn

Leah (Hebrew) One who is weary; in the Bible, Jacob's first wife
Leia, Leigha, Lia, Liah, Leeya

Leanna (Gaelic) Form of Helen, meaning "the shining light"
Leana, Leann, Leanne, Lee-Ann, Leeann, Leeanne, Leianne, Leyanne

Lecia (English) Form of Alice, meaning "woman of the nobility; truthful; having high moral character"
Licia, Lecea, Licea, Lisha, Lysha, Lesha

Ledell (Greek) One who is queenly
Ledelle, Ledele, Ledella, Ledela, Ledel

Legend (American) One who is memorable
Legende, Legund, Legunde

Legia (Spanish) A bright woman
Legiah, Legea, Legeah, Legiya, Legiyah, Legya, Legyah

Leila (Persian) Night, dark beauty
Leela, Lela

Lenis (Latin) One who has soft and silky skin
Lene, Leneta, Lenice, Lenita, Lennice, Lenos, Lenys, Lenisse

Leona (Latin) Feminine form of Leon; having the strength of a lion
Leeona, Leeowna, Leoine, Leola, Leone, Leonelle, Leonia, Leonie

Lequoia (Native American) Form of Sequoia, meaning "of the giant redwood tree"
Lequoya, Lequoiya, Lekoya

Lerola (Latin) Resembling a blackbird
Lerolla, Lerolah, Lerolia, Lerolea

Leslie (Gaelic) From the holly garden; of the gray fortress
Leslea, Leslee, Lesleigh, Lesley, Lesli, Lesly, Lezlee, Lezley

Leucothea (Greek) In mythology, a sea nymph
Leucothia, Leucothiah, Leucotheah

Levora (American) A homebody
Levorah, Levorra, Levorrah, Levoria, Levoriah, Levorea, Levoreah, Levorya

Lewa (African) A very beautiful woman
Lewah

Lewana (Hebrew) Of the white moon
Lewanah, Lewanna, Lewannah

Lia (Italian) Form of Leah, meaning "one who is weary"

Libby (English) Form of Elizabeth, meaning "my God is bountiful; God's promise"
Libba, Libbee, Libbey, Libbie, Libet, Liby, Lilibet, Lilibeth

Liberty (English) An independent woman; having freedom
Libertey, Libertee, Libertea, Liberti, Libertie, Libertas, Libera, Liber

Libra (Latin) One who is balanced; the seventh sign of the zodiac
Leebra, Leibra, Liebra, Leabra, Leighbra, Lybra

Librada (Spanish) One who is free
Libradah, Lybrada, Lybradah

Lieu (Vietnamese) Of the willow tree

Ligia (Greek) One who is musically talented
Ligiah, Ligya, Ligiya, Lygia, Ligea, Lygea, Lygya, Lygiya

Lila (Arabic / Greek) Born at night / resembling a lily
Lilah, Lyla, Lylah

Lilac (Latin) Resembling the bluish-purple flower
Lilack, Lilak, Lylac, Lylack, Lylak, Lilach

Lilette (Latin) Resembling a budding lily
Lilett, Lilete, Lilet, Lileta, Liletta, Lylette, Lylett, Lylete

Liliana (Italian, Spanish) Form of Lillian, meaning "resembling the lily"
Lilliana, Lillianna, Liliannia, Lilyana, Lilia

Lilith (Babylonian) Woman of the night
Lilyth, Lillith, Lillyth, Lylith, Lyllith, Lylyth, Lyllyth, Lilithe

Lillian (Latin) Resembling the lily
Lilian, Liliane, Lilianne, Lilias, Lilas, Lillas, Lillias

Lilo (Hawaiian) One who is generous
Lylo, Leelo, Lealo, Leylo, Lielo, Leilo

Lily (English) Resembling the flower; one who is innocent and beautiful
Leelee, Lil, Lili, Lilie, Lilla, Lilley, Lilli, Lillie, Lilly

Limor (Hebrew) Refers to myrrh
Limora, Limoria, Limorea, Leemor, Leemora, Leemoria, Leemorea

Lin (Chinese) Resembling jade; from the woodland

Linda (Spanish) One who is soft and beautiful
Lindalee, Lindee, Lindey, Lindi, Lindie, Lindira, Lindka, Lindy, Lynn

Linden (English) From the hill of lime trees
Lindenn, Lindon, Lindynn, Lynden, Lyndon, Lyndyn, Lyndin, Lindin

Lindley (English) From the pastureland
Lindly, Lindlee, Lindleigh, Lindli, Lindlie, Leland, Lindlea

Lindsay (English) From the island of linden trees; from Lincoln's wetland
Lind, Lindsea, Lindsee, Lindseigh, Lindsey, Lindsy, Linsay, Linsey

Lisa (English) Form of Elizabeth, meaning "my God is bountiful; God's promise"
Leesa, Liesa, Lisebet, Lise, Liseta, Lisette, Liszka, Lisebeth

Lishan (African) One who is awarded a medal
Lishana, Lishanna, Lyshan, Lyshana, Lyshanna

Lissie (American) Resembling a flower
Lissi, Lissy, Lissey, Lissee, Lissea

Liv (Scandinavian / Latin) One who protects others / from the olive tree
Livia, Livea, Liviya, Livija, Livvy, Livy, Livya, Lyvia

Liya (Hebrew) The Lord's daughter
Liyah, Leeya, Leeyah, Leaya, Leayah

Lo (American) A fiesty woman
Loe, Low, Lowe

Lokelani (Hawaiian) Resembling a small red rose
Lokelanie, Lokelany, Lokelaney, Lokelanee, Lokelanea

Loki (Norse) In mythology, a trickster god
Lokie, Lokee, Lokey, Loky, Lokea, Lokeah, Lokia, Lokiah

Lola (Spanish) Form of Dolores, meaning "woman of sorrow"
Lolah, Loe, Lolo

London (English) From the capital of England
Londyn

Lorelei (German) From the rocky cliff; in mythology, a siren who lured sailors to their deaths
Laurelei, Laurelie, Loralee, Loralei, Loralie, Loralyn

Loretta (Italian) Form of Laura, meaning "crowned with laurel; from the laurel tree"
Laretta, Larretta, Lauretta, Laurette, Leretta, Loreta, Lorette, Lorretta

Lorraine (French) From the kingdom of Lothair
Laraine, Larayne, Laurraine, Leraine, Lerayne, Lorain, Loraina, Loraine

Love (English) One who is full of affection
Lovey, Loveday, Lovette, Lovi, Lovie, Lov, Luv, Luvey

Lovely (American) An attractive and pleasant woman
Loveli, Loveley, Lovelie, Lovelee, Loveleigh, Lovelea

Luana (Hawaiian) One who is content and enjoys life
Lewanna, Lou-Ann, Louann, Louanna, Louanne, Luanda, Luane, Luann

Lucretia (Latin) A bringer of light; a successful woman; in mythology, a maiden who was raped by the prince of Rome
Lacretia, Loucrecia, Loucrezia, Loucresha, Loucretia, Lucrece, Lucrecia, Lucreecia

Lucy (Latin) Feminine form of Lucius; one who is illuminated
Luce, Lucetta, Lucette, Luci, Lucia, Luciana, Lucianna, Lucida, Lucille

Lucylynn (American) A lighthearted woman
Lucylyn, Lucylynne, Lucilynn, Lucilyn, Lucilynne

Luna (Latin) Of the moon
Lunah

Lunet (English) Of the crescent moon
Lunett, Lunette, Luneta, Lunete, Lunetta

Lupita (Spanish) Form of Guadalupe, meaning "from the valley of wolves"
Lupe, Lupyta, Lupelina, Lupeeta, Lupieta, Lupeita, Lupeata

Lurissa (American) A beguiling woman
Lurisa, Luryssa, Lurysa, Luressa, Luresa

Luyu (Native American) Resembling the dove

Lydia (Greek) A beautiful woman from Lydia
Lidia, Lidie, Lidija, Lyda, Lydie, Lydea, Liddy, Lidiy

Lyla (Arabic) Form of Lila, meaning "born at night, resembling a lily"
Lylah

Lynn (English) Woman of the lake; form of Linda, meaning "one who is soft and beautiful"
Linell, Linnell, Lyn, Lynae, Lyndel, Lyndell, Lynell, Lynelle

Lyric (French) Of the lyre; the words of a song
Lyrica, Lyricia, Lyrik, Lyrick, Lyrika, Lyricka

M

Macanta (Gaelic) A kind and gentle woman
Macan, Macantia, Macantea, Macantah

Mackenna (Gaelic) Daughter of the handsome man
Mackendra, Mackennah, McKenna, McKendra, Makenna, Makennah

Mackenzie (Gaelic) Daughter of a wise leader; a fiery woman; one who is fair
Mckenzie, Mackenzey, Makensie, Makenzie, M'Kenzie, McKenzie, Meckenzie, Mackenzee, Mackenzy

McKinley (English) Offspring of the fair hero

Macy (French) One who wields a weapon
Macee, Macey, Maci, Macie, Maicey, Maicy, Macea, Maicea

Madana (Ethiopian) One who heals others
Madayna, Madaina, Madania, Madaynia, Madainia

Maddox (English) Born into wealth and prosperity
Madox, Madoxx, Maddoxx

Madeline (Hebrew) Woman from Magdala
Mada, Madalaina, Madaleine, Madalena, Madalene, Madelyn, Madalyn, Madelynn, Madilyn

Madhavi (Indian) Feminine form of Madhav; born in the springtime
Madhavie, Madhavee, Madhavey, Madhavy, Madhavea

Madini (Swahili) As precious as a gemstone
Madinie, Madiny, Madiney, Madinee, Madyny, Madyni, Madinea, Madynie

Madison (English) Daughter of a mighty warrior
Maddison, Madisen, Madisson, Madisyn, Madyson

Madonna (Italian) My lady; refers to the Virgin Mary
Madonnah, Madona, Madonah

Maeve (Irish) An intoxicating woman
Mave, Meave, Medb, Meabh

Maggie (English) Form of Margaret, meaning "resembling a pearl"
Maggi

Magnolia (French) Resembling the flower
Magnoliya, Magnoliah, Magnolea, Magnoleah, Magnoliyah, Magnolya, Magnolyah

Mahal (Native American) A tender and loving woman
Mahall, Mahale, Mahalle

Mahari (African) One who offers forgiveness
Maharie, Mahary, Maharey

Mahesa (Indian) A powerful and great lady
Maheshvari

Mahira (Arabic) A clever and adroit woman
Mahirah, Mahir, Mahire

Maia (Latin / Maori) The great one; in mythology, the goddess of spring / a brave warrior
Maiah, Mya, Maja

Maida (English) A maiden; a virgin
Maidel, Maidie, Mayda, Maydena, Maydey, Mady, Maegth, Magd

Maiki (Japanese) Resembling the dancing flower
Maikie, Maikei, Maikki, Maikee

Maimun (Arabic) One who is lucky; fortunate
Maimoon, Maimoun

Maine (French) From the mainland; from the state of Maine

Maiolaine (French) As delicate as a flower
Maiolainie, Maiolani

Maisha (African) Giver of life
Maysha, Maishah, Mayshah, Maesha, Maeshah

Maisie (Scottish) Form of Margaret, meaning "resembling a pearl"
Maisee, Maisey, Maisy, Maizie, Mazey, Mazie, Maisi, Maizi

Majaya (Indian) A victorious woman
Majayah

Makala (Hawaiian) Resembling myrtle
Makalah, Makalla, Makallah

Makayla (Celtic / Hebrew / English) Form of Michaela, meaning "who is like God?"
Macaela, MacKayla, Mak, Mechaela, Meeskaela, Mekea, Mekelle

Makani (Hawaiian) Of the wind
Makanie, Makaney, Makany, Makanee

Makareta (Maori) Form of Margaret, meaning "resembling a pearl / the child of light"
Makaretah, Makarita

Makea (Finnish) One who is sweet
Makeah, Makia, Makiah

Makelina (Hawaiian) Form of Madeline, meaning "woman from Magdala"
Makelinah, Makeleena, Makelyna, Makeleana

Makena (African) One who is filled with happiness
Makenah, Makeena, Makeenah, Makeana, Makeanah, Makyna, Makynah, Mackena

Makenna (Irish) Form of McKenna, meaning "of the Irish one"
Makennah

Malak (Arabic) A heavenly messenger; an angel
Malaka, Malaika, Malayka, Malaeka, Malake, Malayk, Malaek, Malakia

Malati (Indian) Resembling a fragrant flower
Malatie, Malaty, Malatey, Malatee, Malatea

Mali (Thai / Welsh) Resembling a flower / form of Molly, meaning "star of the sea / from the sea of bitterness"
Malie, Malee, Maleigh, Maly, Maley

Malia (Hawaiian) Form of Mary, meaning "star of the sea / from the sea of bitterness"
Maliah, Maliyah, Maleah

Malika (Arabic) Destined to be queen
Malikah, Malyka, Maleeka, Maleika, Malieka, Maliika, Maleaka

Malina (Hawaiian) A peaceful woman
Malinah, Maleena, Maleenah, Malyna, Malynah, Maleina, Maliena, Maleana

Malinka (Russian) As sweet as a little berry
Malinkah, Malynka, Maleenka, Malienka, Maleinka, Maleanka

Mana (Polynesian) A charismatic and prestigious woman
Manah

Manal (Arabic) An accomplished woman
Manala, Manall, Manalle, Manalla, Manali

Mandoline (English) One who is accomplished with the stringed instrument
Mandalin, Mandalyn, Mandalynn, Mandelin, Mandellin, Mandellyn, Mandolin, Mandolyn

Mangena (Hebrew) As sweet as a melody
Mangenah, Mangenna, Mangennah

Manyara (African) A humble woman
Manyarah

Maola (Irish) A handmaiden
Maoli, Maole, Maolie, Maolia, Maoly, Maoley, Maolee, Maolea

Maram (Arabic) One who is wished for
Marame, Marama, Marami, Maramie, Maramee, Maramy, Maramey, Maramea

Marcella (Latin) Dedicated to Mars, the God of war
Marcela, Marsela, Marsella, Maricela, Maricel

Marcia (Latin) Feminine form of Marcus; dedicated to Mars, the god of war
Marcena, Marcene, Marchita, Marciana, Marciane, Marcianne, Marcilyn, Marcilynn

Marely (American) form of Marley, "meaning of the marshy meadow"

Margaret (Greek / Persian) Resembling a pearl / the child of light
Maighread, Mairead, Mag, Maggi, Maggie, Maggy, Maiga, Malgorzata, Megan, Marwarid, Marjorie, Marged, Makareta

Margot (French) Form of Margaret, meaning "resembling a pearl / the child of light"
Margo, Margeaux, Margaux

Maria (Spanish) Form of Mary, meaning "star of the sea / from the sea of bitterness"
Mariah, Marialena, Marialinda, Marialisa, Maaria, Mayria, Maeria, Mariabella

Mariah (Latin) Form of Mary, meaning "star of the sea"

Mariana (Italian / Spanish) Form of Mary, meaning "star of the sea"
Marianna

Mariane (French) Blend of Mary, meaning "star of the sea / from the sea of bitterness," and Ann, meaning "a woman graced with God's favor"
Mariam, Mariana, Marian, Marion, Maryann, Maryanne, Maryanna, Maryane

Marietta (French) Form of Mary, meaning "star of the sea / from the sea of bitterness"
Mariette, Maretta, Mariet, Maryetta, Maryette, Marieta

Marika (Danish) Form of Mary, meaning "star of the sea / from the sea of bitterness"

Mariko (Japanese) Daughter of Mari; a ball or sphere
Maryko, Mareeko, Marieko, Mareiko

Marilyn (English) Form of Mary, meaning "star of the sea / from the sea of bitterness"
Maralin, Maralyn, Maralynn, Marelyn, Marilee, Marilin

Marissa (Latin) Woman of the sea
Maressa, Maricia, Marisabel, Marisha, Marisse, Maritza, Mariza, Marrissa

Marjani (African) Of the coral reef
Marjanie, Marjany, Marjaney, Marjanee, Marjean, Marjeani, Marjeanie, Marijani

Marjorie (English) Form of Margaret, meaning "resembling a pearl / the child of light"
Marcharie, Marge, Margeree, Margerie, Margery, Margey, Margi

Marlene (German) Blend of Mary, meaning "star of the sea / from the sea of bitterness," and Magdalene, meaning "woman from Magdala"
Marlaina, Marlana, Marlane, Marlayna

Marley (English) Of the marshy meadow
Marlee, Marleigh, Marli, Marlie, Marly

Marlis (German) Form of Mary, meaning "star of the sea / from the sea of bitterness"
Marlisa, Marliss, Marlise, Marlisse, Marlissa, Marlys, Marlyss, Marlysa

Marlo (English) One who resembles driftwood
Marloe, Marlow, Marlowe, Marlon

Marsala (Italian) From the place of sweet wine
Marsalah, Marsalla, Marsallah

Martha (Aramaic) Mistress of the house; in the Bible, the sister of Lazarus and Mary
Maarva, Marfa, Marhta, Mariet, Marit, Mart, Marta, Marte

Mary (Latin / Hebrew) Star of the sea / from the sea of bitterness
Mair, Mal, Mallie, Manette, Manon, Manya, Mare, Maren, Maria, Marietta, Marika, Marilyn, Marlis, Maureen, May, Mindel, Miriam, Molly, Mia

Masami (African / Japanese) A commanding woman / one who is truthful
Masamie, Masamee, Masamy, Masamey, Masamea

Mashaka (African) A trouble-maker; a mischievous woman
Mashakah, Mashakia

Massachusetts (Native American) From the big hill; from the state of Massachusetts
Massachusets, Massachusette, Massachusetta, Massa, Massachute, Massachusta

Matana (Hebrew) A gift from God
Matanah, Matanna, Matannah, Matai

Matangi (Hindi) In Hinduism, the patron of inner thought
Matangy, Matangie, Matangee, Matangey, Matangea

Matsuko (Japanese) Child of the pine tree

Maureen (Irish) Form of Mary, meaning "star of the sea / from the sea of bitterness"
Maura, Maurene, Maurianne, Maurine, Maurya, Mavra, Maure, Mo

Mauve (French) Of the mallow plant
Mawve

Maven (English) Having great knowledge
Mavin, Mavyn

Maverick (American) One who is wild and free
Maverik, Maveryck, Maveryk, Mavarick, Mavarik

Mavis (French) Resembling a songbird
Mavise, Maviss, Mavisse, Mavys, Mavyss, Mavysse

May (Latin) Born during the month of May; form of Mary, meaning "star of the sea / from the sea of bitterness"
Mae, Mai, Maelynn, Maelee, Maj, Mala, Mayana, Maye

Maya (Indian / Hebrew) An illusion, a dream / woman of the water
Mya

Mayumi (Japanese) One who embodies truth, wisdom, and beauty

Mazarine (French) Having deep-blue eyes
Mazareen, Mazareene, Mazaryn, Mazaryne, Mazine, Mazyne, Mazeene

McKayla (Gaelic) A fiery woman
McKale, McKaylee, McKaleigh, McKay, McKaye, McKaela

Meadow (American) From the beautiful field
Meadow, Meado, Meadoe, Medow, Medowe, Medoe

Meara (Gaelic) One who is filled with happiness
Mearah

Medea (Greek) A cunning ruler; in mythology, a sorceress
Madora, Medeia, Media, Medeah, Mediah, Mediya

Medini (Indian) Daughter of the earth
Medinie, Mediny, Mediney, Medinee, Medinea

Meditrina (Latin) The healer; in mythology, goddess of health and wine
Meditreena, Meditryna, Meditriena

Medora (Greek) A wise ruler
Medoria, Medorah, Medorra, Medorea

Medusa (Greek) In mythology, a Gorgon with snakes for hair
Medoosa, Medusah, Medoosah, Medousa, Medousah

Meenakshi (Indian) Having beautiful eyes

Megan (Welsh) Form of Margaret, meaning "resembling a pearl / the child of light"
Maegan, Meg, Magan, Magen, Megin, Maygan, Meagan, Meaghan, Meghan

Mehalia (Hebrew) An affectionate woman
Mehaliah, Mehalea, Mehaleah, Mehaliya, Mehaliyah

Melanie (Greek) A dark-skinned beauty
Malaney, Malanie, Mel, Mela, Melaina, Melaine, Melainey, Melany

Meli (Native American) One who is bitter
Melie, Melee, Melea, Meleigh, Mely, Meley

Melia (Hawaiian / Greek) Resembling the plumeria / of the ash tree; in mythology, a nymph
Melidice, Melitine, Meliah, Meelia, Melya

Melika (Turkish) A great beauty
Melikah, Melicka, Melicca, Melyka, Melycka, Meleeka, Meleaka

Melinda (Latin) One who is sweet and gentle
Melynda, Malinda, Malinde, Mallie, Mally, Malynda, Melinde, Mellinda, Mindy

Melisande (French) Having the strength of an animal
Malisande, Malissande, Malyssandre, Melesande, Melisandra, Melisandre

Melissa (Greek) Resembling a honeybee; in mythology, a nymph
Malissa, Mallissa, Mel, Melesa, Melessa, Melisa, Melise, Melisse

Melita (Greek) As sweet as honey
Malita, Malitta, Melida, Melitta, Melyta, Malyta, Meleeta, Meleata

Melody (Greek) A beautiful song
Melodee, Melodey, Melodi, Melodia, Melodie, Melodea

Merana (American) Woman of the waters
Meranah, Meranna, Merannah

Mercer (English) A prosperous merchant

Meredith (Welsh) A great ruler; protector of the sea
Maredud, Meridel, Meredithe, Meredyth, Meridith, Merridie, Meradith, Meredydd

Meribah (Hebrew) A quarrelsome woman
Meriba

Meroz (Hebrew) From the cursed plains
Meroza, Merozia, Meroze

Merry (English) One who is lighthearted and joyful
Merree, Merri, Merrie, Merrielle, Merrile, Merrilee, Merrili, Merrily

Mertice (English) A well-known lady

Metea (Greek) A gentle
woman
Meteah, Metia, Metiah

Metin (Greek) A wise counselor
Metine, Metyn, Metyne

Metis (Greek) One who is
industrious
*Metiss, Metisse, Metys, Metyss,
Metysse*

Mettalise (Danish) As graceful
as a pearl
*Metalise, Mettalisse, Mettalisa,
Mettalissa*

Mia (Israeli / Latin) Who is
like God? / form of Mary,
meaning "star of the sea /
from the sea of bitterness"
Miah, Mea, Meah, Meya

Michaela (Celtic, Gaelic,
Hebrew, English, Irish)
Feminine form of Michael;
who is like God?
*Macaela, MacKayla, Mak,
Mechaela, Meeskaela, Mekea,
Micaela, Mikaela*

Michelle (French) Feminine
form of Michael; who is like
God?
*Machelle, Mashelle, M'chelle,
Mechelle, Meechelle, Me'Shell,
Meshella, Mischa*

Michewa (Tibetan) Sent from
heaven
Michewah

Mide (Irish) One who is thirsty
Meeda, Mida

Midori (Japanese) Having
green eyes
*Midorie, Midory, Midorey,
Midoree, Midorea*

Mignon (French) One who is
cute and petite

Mikayla (English) Feminine
form of Michael, meaning
"who is like God?"

Mila (Slavic) One who is
industrious and hardworking
Milaia, Milaka, Milla, Milia

Milan (Latin) From the city in
Italy; one who is gracious
Milaana

Milena (Slavic) The favored
one
*Mileena, Milana, Miladena,
Milanka, Mlada, Mladena*

Miley (American) Form of
Mili, meaning "a virtuous
woman"
Milee, Mylee, Mareli

Miliana (Latin) Feminine of
Emeliano; one who is eager
and willing
*Milianah, Milianna, Miliane,
Miliann, Milianne*

Millo (Hebrew) Defender of the sacred city
Milloh, Millowe, Milloe

Mima (Hebrew) Form of Jemima, meaning "our little dove"
Mimah, Mymah, Myma

Minda (Native American / Hindi) Having great knowledge
Mindah, Mynda, Myndah, Menda, Mendah

Mindel (Hebrew) Form of Mary, meaning "star of the sea / from the sea of bitterness"
Mindell, Mindelle, Mindele, Mindela, Mindella

Mindy (English) Form of Melinda, meaning "one who is sweet and gentle"
Minda, Mindee, Mindi, Mindie, Mindey, Mindea

Ming Yue (Chinese) Born beneath the bright moon

Minka (Teutonic) One who is resolute; having great strength
Minkah, Mynka, Mynkah, Minna, Minne

Minowa (Native American) One who has a moving voice
Minowah, Mynowa, Mynowah

Minuit (French) Born at midnight
Minueet

Miracle (American) An act of God's hand
Mirakle, Mirakel, Myracle, Myrakle

Mirai (Basque / Japanese) A miracle child / future
Miraya, Mirari, Mirarie, Miraree, Mirae

Miranda (Latin) Worthy of admiration
Maranda, Myranda, Randi

Miremba (Ugandan) A promoter of peace
Mirembe, Mirem, Mirembah, Mirembeh, Mirema

Miriam (Hebrew) Form of Mary, meaning "star of the sea / from the sea of bitterness"
Mariam, Maryam, Meriam, Meryam, Mirham, Mirjam, Mirjana, Mirriam

Mirinesse (English) Filled with joy
Miriness, Mirinese, Mirines, Mirinessa, Mirinesa

Mirit (Hebrew) One who is strong-willed

Mischa (Russian) Form of Michelle, meaning "who is like God?"
Misha

Mistico (Italian) A mystical woman
Mistica, Mystico, Mystica, Mistiko, Mystiko

Mitali (Indian) A friendly and sweet woman
Mitalie, Mitalee, Mitaleigh, Mitaly, Mitaley, Meeta, Mitalea

Miya (Japanese) From the sacred temple
Miyah

Miyo (Japanese) A beautiful daughter
Miyoko

Mizar (Hebrew) A little woman; petite
Mizarr, Mizarre, Mizare, Mizara, Mizaria, Mizarra

Mliss (Cambodian) Resembling a flower
Mlissa, Mlisse, Mlyss, Mlysse, Mlyssa

Mocha (Arabic) As sweet as chocolate
Mochah

Modesty (Latin) One who is without conceit
Modesti, Modestie, Modestee, Modestus, Modestey, Modesta, Modestia, Modestina

Moesha (American) Drawn from the water
Moisha, Moysha, Moeesha, Moeasha, Moeysha

Mohini (Indian) The most beautiful
Mohinie, Mohinee, Mohiny

Moladah (Hebrew) A giver of life
Molada

Molly (Irish) Form of Mary, meaning "star of the sea / from the sea of bitterness"
Moll, Mollee, Molley, Molli, Mollie, Molle, Mollea, Mali

Mona (Gaelic) One who is born into the nobility
Moina, Monah, Monalisa, Monalissa, Monna, Moyna, Monalysa, Monalyssa

Moncha (Irish) A solitary woman
Monchah

Monica (Greek / Latin) A solitary woman / one who advises others
Monnica, Monca, Monicka, Monika, Monike

Monique (French) One who provides wise counsel
Moniqua, Moneeque, Moneequa, Moneeke, Moeneek, Moneaque, Moneaqua, Moneake

Monisha (Hindi) Having great intelligence
Monishah, Monesha, Moneisha, Moniesha, Moneysha, Moneasha

Monroe (Gaelic) Woman from the river
Monrow, Monrowe, Monro

Monserrat (Latin) From the jagged mountain
Montserrat

Montana (Latin) Woman of the mountains; from the state of Montana
Montanna, Montina, Monteene, Montese

Morcan (Welsh) Of the bright sea
Morcane, Morcana, Morcania, Morcanea

Moreh (Hebrew) A great archer; a teacher

Morgan (Welsh) Circling the bright sea; a sea dweller
Morgaine, Morgana, Morgance, Morgane, Morganica, Morgann, Morganne, Morgayne

Morguase (English) In Arthurian legend, the mother of Gawain
Marguase, Margawse, Morgawse, Morgause, Margause

Morina (Japanese) From the woodland town
Morinah, Moreena, Moryna, Moriena, Moreina, Moreana

Mubarika (Arabic) One who is blessed
Mubaarika, Mubaricka, Mubaryka, Mubaricca, Mubarycca

Mubina (Arabic) One who displays her true image
Mubeena, Mubinah, Mubyna, Mubeana, Mubiena

Mudan (Mandarin) Daughter of a harmonious family
Mudane, Mudana, Mudann, Mudaen, Mudaena

Mufidah (Arabic) One who is helpful to others
Mufeeda, Mufeyda, Mufyda, Mufeida, Mufieda, Mufeada

Muirne (Irish) One who is dearly loved
Muirna

Munay (African) One who loves and is loved
Manay, Munaye, Munae, Munai

Munazza (Arabic) An independent woman; one who is free
Munazzah, Munaza, Munazah

Muriel (Irish) Of the shining sea
Merial, Meriel, Merrill

Murphy (Celtic) Daughter of a great sea warrior
Murphi, Murphie, Murphey

Musoke (African) Having the beauty of a rainbow

Mya (American) Form of Maya, meaning "an illusion, woman of the water"
Myah

Myisha (Arabic) Form of Aisha, meaning "lively; womanly"
Myesha, Myeisha, Myeshia, Myiesha, Myeasha

Myka (Hebrew) Feminine of Micah, meaning "who is like God?"
Micah, Mika

Myrina (Latin) In mythology, an Amazon
Myrinah, Myreena, Myreina, Myriena, Myreana

Myrrh (Egyptian) Resembling the fragrant oil

N

Naama (Hebrew) Feminine form of Noam; an attractive woman; good-looking
Naamah

Naava (Hebrew) A lovely and pleasant woman
Naavah, Nava, Navah, Navit

Nabila (Arabic) Daughter born into nobility; a highborn daughter
Nabilah, Nabeela, Nabyla, Nabeelah, Nabylah, Nabeala, Nabealah

Nadda (Arabic) A very generous woman
Naddah, Nada, Nadah

Nadia (Slavic) One who is full of hope
Nadja, Nadya, Naadiya, Nadine, Nadie, Nadiyah, Nadea, Nadija

Nadirah (Arabic) One who is precious; rare
Nadira, Nadyra, Nadyrah, Nadeera, Nadeerah, Nadra

Naeva (French) Born in the evening
Naevah, Naevia, Naevea, Nayva, Nayvah

Nagge (Hebrew) A radiant woman

Nailah (Arabic) Feminine form of Nail; a successful woman; the acquirer
Na'ila, Na'ilah, Naa'ilah, Naila, Nayla, Naylah, Naela, Naelah

Najia (Arabic) An independent woman; one who is free
Naajia

Najja (African) The second-born child
Najjah

Namid (Native American) A star dancer
Namide, Namyd, Namyde

Namita (Papuan) In mythology, a mother goddess
Namitah, Nameeta, Namyta

Nana (Hawaiian / English) Born during the spring; a star / a grandmother or one who watches over children

Nancy (English) Form of Anna, meaning "a woman graced with God's favor"
Nainsey, Nainsi, Nance, Nancee, Nancey, Nanci, Nancie, Nancsi

Nandalia (Australian) A fiery woman
Nandaliah, Nandalea, Nandaleah, Nandali, Nandalie, Nandalei, Nandalee, Nandaleigh

Nandita (Indian) A delightful daughter
Nanditah, Nanditia, Nanditea

Naomi (Hebrew / Japanese) One who is pleasant / a beauty above all others
Namoie, Nayomi, Naomee

Narella (Greek) A bright woman; intelligent
Narellah, Narela, Narelah, Narelle, Narell, Narele

Nascio (Latin) In mythology, goddess of childbirth

Natalia (Spanish / Latin) form of Natalie; born on Christmas day
Natalya, Natalja

Natalie (Latin) Refers to Christ's birthday; born on Christmas Day
Natala, Natalee, Nathalie, Nataline, Nataly, Natasha

Natane (Native American) Her father's daughter
Natanne

Natasha (Russian) Form of Natalie, meaning "born on Christmas Day"
Nastaliya, Nastalya, Natacha, Natascha, Natashenka, Natashia, Natasia, Natosha

Navida (Iranian) Feminine form of Navid; bringer of good news
Navyda, Navidah, Navyda, Naveeda, Naveedah, Naveada, Naveadah

Navya (Indian) One who is youthful
Navyah, Naviya, Naviyah

Nawal (Arabic) A gift of God
Nawall, Nawalle, Nawala, Nawalla

Nawar (Arabic) Resembling a flower
Nawaar

Nazahah (Arabic) One who is pure and honest
Nazaha, Nazihah, Naziha

Nechama (Hebrew) One who provides comfort
Nehama, Nehamah, Nachmanit, Nachuma, Nechamah, Nechamit

Neda (Slavic) Born on a Sunday
Nedda, Nedah, Nedi, Nedie, Neddi, Neddie, Nedaa

Neena (Hindi) A woman who has beautiful eyes
Neenah, Neanah, Neana, Neyna, Neynah

Nefertiti (Egyptian) A queenly woman
Nefertari, Nefertyty, Nefertity, Nefertitie, Nefertitee, Nefertytie, Nefertitea

Neith (Egyptian) In mythology, goddess of war and hunting
Neitha, Neytha, Neyth, Neit, Neita, Neitia, Neitea, Neithe, Neythe

Nekana (Spanish) Woman of sorrow
Nekane, Nekania, Nekanea

Neo (African) A gift from God

Nerissa (Italian / Greek) A black-haired beauty / sea nymph
Narissa, Naryssa, Nericcia, Neryssa, Narice, Nerice, Neris

Nessa (Hebrew / Greek) A miracle child / form of Agnes, meaning "one who is pure; chaste"
Nesha, Nessah, Nessia, Nessya, Nesta, Neta, Netia, Nessie

Netis (Native American) One who is trustworthy
Netiss, Netisse, Netys, Netyss, Netysse

Nevaeh (American) Child from heaven

Nevina (Scottish) Feminine form of Nevin; daughter of a saint
Nevinah, Neveena, Nevyna, Nevinne, Nevynne, Neveene, Neveana, Neveane

Newlyn (Gaelic) Born during the spring
Newlynn, Newlynne, Newlin, Newlinn, Newlinne, Newlen, Newlenn, Newlenne

Neziah (Hebrew) One who is pure; a victorious woman
Nezia, Nezea, Nezeah, Neza, Nezah, Neziya, Neziyah

Niabi (Native American) Resembling a fawn
Niabie, Niabee, Niabey, Niaby

Niagara (English) From the famous waterfall
Niagarah, Niagarra, Niagarrah, Nyagara, Nyagarra

Nicole (Greek) Feminine form of Nicholas; of the victorious people
Necole, Niccole, Nichol, Nichole, Nicholle, Nickol, Nickole, Nicol

Nicosia (English) Woman from the capital of Cyprus
Nicosiah, Nicosea, Nicoseah, Nicotia, Nicotea

Nidia (Spanish) One who is gracious
Nydia, Nidiah, Nydiah, Nidea, Nideah, Nibia, Nibiah, Nibea

Nike (Greek) One who brings victory; in mythology, goddess of victory
Nikee, Nikey, Nykee, Nyke

Nilam (Arabic) Resembling a precious blue stone
Neelam, Nylam, Nilima, Nilyma, Nylyma, Nylima, Nealam, Nealama

Nilsine (Scandinavian) Feminine form of Neil; a champion

Nimeesha (African) A princess; daughter born to royalty
Nimeeshah, Nimiesha

Nini (African) As solid as a stone
Ninie, Niny, Niney, Ninee, Ninea

Nishan (African) One who wins awards
Nishann, Nishanne, Nishana, Nishanna, Nyshan, Nyshana

Nitya (Indian) An eternal beauty
Nithya, Nithyah, Nityah

Nixie (German) A beautiful water sprite
Nixi, Nixy, Nixey, Nixee, Nixea

Noelle (French) Born at Christmastime
Noel, Noela, Noele, Noe

Nolcha (Native American) Of the sun
Nolchia, Nolchea

Nomusa (African) One who is merciful
Nomusah, Nomusha, Nomusia, Nomusea, Nomushia, Nomushea

Nora (English) Form of Eleanor, meaning "the shining light"
Norah, Noora, Norella, Norelle, Norissa, Norri, Norrie, Norry

Nyala (African) Resembling an antelope
Nyalah, Nyalla, Nyallah

Nylah (Gaelic) Cloud or champion

Oaisara (Arabic) A great ruler; an empress
Oaisarah, Oaisarra, Oaisarrah

Oamra (Arabic) Daughter of the moon
Oamrah, Oamira, Oamyra, Oameera

Oba (African) In mythology, the goddess of rivers
Obah, Obba, Obbah

Octavia (Latin) Feminine form of Octavius; the eighth-born child
Octaviana, Octavianne, Octavie, Octiana, Octoviana, Ottavia, Octavi, Octavy

Ode (Egyptian / Greek) Traveler of the road / a lyric poem
Odea

Odessa (Greek) Feminine form of Odysseus; one who wanders; an angry woman
Odissa, Odyssa, Odessia, Odissia, Odyssia, Odysseia

Odina (Latin / Scandinavian)
From the mountain / feminine form of Odin, the highest of the gods
Odinah, Odeena, Odeene, Odeen, Odyna, Odyne, Odynn, Odeana

Oheo (Native American) A beautiful woman

Oira (Latin) One who prays to God
Oyra, Oirah, Oyrah

Okalani (Hawaiian) Form of Kalani, meaning "from the heavens"
Okalanie, Okalany, Okalaney, Okalanee, Okaloni, Okalonie, Okalonee, Okalony, Okaloney, Okeilana, Okelani, Okelani, Okelanie, Okelany, Okelaney, Okelanee, Okalanea, Okalonea, Okelanea

Okei (Japanese) Woman of the ocean

Oksana (Russian) Hospitality
Oksanah, Oksie, Aksana

Ola (Nigerian / Hawaiian / Norse) One who is precious / giver of life; well-being / a relic of one's ancestors
Olah, Olla, Ollah

Olaide (American) A thoughtful woman
Olaid, Olaida, Olayd, Olayde, Olayda, Olaed, Olaede, Olaeda

Olathe (Native American) A lovely young woman

Olayinka (Yoruban)
Surrounded by wealth and honor
Olayenka, Olayanka

Oleda (English) Resembling a winged creature
Oldedah, Oleta, Olita, Olida, Oletah, Olitah, Olidah

Olethea (Latin) Form of Alethea, meaning "one who is truthful"
Oletheia, Olethia, Oletha, Oletea, Olthaia, Olithea, Olathea, Oletia

Olina (Hawaiian) One who is joyous
Oline, Oleen, Oleene, Olyne, Oleena, Olyna, Olin

Olivia (Latin) Feminine form of Oliver; of the olive tree; one who is peaceful
Oliviah, Oliva, Olive, Oliveea, Olivet, Olivetta, Olivette, Olivija

Olwen (Welsh) One who leaves a white footprint
Olwynn, Olvyen, Olvyin

Olympia (Greek) From Mount Olympus; a goddess
Olympiah, Olimpe, Olimpia, Olimpiada, Olimpiana, Olypme, Olympie, Olympi

Omri (Arabic) A red-haired woman
Omrie, Omree, Omrea, Omry, Omrey

Ona (Hebrew) Filled with grace
Onit, Onat, Onah

Ondrea (Slavic) Form of Andrea, meaning "courageous and strong / womanly"
Ondria, Ondrianna, Ondreia, Ondreina, Ondreya, Ondriana, Ondreana, Ondera

Oneida (Native American) Our long-awaited daughter
Onieda, Oneyda, Onida, Onyda

Onida (Native American) The one who has been expected
Onidah, Onyda, Onydah

Ontina (American) An open-minded woman
Ontinah, Onteena, Onteenah, Onteana, Onteanah, Ontiena, Ontienah, Onteina

Oona (Gaelic) Form of Agnes, meaning "one who is pure; chaste"

Opal (Sanskrit) A treasured jewel; resembling the iridescent gemstone
Opall, Opalle, Opale, Opalla, Opala, Opalina, Opaline, Opaleena

Ophelia (Greek) One who offers help to others
Ofelia, Ofilia, OphÈlie, Ophelya, Ophilia, Ovalia, Ovelia, Opheliah

Ophrah (Hebrew) Resembling a fawn; from the place of dust
Ofra, Ofrit, Ophra, Oprah, Orpa, Orpah, Ofrat, Ofrah

Orange (Latin) Resembling the sweet fruit
Orangetta, Orangia, Orangina, Orangea

Orbelina (American) One who brings excitement
Orbelinah, Orbeleena

Orea (Greek) From the mountains
Oreah

Orenda (Iroquois) A woman with magical powers

Oriana (Latin) Born at sunrise
Oreana, Orianna, Oriane, Oriann, Orianne

Oribel (Latin) A beautiful
golden child
*Orabel, Orabelle, Orabell,
Orabela, Orabella, Oribell,
Oribelle, Oribele*

Orin (Irish) A dark-haired
beauty
*Orine, Orina, Oryna, Oryn,
Oryne*

Orinthia (Hebrew / Gaelic) Of
the pine tree / a fair lady
*Orrinthia, Orenthia, Orna,
Ornina, Orinthea, Orenthea,
Orynthia, Orynthea*

Oriole (Latin) Resembling the
gold-speckled bird
*Oreolle, Oriolle, Oreole, Oriola,
Oriolla, Oriol, Oreola, Oreolla*

Orion (Greek) The huntress; a
constellation

Orithna (Greek) One who is
natural
*Orithne, Orythna, Orythne,
Orithnia, Orythnia, Orithnea,
Orythnea*

Orla (Gaelic) The golden
queen
*Orlah, Orrla, Orrlah, Orlagh,
Orlaith, Orlaithe, Orghlaith,
Orghlaithe*

Ornella (Italian) Of the flowering
ash tree

Ornice (Irish) A pale-skinned
woman
*Ornyce, Ornise, Orynse,
Orneice, Orneise, Orniece,
Orniese, Orneece*

Orva (Anglo-Saxon / French)
A courageous friend / as precious as gold

Orynko (Ukrainian) A peaceful
woman
Orinko, Orynka, Orinka

Osaka (Japanese) From the
city of industry
*Osaki, Osakie, Osakee, Osaky,
Osakey, Osakea*

Osma (English) Feminine
form of Osmond; protected
by God
Osmah, Ozma, Ozmah

Otina (American) A fortunate
woman
*Otinah, Otyna, Otynah,
Oteena, Oteenah, Oteana,
Oteanah, Otiena*

Owena (Welsh) A high-born
woman
*Owenah, Owenna, Owennah,
Owenia, Owenea*

Ozora (Hebrew) One who is
wealthy
Ozorah, Ozorra, Ozorrah

P

Pace (American) A charismatic young woman
Paice, Payce, Paece, Pase, Paise, Payse, Paese

Pacifica (Spanish) A peaceful woman
Pacifika, Pacyfyca, Pacyfyka, Pacifyca, Pacifyka, Pacyfica, Pacyfika

Pageant (American) A dramatic woman
Pagent, Padgeant, Padgent

Paige (English) A young assistant
Page, Payge, Paege

Paisley (English) Woman of the church
Paislee

Paki (African) A witness of God
Pakki, Packi, Pacci, Pakie, Pakkie, Paky, Pakky, Pakey

Palba (Spanish) A fair-haired woman

Palesa (African) Resembling a flower
Palessa, Palesah, Palysa, Palisa, Paleesa

Paloma (Spanish) Dove-like
Palloma, Palomita, Palometa, Peloma, Aloma

Pamela (English) A woman who is as sweet as honey
Pamelah, Pamella, Pammeli, Pammelie, Pameli, Pamelie, Pamelia, Pamelea

Panagiota (Greek) Feminine form of Panagiotis; a holy woman

Panchali (Indian) A princess; a high-born woman
Panchalie, Panchaly, Panchalli

Pandara (Indian) A good wife
Pandarah, Pandarra, Pandaria, Pandarea

Pandora (Greek) A gifted, talented woman; in mythology, the first mortal woman, who unleashed evil upon the world
Pandorah, Pandorra, Pandoria, Pandorea, Pandoriya

Pantxike (Latin) A woman who is free
Pantxikey, Pantxikye, Pantxeke, Pantxyke

Paras (Indian) A woman against whom others are measured

Paris (English) Woman of the city in France
Pariss, Parisse, Parys, Paryss, Parysse

Parker (English) The keeper of the park
Parkyr

Parry (Welsh) Daughter of Harry
Parri, Parrie, Parrey, Parree, Parrea

Parvani (Indian) Born during a full moon
Parvanie, Parvany, Parvaney, Parvanee, Parvanea

Parvati (Hindi) Daughter of the mountain; in Hinduism, a name for the wife of Shiva
Parvatie, Parvaty, Parvatey, Parvatee, Pauravi, Parvatea, Pauravie, Pauravy

Paterekia (Hawaiian) An upper-class woman
Paterekea, Pakelekia, Pakelekea

Patience (English) One who is patient; an enduring woman
Patiencia, Paciencia, Pacencia, Pacyncia, Pacincia, Pacienca

Patricia (English) Feminine form of Patrick; of noble descent
Patrisha, Patrycia, Patrisia, Patsy, Patti, Patty, Patrizia, Pattie, Trisha

Patrina (American) Born into the nobility
Patreena, Patriena, Patreina, Patryna, Patreana

Paula (English) Feminine form of Paul; a petite woman
Paulina, Pauline, Paulette, Paola, Pauleta, Pauletta, Pauli, Paulete

Pausha (Hindi) Resembling the moon
Paushah

Pax (Latin) One who is peaceful; in mythology, the goddess of peace
Paxi, Paxie, Paxton, Paxten, Paxtan, Paxy, Paxey, Paxee

Payton (English) From the warrior's village
Paton, Paeton, Paiton, Payten, Paiten

Pearl (Latin) A precious gem of the sea
Pearla, Pearle, Pearlie, Pearly, Pearline, Pearlina, Pearli, Pearley

Pelopia (Greek) In mythology, the wife of Thyestes and mother of Aegisthus
Pelopiah, Pelopea, Pelopeah, Pelopiya

Pembroke (English) From the broken hill
Pembrook, Pembrok, Pembrooke

Pendant (French) A decorated woman
Pendent, Pendante, Pendente

Penelope (Greek) Resembling a duck; in mythology, the faithful wife of Odysseus
Peneloppe, Penelopy, Penelopey, Penelopi, Penelopie, Penelopee, Penella, Penelia, Penny

Penthesilea (Greek) In mythology, a queen of the Amazons

Peony (Greek) Resembling the flower
Peoney, Peoni, Peonie, Peonee, Peonea

Pepin (French) An awe-inspiring woman
Peppin, Pepine, Peppine, Pipin, Pippin, Pepen, Pepan, Peppen

Pepita (Spanish) Feminine form of Joseph; God will add
Pepitah, Pepitta, Pepitia, Pepitina

Perdita (Latin) A lost woman
Perditah, Perditta, Perdy, Perdie, Perdi, Perdee, Perdea, Perdeeta

Perdix (Latin) Resembling a partridge
Perdixx, Perdyx, Perdyxx

Peri (Persian / English) In mythology, a fairy / from the pear tree
Perry, Perri, Perie, Perrie, Pery, Perrey, Perey, Peree

Perpetua (Latin) One who is constant; steadfast

Persephone (Greek) In mythology, the daughter of Demeter and Zeus who was abducted to the underworld
Persephoni, Persephonie, Persephony, Persephoney, Persephonee, Persefone, Persefoni, Persefonie

Persis (Greek) Woman of Persia
Persiss, Persisse, Persys, Persyss, Persysse

Pesha (Hebrew) A flourishing woman
Peshah, Peshia, Peshiah, Peshea, Pesheah, Peshe

Petronela (Latin) Feminine form of Peter, as solid and strong as a rock
Petronella, Petronelle, Petronia, Petronilla, Petronille, Petrona, Petronia, Petronel

Petunia (English) Resembling the flower
Petuniah, Petuniya, Petunea, Petoonia, Petounia

Peyton (English) From the warrior's village
Peyten

Phaedra (Greek) A bright woman; in mythology, the wife of Theseus
Phadra, Phaidra, Phedra, Phaydra, Phedre, Phaedre

Phailin (Thai) Resembling a sapphire
Phaylin, Phaelin, Phalin

Pheakkley (Vietnamese) A faithful woman
Pheakkly, Pheakkli, Pheakklie, Pheakklee, Pheakkleigh, Pheakklea

Pheodora (Greek) A supreme gift
Pheodorah, Phedora, Phedorah

Phernita (American) A well-spoken woman
Pherneeta, Phernyta, Phernieta, Pherneita, Pherneata

Phia (Italian) A saintly woman
Phiah, Phea, Pheah

Philippa (English) Feminine form of Phillip; a friend of horses
Phillippa, Philipa, Phillipa, Philipinna, Philippine, Phillipina, Phillipine, Pilis

Philomena (Greek) A friend of strength
Filomena, Philomina, Mena

Phoebe (Greek) A bright, shining woman; in mythology, another name for the goddess of the moon
Phebe, Phoebi, Phebi, Phoebie, Phebie, Pheobe, Phoebee, Phoebea

Phoena (Greek) Resembling a mystical bird
Phoenah, Phoenna, Phena, Phenna

Phoenix (Greek) A dark-red color; in mythology, an immortal bird
Phuong, Phoenyx

Phyllis (Greek) Of the foliage; in mythology, a girl who was turned into an almond tree
Phylis, Phillis, Philis, Phylys, Phyllida, Phylida, Phillida, Philida

Pili (Egyptian) The second-born child
Pilie, Pily, Piley, Pilee, Pilea, Pileigh

Pililani (Hawaiian) Having great strength
Pililanie, Pililany, Pililaney, Pililanee, Pililanea

Piluki (Hawaiian) Resembling a small leaf
Pilukie, Piluky, Pilukey, Pilukee, Pilukea

Pineki (Hawaiian) Resembling a peanut
Pinekie, Pineky, Pinekey, Pinekee, Pinekea

Ping (Chinese) One who is peaceful
Pyng

Pinga (Inuit) In mythology, goddess of the hunt, fertility, and healing
Pingah, Pyngah, Pyngah

Pinquana (Native American) Having a pleasant fragrance
Pinquan, Pinquann, Pinquanne, Pinquanna, Pinquane

Piper (English) One who plays the flute
Pipere, Piperel, Piperell, Piperele, Piperelle, Piperela, Piperella, Pyper

Pippi (French / English) A friend of horses / a blushing young woman
Pippie, Pippy, Pippey, Pippee, Pippea

Pirouette (French) A ballet dancer
Piroette, Pirouett, Piroett, Piroueta, Piroeta, Pirouetta, Piroetta, Pirouet

Pisces (Latin) The twelfth sign of the zodiac; the fishes
Pysces, Piscees, Pyscees, Piscez, Pisceez

Pithasthana (Hindi) In Hinduism, a name for the wife of Shiva

Platt (French) From the plains
Platte

Pleshette (American) An extravagent woman
Pleshett, Pleshet, Pleshete, Plesheta, Pleshetta

Pleun (American) One who is good with words
Pleune

Po (Italian) A lively woman

Podarge (Greek) In mythology, one of the Harpies

Poetry (American) A romantic woman
Poetrey, Poetri, Poetrie, Poetree, Poetrea

Polete (Hawaiian) A kind young woman
Polet, Polett, Polette, Poleta, Poletta

Polina (Russian) A small woman
Polinah, Poleena, Poleenah, Poleana, Poleanah, Poliena, Polienah, Poleina

Pomona (Latin) In mythology, goddess of fruit trees
Pomonah, Pomonia, Pomonea, Pamona, Pamonia, Pamonea

Poodle (American) Resembling the dog; one with curly hair
Poudle, Poodel, Poudel

Porter (Latin) The doorkeeper

Posala (Native American) Born at the end of spring
Posalah, Posalla, Posallah

Posh (American) A fancy young woman
Poshe, Posha

Potina (Latin) In mythology, goddess of children's food and drink
Potinah, Potyna, Potena, Poteena, Potiena, Poteina, Poteana

Powder (American) A light-hearted woman
Powdar, Powdir, Powdur, Powdor, Powdi, Powdie, Powdy, Powdey

Praise (Latin) One who expresses admiration
Prayse, Praize, Prayze, Praze, Praese, Praeze

Pramada (Indian) One who is indifferent

Pramlocha (Hindi) In Hinduism, a celestial nymph

Precious (American) One who is treasured
Preshis, Preshys

Presley (English) Of the priest's town
Presly, Preslie, Presli, Preslee

Primola (Latin) Resembling a primrose
Primolah, Primolia, Primoliah, Primolea, Primoleah

Princess (English) A high-born daughter; born to royalty
Princessa, Princesa, Princie, Princi, Princy, Princee, Princey, Princea

Prisca (Latin) From an ancient family
Priscilla, Priscella, Precilla, Presilla, Prescilla, Prisilla, Prisella, Prissy, Prissi

Promise (American) A faithful woman
Promice, Promyse, Promyce, Promis, Promiss, Promys, Promyss

Prudence (English) One who is cautious and exercises good judgment
Prudencia, Prudensa, Prudensia, Prudentia, Predencia, Predentia, Prue, Pru

Pryce (American / Welsh) One who is very dear / an enthusiastic child
Price, Prise, Pryse

Pulcheria (Italian) A chubby baby
Pulcheriah, Pulcherea, Pulchereah, Pulcherya, Pulcheryah, Pulcheriya

Pulika (African) An obedient and well-behaved girl
Pulikah, Pulicca, Pulicka, Pulyka, Puleeka, Puleaka

Pyrena (Greek) A fiery woman
Pyrenah, Pyrina, Pyrinah, Pyryna, Pyrynah, Pyreena, Pyreenah, Pyriena

Pyria (American) One who is cherished
Pyriah, Pyrea, Pyreah, Pyriya, Pyriyah, Pyra

Qadesh (Syrian) In mythology, goddess of love and sensuality
Quedesh, Qadesha, Quedesha, Qadeshia, Quedeshia, Quedeshiya

Qamra (Arabic) Of the moon
Qamrah, Qamar, Qamara, Qamrra, Qamaria, Qamrea, Qamria

Qimat (Indian) A valuable woman
Qimate, Qimatte, Qimata, Qimatta

Qitarah (Arabic) Having a nice fragrance
Qitara, Qytarah, Qytara, Qitaria, Qitarra, Qitarria, Qytarra, Qytarria

Quana (Native American) One who is aromatic; sweet-smelling
Quanah, Quanna, Quannah, Quania, Quaniya, Quanniya, Quannia, Quanea

Querida (Spanish) One who is
dearly loved; beloved
*Queridah, Queryda, Querydah,
Querrida, Queridda,
Querridda, Quereeda,
Quereada*

Queta (Spanish) Head of the
household
Quetah, Quetta, Quettah

Quiana (American) Living
with grace; heavenly
*Quianah, Quianna, Quiane,
Quian, Quianne, Quianda,
Quiani, Quianita*

Quincy (English) The fifth-
born child
*Quincey, Quinci, Quincie,
Quincee, Quincia, Quinncy,
Quinnci, Quyncy*

Quinn (English / Irish)
Woman who is queenly
Quin, Quinne

Quintana (Latin / English) The
fifth girl / queen's lawn
*Quintanah, Quinella, Quinta,
Quintina, Quintanna,
Quintann, Quintara, Quintona*

Quintessa (Latin) Of the
essence
*Quintessah, Quintesa,
Quintesha, Quintisha,
Quintessia, Quyntessa,
Quintosha, Quinticia*

Quinyette (American) The
fifth-born child
*Quinyett, Quinyet, Quinyeta,
Quinyette, Quinyete*

Quirina (Latin) One who is
contentious
*Quirinah, Quiryna, Quirynah,
Quireena, Quireenah,
Quireina, Quireinah, Quiriena*

Quiritis (Latin) In mythology,
goddess of motherhood
*Quiritiss, Quiritisse, Quirytis,
Quirytys, Quiritys, Quirityss*

R

Rabiah (Egyptian / Arabic)
Born in the springtime / of
the gentle wind
Rabia, Raabia, Rabi'ah, Rabi

Rachana (Hindi) Born of the
creation
*Rachanna, Rashana,
Rashanda, Rachna*

Rachel (Hebrew) The innocent
lamb; in the Bible, Jacob's wife
*Rachael, Racheal, Rachelanne,
Rachelce, Rachele, Racheli,
Rachell, Rachelle, Raquel*

Radcliffe (English) Of the red cliffs
Radcleff, Radclef, Radclif, Radclife, Radclyffe, Radclyf, Radcliphe, Radclyphe

Radella (English) An elfin counselor
Radell, Radel, Radele, Radela, Raedself, Radself, Raidself

Radmilla (Slavic) Hard-working for the people
Radilla, Radinka, Radmila, Redmilla, Radilu

Rafi'a (Arabic) An exalted woman
Rafia, Rafi'ah, Rafee'a, Rafeea, Rafeeah, Rafiya, Rafiyah

Ragnara (Swedish) Feminine form of Ragnar; one who provides counsel to the army
Ragnarah, Ragnarra, Ragnaria, Ragnarea, Ragnari, Ragnarie, Ragnary, Ragnarey

Rahi (Arabic) Born during the springtime
Rahii, Rahy, Rahey, Rahee, Rahea, Rahie

Rahimah (Arabic) A compassionate woman; one who is merciful
Rahima, Raheema, Raheemah, Raheima, Rahiema, Rahyma, Rahymah, Raheama

Raina (Polish) Form of Regina, meaning "a queenly woman"
Raenah, Raene, Rainah, Raine, Rainee, Rainey, Rainelle, Rainy

Raja (Arabic) One who is filled with hope
Rajah

Raleigh (English) From the clearing of roe deer
Raileigh, Railey, Raley, Rawleigh, Rawley, Raly, Rali, Ralie

Ramona (Spanish) Feminine form of Ramon; a wise protector
Ramee, Ramie, Ramoena, Ramohna, Ramonda, Ramonde, Ramonita, Ramonna

Randi (English) Feminine form of Randall; shielded by wolves; form of Miranda, meaning "worthy of admiration"
Randa, Randee, Randelle, Randene, Randie, Randy, Randey, Randilyn

Raquel (Spanish) Form of Rachel, meaning "the innocent lamb"
Racquel, Racquell, Raquela, Raquelle, Roquel, Roquela, Rakel, Rakell

Rasha (Arabic) Resembling a young gazelle
Rashah, Raisha, Raysha, Rashia, Raesha

Ratana (Thai) Resembling a crystal
Ratanah, Ratanna, Ratannah, Rathana, Rathanna

Rati (Hindi) In Hinduism, goddess of passion and lust
Ratie, Ratea, Ratee, Raty, Ratey

Ratri (Indian) Born in the evening
Ratrie, Ratry, Ratrey, Ratree, Ratrea

Rawiyah (Arabic) One who recites ancient poetry
Rawiya, Rawiyya, Rawiyyah

Rawnie (English) An elegant lady
Rawni, Rawny, Rawney, Rawnee, Rawnea

Raya (Israeli) A beloved friend
Rayah

Raymonde (German) Feminine form of Raymond; one who offers wise protection
Raymondi, Raymondie, Raymondee, Raymondea, Raymonda, Raymunde, Raymunda

Rayna (Hebrew / Scandinavian) One who is pure / one who provides wise counsel
Raynah, Raynee, Rayni, Rayne, Raynea, Raynie

Reba (Hebrew) Form of Rebecca, meaning "one who is bound to God"
Rebah, Reeba, Rheba, Rebba, Ree, Reyba, Reaba

Rebecca (Hebrew) One who is bound to God; in the Bible, the wife of Isaac
Rebakah, Rebbeca, Rebbecca, Rebbecka, Rebeca, Rebeccah, Rebeccea, Becky, Reba

Reese (American) Form of Rhys, meaning "having great enthusiasm for life"
Rhyss, Rhysse, Reece, Reice, Reise, Reace, Rease, Riece

Reagan (Gaelic) Born into royalty; the little ruler
Raegan, Ragan, Raygan, Reganne, Regann, Regane, Reghan, Regan

Regina (Latin) A queenly woman
Regeena, Regena, Reggi, Reggie, Régine, Regine, Reginette, Reginia, Raina

Rehan (Armenian) Resembling a flower
Rehane, Rehann, Rehanne, Rehana, Rehanna, Rehanan, Rehannan, Rehania

Rehoboth (Hebrew) From the city by the river
Rehobothe, Rehobotha, Rehobothia

Rekha (Indian) One who walks a straight line
Rekhah, Reka, Rekah

Remy (French) Woman from the town of Rheims
Remi, Remie, Remmy, Remmi, Remmie, Remmey, Remey

Ren (Japanese) Resembling a water lily

Renée (French) One who has been reborn
Ranae, Ranay, Ranée, Renae, Renata, Renay, Renaye, René

Reseda (Latin) Resembling the mignonette flower
Resedah, Reselda, Resedia, Reseldia

Resen (Hebrew) From the head of the stream; refers to a bridle

Reshma (Arabic) Having silky skin
Reshmah, Reshman, Reshmane, Reshmann, Reshmanne, Reshmana, Reshmanna, Reshmaan

Reya (Spanish) A queenly woman
Reyah, Reyeh, Reye, Reyia, Reyiah, Reyea, Reyeah

Reza (Hungarian) Form of Theresa, meaning "a harvester"
Rezah, Rezia, Reziah, Rezi, Rezie, Rezy, Rezee, Resi

Rhea (Greek) Of the flowing stream; in mythology, the wife of Cronus and mother of gods and goddesses
Rea, Rhae, Rhaya, Rhia, Rhiah, Rhiya, Rheya

Rheda (Anglo-Saxon) A divine woman; a goddess
Rhedah

Rhiannon (Welsh) The great and sacred queen
Rheanna, Rheanne, Rhiana, Rhiann, Rhianna, Rhiannan, Rhianon, Rhyan

Rhonda (Welsh) Wielding a good spear
Rhondelle, Rhondene, Rhondiesha, Rhonette, Rhonnda, Ronda, Rondel, Rondelle

Rhys (Welsh) Having great enthusiasm for life
Rhyss, Rhysse, Reece, Reese, Reice, Reise, Reace, Rease

Ria (Spanish) From the river's mouth
Riah

Riane (Gaelic) Feminine form of Ryan; little ruler
Riana, Rianna, Rianne, Ryann, Ryanne, Ryana, Ryanna, Riann

Rica (English) Form of Frederica, meaning "peaceful ruler"; form of Erica, meaning "ever the ruler / resembling heather"
Rhica, Ricca, Ricah, Rieca, Riecka, Rieka, Riqua, Ryca

Riddhi (Indian) A prosperous woman
Riddhie, Riddhy, Riddhey, Riddhee, Riddhea

Rihanna (Arabic) Resembling sweet basil
Rihana

Riley (Gaelic) From the rye clearing; a courageous woman
Reilley, Reilly, Rilee, Rileigh, Ryley, Rylee, Ryleigh, Rylie

Rini (Japanese) Resembling a young rabbit
Rinie, Rinee, Rinea, Riny, Riney

Rio (Spanish) Woman of the river
Rhio

Risa (Latin) One who laughs often
Risah, Reesa, Riesa, Rise, Rysa, Rysah, Riseh, Risako

Rita (Greek) Precious pearl
Ritta, Reeta, Reita, Rheeta, Riet, Rieta, Ritah, Reta

Roberta (English) Feminine form of Robert; one who is bright with fame
Robertah, Robbie, Robin

Rochelle (French) From the little rock
Rochel, Rochele, Rochell, Rochella, Rochette, Roschella, Roschelle, Roshelle

Roja (Spanish) A red-haired lady
Rojah

Rolanda (German) Feminine form of Roland; well-known throughout the land
Rolandah, Rolandia, Roldandea, Rolande, Rolando, Rollanda, Rollande

Romhilda (German) A glorious battle maiden
Romhilde, Romhild, Romeld, Romelde, Romelda, Romilda, Romild, Romilde

Ronli (Hebrew) My joy is the Lord
Ronlie, Ronlee, Ronleigh, Ronly, Ronley, Ronlea, Ronia, Roniya

Ronni (English) Form of Veronica, meaning "displaying her true image"
Ronnie, Ronae, Ronay, Ronee, Ronelle, Ronette, Roni, Ronica, Ronika

Rosalind (German / English) Resembling a gentle horse / form of Rose, meaning "resembling the beautiful and meaningful flower"
Ros, Rosaleen, Rosalen, Rosalin, Rosalina, Rosalinda, Rosalinde, Rosaline, Chalina

Rose (Latin) Resembling the beautiful and meaningful flower
Rosa, Rosie, Rosalind, Rosalyn

Roseanne (English) Resembling the graceful rose
Ranna, Rosana, Rosanagh, Rosanna, Rosannah, Rosanne, Roseann, Roseanna

Rosemary (Latin / English) The dew of the sea / resembling a bitter rose
Rosemaree, Rosemarey, Rosemaria, Rosemarie, Rosmarie, Rozmary, Rosamaria, Rosamarie

Rowan (Gaelic) Of the red-berry tree
Rowann, Rowane, Rowanne, Rowana, Rowanna

Rowena (Welsh / German) One who is fair and slender / having much fame and happiness
Rhowena, Roweena, Roweina, Rowenna, Rowina, Rowinna, Rhonwen, Rhonwyn

Ruana (Indian) One who is musically inclined
Ruanah, Ruanna, Ruannah, Ruane, Ruann, Ruanne

Ruby (English) As precious as the red gemstone
Rubee, Rubi, Rubie, Rubyna, Rubea

Rudella (German) A well-known woman
Rudela, Rudelah, Rudell, Rudelle, Rudel, Rudele, Rudy, Rudie

Rue (English, German) A medicinal herb
Ru, Larue

Rufina (Latin) A red-haired woman
Rufeena, Rufeine, Ruffina, Rufine, Ruffine, Rufyna, Ruffyna, Rufyne

Ruhi (Arabic) A spiritual woman
Roohee, Ruhee, Ruhie, Ruhy, Ruhey, Roohi, Roohie, Ruhea

Rumah (Hebrew) One who has been exalted
Ruma, Rumia, Rumea, Rumiah, Rumeah, Rumma, Rummah

Rumina (Latin) In mythology, a protector goddess of mothers and babies
Ruminah, Rumeena, Rumeenah, Rumeina, Rumiena, Rumyna, Rumeinah, Rumienah

Rupali (Indian) A beautiful woman
Rupalli, Rupalie, Rupalee, Rupallee, Rupal, Rupa, Rupaly, Rupaley

Ruth (Hebrew) A beloved companion
Ruthe, Ruthelle, Ruthellen, Ruthetta, Ruthi, Ruthie, Ruthina, Ruthine

Ryba (Slavic) Resembling a fish
Rybah, Rybba, Rybbah

Ryder (American) An accomplished horsewoman
Rider

Rylee (American) Form of Riley, meaning "from the rye clearing / a courageous woman"

Saba (Greek / Arabic) Woman from Sheba / born in the morning
Sabah, Sabaa, Sabba, Sabbah, Sabaah

Sabi (Arabic) A lovely young lady
Sabie, Saby, Sabey, Sabee, Sabbi, Sabbee, Sabea

Sabirah (Arabic) Having great patience
Sabira, Saabira, Sabeera, Sabiera, Sabeira, Sabyra, Sabirra, Sabyrra

Sabrina (English) A legendary princess
Sabrinah, Sabrinna, Sabreena, Sabriena, Sabreina, Sabryna, Sabrine, Sabryne, Cabrina, Zabrina

Sachet (Hindi) Having consciousness
Sachett, Sachette

Sada (Japanese) The pure one
Sadda, Sadaa, Sadako, Saddaa

Sadella (American) A beautiful fairylike princess
Sadel, Sadela, Sadelah, Sadele, Sadell, Sadellah, Sadelle, Sydel

Sadhana (Hindi) A devoted woman
Sadhanah, Sadhanna, Sadhannah, Sadhane, Sadhanne, Sadhann, Sadhan

Sadie (English) Form of Sarah, meaning "a princess; lady"
Sadi, Sady, Sadey, Sadee, Saddi, Saddee, Sadiey, Sadye

Sadiya (Arabic) One who is fortunate; lucky
Sadiyah, Sadiyyah, Sadya, Sadyah

Sadzi (American) Having a sunny disposition
Sadzee, Sadzey, Sadzia, Sadziah, Sadzie, Sadzya, Sadzyah, Sadzy

Safa (Arabic) One who is innocent and pure
Safah, Saffa, Sapha, Saffah, Saphah

Saffron (English) Resembling the yellow flower
Saffrone, Saffronn, Saffronne, Safron, Safronn, Safronne, Saffronah, Safrona

Saheli (Indian) A beloved friend
Sahelie, Sahely, Saheley, Sahelee, Saheleigh, Sahyli, Sahelea

Sahila (Indian) One who provides guidance
Sahilah, Saheela, Sahyla, Sahiela, Saheila, Sahela, Sahilla, Sahylla

Sahkyo (Native American) Resembling the mink
Sakyo

Saida (Arabic) Fortunate one; one who is happy
Saidah, Sa'ida, Sayida, Saeida, Saedah, Said, Sayide, Sayidea

Saihah (Arabic) One who is useful; good
Saiha, Sayiha

Sailor (American) One who sails the seas
Sailer, Sailar, Saylor, Sayler, Saylar, Saelor, Saeler, Saelar

Saima (Arabic) A fasting woman
Saimah, Saimma, Sayima

Sajni (Indian) One who is dearly loved
Sajnie, Sajny, Sajney, Sajnee, Sajnea

Sakae (Japanese) One who is prosperous
Sakai, Sakaie, Sakay, Sakaye

Sakari (Native American) A sweet girl
Sakarie, Sakary, Sakarri, Sakarey, Sakaree, Sakarree, Sakarah, Sakarrie

Sakina (Indian / Arabic) A beloved friend / having God-inspired peace of mind
Sakinah, Sakeena, Sakiena, Sakeina, Sakyna, Sakeyna, Sakinna, Sakeana

Sakti (Hindi) In Hinduism, the divine energy
Saktie, Sakty, Sakkti, Sackti, Saktee, Saktey, Saktia, Saktiah

Saku (Japanese) Remembrance of the Lord
Sakuko

Sakura (Japanese) Resembling a cherry blossom
Sakurah, Sakurako, Sakurra

Sala (Hindi) From the sacred sala tree
Salah, Salla, Sallah

Salal (English) An evergreen shrub with flowers and berries
Sallal, Salall, Sallall, Salalle, Salale, Sallale

Salamasina (Samoan) A princess; born to royalty
Salamaseena, Salamasyna, Salamaseana, Salamaseina, Salamasiena

Salina (French) One of a solemn, dignified character
Salin, Salinah, Salinda, Salinee, Sallin, Sallina, Sallinah, Salline

Saloma (Hebrew) One who offers peace and tranquility
Salomah, Salome, Salomia, Salomiah, Schlomit, Shulamit, Salomeaexl, Salomma

Salus (Latin) In mythology, goddess of health and prosperity; salvation
Saluus, Salusse, Saluss

Salwa (Arabic) One who provides comfort; solace
Salwah

Samah (Arabic) A generous, forgiving woman
Sama, Samma, Sammah

Samantha (Aramaic) One who listens well
Samanthah, Samanthia, Samanthea, Samantheya, Samanath, Samanatha, Samana, Samanitha

Sameh (Arabic) One who forgives
Sammeh, Samaya, Samaiya

Samina (Arabic) A healthy woman
Saminah, Samine, Sameena, Samyna, Sameana, Sameina, Samynah

Samone (Hebrew) Form of Simone, meaning "one who listens well"
Samoan, Samoane, Samon, Samona, Samonia

Samuela (Hebrew) Feminine form of Samuel; asked of God
Samuelah, Samuella, Samuell, Samuelle, Sammila, Sammile, Samella, Samielle

Sana (Persian / Arabic) One who emanates light / brilliance; splendor
Sanah, Sanna, Sanako, Sanaah, Sane, Saneh

Sandeep (Punjabi) One who is enlightened
Sandeepe, Sandip, Sandipp, Sandippe, Sandeyp, Sandeype

Sandhya (Hindi) Born at twilight; name of the daughter of the god Brahma
Sandhiya, Sandhyah, Sandya, Sandyah

Sandra (Greek) Form of Alexandra, meaning "a helper and defender of mankind"
Sandrah, Sandrine, Sandy, Sandi, Sandie, Sandey, Sandee, Sanda, Sandrica

Sandrica (Greek) Form of Alexandra, meaning "a helper and defender of mankind"
Sandricca, Sandricah, Sandricka, Sandrickah, Sandrika, Sandrikah, Sandryca, Sandrycah

Sandrine (Greek) Form of Alexandra, meaning "a helper and defender of mankind"
Sandrin, Sandreana, Sandreanah, Sandreane, Sandreen, Sandreena, Sandreenah, Sandreene

Sangita (Indian) One who is musical
Sangitah, Sangeeta, Sangeita, Sangyta, Sangieta, Sangeata

Saniya (Indian) A moment in time preserved
Saniyah, Sanya, Sanea, Sania

Sanjna (Indian) A conscientious woman

Santana (Spanish) A saintly woman
Santa, Santah, Santania, Santaniah, Santaniata, Santena, Santenah, Santenna

Saoirse (Gaelic) An independent woman; having freedom
Saoyrse

Sapna (Hindi) A dream come true
Sapnah, Sapnia, Sapniah, Sapnea, Sapneah, Sapniya, Sapniyah

Sarah (Hebrew) A princess; lady; in the Bible, wife of Abraham
Sara, Sari, Sariah, Sarika, Saaraa, Sarita, Sarina, Sarra, Kala, Sadie

Saraid (Irish) One who is excellent; superior
Saraide, Saraed, Saraede, Sarayd, Sarayde

Sarama (African / Hindi) A kind woman / in Hinduism, Indra's dog
Saramah, Saramma, Sarrama, Sarramma

Saran (African) One who brings joy to others
Sarane, Sarran, Saranne, Saranna, Sarana, Sarann

Sarasvati (Hindi) In Hinduism, goddess of learning and the arts
Sarasvatti, Sarasvatie, Sarasvaty, Sarasvatey, Sarasvatee, Sarasvatea

Saraswati (Hindi) Owning water; in Hinduism, a river goddess
Saraswatti, Saraswatie, Saraswaty, Saraswatey, Saraswatee, Saraswatea

Sardinia (Italian) Woman from a mountainous island
Sardiniah, Sardinea, Sardineah, Sardynia, Sardyniah, Sardynea, Sardyneah

Sasa (Japanese) One who is helpful; gives aid
Sasah

Sasha (Russian) Form of Alexandra, meaning "a helper and defender of mankind"
Sascha, Sashenka, Saskia

Sauda (Swahili) A dark beauty
Saudaa, Sawda, Saudda

Savannah (English) From the open grassy plain
Savanna, Savana, Savanne, Savann, Savane, Savanneh

Savarna (Hindi) Daughter of the ocean
Savarnia, Savarnea, Savarniya, Savarneia

Savitri (Hindi) In Hinduism, the daughter of the god of the sun
Savitari, Savitrie, Savitry, Savitarri, Savitarie, Savitree, Savitrea, Savitrey

Savvy (American) Smart and perceptive woman
Savy, Savvi, Savvie, Savvey, Savee, Savvee, Savvea, Savea

Sayyida (Arabic) A mistress
Sayyidah, Sayida, Sayyda, Seyyada, Seyyida, Seyada, Seyida

Scarlett (English) Vibrant red color; a vivacious woman
Scarlet, Scarlette, Skarlet

Scota (Irish) Woman of Scotland
Scotta, Scotah, Skota, Skotta, Skotah

Season (Latin) A fertile woman; one who embraces change
Seazon, Seeson, Seezon, Seizon, Seasen, Seasan, Seizen, Seizan

Sebille (English) In Arthurian legend, a fairy
Sebylle, Sebill, Sebile, Sebyle, Sebyl

Secunda (Latin) The second-born child
Secundah, Secuba, Secundus, Segunda, Sekunda

Seda (Armenian) Voices of the forest
Sedda, Sedah, Seddah

Sedona (American) Woman from a city in Arizona
Sedonah, Sedonna, Sedonnah, Sedonia, Sedonea

Seema (Greek) A symbol; a sign
Seyma, Syma, Seama, Seima, Siema

Sefarina (Greek) Of a gentle wind
Sefarinah, Sefareena, Sefareenah, Sefaryna, Sefarynah, Sefareana, Sefareanah

Seiko (Japanese) The force of truth

Selene (Greek) Of the moon
Sela, Selena, Selina, Celina, Zalina

Sema (Arabic) A divine omen; a known symbol
Semah

Senalda (Spanish) A sign; a symbol
Senaldah, Senaldia, Senaldiya, Senaldea, Senaldya

September (American) Born in the month of September
Septimber, Septymber, Septemberia, Septemberea

Sequoia (Native American) Of the giant redwood tree
Sekwoya, Lequoia

Serafina (Latin) A seraph; a heavenly winged angel
Serafinah, Serafine, Seraphina, Serefina, Seraphine, Sera

Serena (Latin) Having a peaceful disposition
Serenah, Serene, Sereena, Seryna, Serenity, Serenitie, Serenitee, Serepta, Cerina, Xerena

Serendipity (American) A fateful meeting; having good fortune
Serendipitey, Serendipitee, Serendipiti, Serendipitie, Serendypyty

Serenity (Latin) Peaceful

Sevati (Indian) Resembling the white rose
Sevatie, Sevatti, Sevate, Sevatee, Sevatea, Sevaty, Sevatey, Sevti

Shabana (Arabic) A maiden belonging to the night
Shabanah, Shabanna, Shabaana, Shabanne, Shabane

Shabnan (Persian) A falling raindrop
Shabnane, Shabnann, Shabnanne

Shadha (Arabic) An aromatic fragrance
Shadhah

Shafiqa (Arabic) A compassionate woman
Shafiqah, Shafiqua, Shafeeqa, Shafeequa

Shai (Gaelic) A gift of God
Shay, Shae, Shayla, Shea, Shaye

Sha'ista (Arabic) One who is polite and well-behaved
Shaistah, Shaista, Shaa'ista, Shayista, Shaysta

Shakila (Arabic) Feminine form of Shakil; beautiful one
Shakilah, Shakela, Shakeela, Shakeyla, Shakyla, Shakeila, Shakiela, Shakina

Shakira (Arabic) Feminine form of Shakir; grateful; thankful
Shakirah, Shakiera, Shaakira, Shakeira, Shakyra, Shakeyra, Shakura, Shakirra

Shakti (Indian) A divine woman; having power
Shaktie, Shakty, Shaktey, Shaktee, Shaktye, Shaktea

Shaliqa (Arabic) One who is sisterly
Shaliqah, Shaliqua, Shaleeqa, Shaleequa, Shalyqa, Shalyqua

Shamima (Arabic) A woman full of flavor
Shamimah, Shameema, Shamiema, Shameima, Shamyma, Shameama

Shandy (English) One who is rambunctious; boisterous
Shandey, Shandee, Shandi, Shandie, Shandye, Shandea

Shani (African) A marvelous woman
Shanie, Shany, Shaney, Shanee, Shanni, Shanea, Shannie, Shanny

Shanley (Gaelic) Small and ancient woman
Shanleigh, Shanlee, Shanly, Shanli, Shanlie, Shanlea

Shannon (Gaelic) Having ancient wisdom; river name
Shanon, Shannen, Shannan, Shannin, Shanna, Shannae, Shannun, Shannyn

Shaquana (American) Truth in life
Shaqana, Shaquanah, Shaquanna, Shaqanna, Shaqania

Sharifah (Arabic) Feminine form of Sharif; noble; respected; virtuous
Sharifa, Shareefa, Sharufa, Sharufah, Sharyfa, Sharefa, Shareafa, Shariefa

Sharik (African) One who is a child of God
Shareek, Shareake, Sharicke, Sharick, Sharike, Shareak, Sharique, Sharyk

Sharikah (Arabic) One who is a good companion
Sharika, Shareeka, Sharyka, Shareka, Shariqua, Shareaka

Sharlene (French) Feminine form of Charles; petite and womanly
Sharleene, Sharleen, Sharla, Sharlyne, Sharline, Sharlyn, Sharlean, Sharleane

Sharon (Hebrew) From the plains; a flowering shrub
Sharron, Sharone, Sharona, Shari, Sharis, Sharne, Sherine, Sharun

Shasta (Native American) From the triple-peaked mountain
Shastah, Shastia, Shastiya, Shastea, Shasteya

Shawnee (Native American) A tribal name
Shawni, Shawnie, Shawnea, Shawny, Shawney, Shawnea

Shayla (Irish) Of the fairy palace; form of Shai, meaning "a gift of God"
Shaylah, Shaylagh, Shaylain, Shaylan, Shaylea, Shayleah, Shaylla, Sheyla

Shaylee (Gaelic) From the fairy palace; a fairy princess
Shalee, Shayleigh, Shailee, Shaileigh, Shaelee, Shaeleigh, Shayli, Shaylie

Sheehan (Celtic) Little peaceful one; peacemaker
Shehan, Sheyhan, Shihan, Shiehan, Shyhan, Sheahan

Sheela (Indian) One of cool conduct and character
Sheelah, Sheetal

Sheena (Gaelic) God's gracious gift
Sheenah, Shena, Shiena, Sheyna, Shyna, Sheana, Sheina

Sheila (Irish) Form of Cecilia, meaning "one who is blind"
Sheilah, Sheelagh, Shelagh, Shiela, Shyla, Selia, Sighle, Sheiletta

Shelby (English) From the willow farm
Shelbi, Shelbey, Shelbie, Shelbee, Shelbye, Shelbea

Sheridan (Gaelic) One who is wild and untamed; a searcher
Sheridann, Sheridanne, Sherydan, Sherridan, Sheriden, Sheridon, Sherrerd, Sherida

Shifra (Hebrew) A beautiful midwife
Shifrah, Shiphrah, Shiphra, Shifria, Shifriya, Shifrea

Shikha (Indian) Flame burning brightly
Shikhah, Shikkha, Shekha, Shykha

Shima (Native American) Little mother
Shimah, Shimma, Shyma, Shymah

Shina (Japanese) A virtuous woman; having goodness
Shinah, Shinna, Shyna, Shynna

Shobha (Indian) An attractive woman
Shobhah, Shobbha, Shoba, Shobhan, Shobhane

Shoshana (Arabic) Form of Susannah, meaning "white lily"
Shosha, Shoshan, Shoshanah, Shoshane, Shoshanha, Shoshann, Shoshanna, Shoshannah

Shradhdha (Indian) One who is faithful; trusting
Shraddha, Shradha, Shradhan, Shradhane

Shruti (Indian) Having good hearing
Shrutie, Shruty, Shrutey, Shrutee, Shrutye, Shrutea

Shunnareh (Arabic) Pleasing in manner and behavior
Shunnaraya, Shunareh, Shunarreh

Shyann (English) Form of Cheyenne, meaning "unintelligible speaker"
Shyanne, Shyane, Sheyann, Sheyanne, Sheyenne, Sheyene

Shysie (Native American) A quiet child
Shysi, Shysy, Shysey, Shysee, Shycie, Shyci, Shysea, Shycy

Sibyl (English) A prophetess; a seer
Sybil, Sibyla, Sybella, Sibil, Sibella, Sibilla, Sibley, Sibylla

Siddhi (Hindi) Having spiritual power
Sidhi, Syddhi, Sydhi

Sidero (Greek) In mythology, stepmother of Pelias and Neleus
Siderro, Sydero, Sideriyo

Sieglinde (German) Winning a gentle victory

Sienna (Italian) Woman with reddish-brown hair
Siena, Siennya, Sienya, Syenna, Syinna

Sierra (Spanish) From the jagged mountain range
Siera, Syerra, Syera, Seyera, Seeara

Sigfreda (German) A woman who is victorious
Sigfreeda, Sigfrida, Sigfryda, Sigfreyda, Sigfrieda, Sigfriede, Sigfrede

Signia (Latin) A distinguishing sign
Signiya, Signea, Signeia, Signeya, Signa

Sigyn (Norse) In mythology, the wife of Loki

Sihu (Native American) As delicate as a flower

Silka (Latin) Form of Cecelia, meaning "one who is blind"
Silke, Silkia, Silkea, Silkie, Silky, Silkee, Sylka, Sylke

Sima (Arabic) One who is treasured; a prize
Simma, Syma, Simah, Simia, Simiya

Simone (French) One who listens well
Sim, Simonie, Symone, Samone

Sine (Scottish) Form of Jane, meaning "God is gracious"
Sinead, Sineidin, Sioned, Sionet, Sion, Siubhan, Siwan, Sineh

Sinobia (Greek) Form of Zenobia, meaning "child of Zeus"
Sinobiah, Sinobya, Sinobe, Sinobie, Sinovia, Senobia, Senobya, Senobe

Sinopa (Native American) Resembling a fox

Sinope (Greek) In mythology, one of the daughters of Asopus

Siran (Armenian) An alluring and lovely woman

Siren (Greek) In mythology, a sea nymph whose beautiful singing lured sailors to their deaths; refers to a seductive and beautiful woman
Sirene, Sirena, Siryne, Siryn, Syren, Syrena, Sirine, Sirina

Siria (Spanish / Persian) Bright like the sun / a glowing woman
Siriah, Sirea, Sireah, Siriya, Siriyah, Sirya, Siryah

Siroun (Armenian) A lovely woman
Sirune

Sirpuhi (Armenian) One who is holy; pious
Sirpuhie, Sirpuhy, Sirpuhey, Sirpuhea, Sirpuhee

Sissy (English) Form of Cecilia, meaning "one who is blind"
Sissey, Sissie, Sisley, Sisli, Sislee, Sissel, Sissle, Syssy

Sita (Hindi) In Hinduism, goddess of the harvest and wife of Rama

Sive (Irish) A good and sweet girl
Sivney, Sivny, Sivni, Sivnie, Sivnee, Sivnea

Skylar (English) One who is learned, a scholar
Skylare, Skylarr, Skyler, Skylor, Skylir

Sloane (Irish) A strong protector; a woman warrior
Sloan, Slone

Smita (Indian) One who smiles a lot

Snow (American) Frozen rain
Snowy, Snowie, Snowi, Snowey, Snowee, Snowea, Sno

Snowdrop (English) Resembling a small white flower

Solana (Latin / Spanish) Wind from the east / of the sun-shine
Solanah, Solanna, Solann, Solanne

Solange (French) One who is religious and dignified

Solaris (Greek) Of the sun
Solarise, Solariss, Solarisse, Solarys, Solaryss, Solarysse, Sol, Soleil

Solita (Latin) One who is solitary
Solitah, Solida, Soledad, Soledada, Soledade

Somatra (Indian) Of the excellent moon

Sona (Arabic) The golden one
Sonika, Sonna

Sonora (Spanish) A pleasant-sounding woman
Sonorah, Sonoria, Sonorya, Sonoriya

Soo (Korean) Having an excellent long life

Sophia (Greek) Form of Sophie, meaning great wisdom and foresight
Sofia, Sofiya

Sophie (Greek) Wisdom
Sophia, Sofiya, Sofie, Sofia, Sofi, Sofiyko, Sofronia, Sophronia, Zofia

Sorina (Romanian) Feminine form of Sorin; of the sun
Sorinah, Sorinna, Sorinia, Soriniya, Sorinya, Soryna, Sorynia, Sorine

Sorrel (French) From the surele plant
Sorrell, Sorrelle, Sorrele, Sorrela, Sorrella

Sparrow (English) Resembling a small songbird
Sparro, Sparroe, Sparo, Sparow, Sparowe, Sparoe

Sslama (Egyptian) One who is peaceful

Stacey (English) Form of Anastasia, meaning "one who shall rise again"
Stacy, Staci, Stacie, Stacee, Stacia, Stasia, Stasy, Stasey

Stella (English) Star of the sea
Stela, Stelle, Stele, Stellah, Stelah

Stephanie (Greek) Feminine form of Stephen; crowned in victory
Stephani, Stephany, Stephaney, Stephanee, Stephene, Stephana, Stefanie, Stefani

Stevonna (Greek) A crowned lady
Stevonnah, Stevona, Stevonah, Stevonia, Stevonea, Stevoniya

Styx (Greek) In mythology, the river of the underworld
Stixx, Styxx, Stix

Suave (American) A smooth and courteous woman
Swave

Subhadra (Hindi) In Hinduism, the sister of Krishna

Subhaga (Indian) A fortunate person

Subhuja (Hindi) An auspicious celestial damsel

Subira (African) One who is patient
Subirah, Subirra, Subyra, Subyrra, Subeera, Subeara, Subeira, Subiera

Suhaila (Arabic) Feminine form of Suhail; the second brightest star
Suhayla, Suhaela, Suhala, Suhailah, Suhaylah, Suhaelah, Suhalah

Sulwyn (Welsh) One who shines as bright as the sun
Sulwynne, Sulwynn, Sulwinne, Sulwin, Sulwen, Sulwenn, Sulwenne

Sumana (Indian) A good-natured woman
Sumanah, Sumanna, Sumane, Sumanne, Sumann

Sumi (Japanese) One who is elegant and refined
Sumie

Sumitra (Indian) A beloved friend
Sumitrah, Sumita, Sumytra, Sumyta, Sumeetra, Sumeitra, Sumietra, Sumeatra

Summer (American) Refers to the season; born in summer
Sommer, Sumer, Somer, Somers

Suna (Turkish) A swan-like woman

Sunanda (Indian) Having a sweet character
Sunandah, Sunandia, Sunandiya, Sunandea, Sunandya

Sunila (Indian) Feminine form of Sunil; very blue
Sunilah, Sunilla, Sunilya, Suniliya

Sunniva (English) Gift of the sun
Synnove, Synne, Synnove, Sunn

Surabhi (Indian) Having a lovely fragrance
Surbhii, Surabhie, Surabhy, Surabhey, Surabhee, Surabhea

Susannah (Hebrew) White lily
Susanna, Susanne, Susana, Susane, Susan, Suzanna, Suzannah, Suzanne, Shoshana, Huhana

Sushanti (Indian) A peaceful woman; tranquil
Sushantie, Sushanty, Sushantey, Sushantee, Sushantea

Suzu (Japanese) One who is long-lived
Suzue, Suzuko

Swanhilda (Norse) A woman warrior; in mythology, the daughter of Sigurd
Swanhild, Swanhilde, Svanhilde, Svanhild, Svenhilde, Svenhilda

Swarupa (Indian) One who is devoted to the truth

Sydney (English) Of the wide meadow
Sydny, Sydni, Sydnie, Sydnea, Sydnee, Sidney, Sidne, Sidnee

T

Taariq (Swahili) Resembling the morning star
Tariq, Taarique, Tarique

Tabia (African / Egyptian) One who makes incantations / a talented woman
Tabiah, Tabya, Tabea, Tabeah, Tabiya

Tabita (African) A graceful woman
Tabitah, Tabyta, Tabytah, Tabeeta, Tabeata, Tabieta, Tabeita

Tabitha (Greek) Resembling a gazelle; known for beauty and grace
Tabithah, Tabbitha, Tabetha, Tabbetha, Tabatha, Tabbatha, Tabotha, Tabbotha

Tabora (Spanish) One who plays a small drum
Taborah, Taborra, Taboria, Taborya

Tacincala (Native American) Resembling a deer
Tacincalah, Tacyncala, Tacyncalah, Tacincalla, Tacyncalla

Tahsin (Arabic) Beautification; one who is praised
Tahseen, Tahsene, Tahsyne, Tasine, Tahseene, Tahsean, Tahseane

Tahzib (Arabic) One who is educated and cultured
Tahzeeb, Tahzebe, Tahzybe, Tazib, Tazyb, Tazeeb, Tahzeab, Tazeab

Taithleach (Gaelic) A quiet and calm young lady

Takako (Japanese) A lofty child

Takoda (Native American) Friend to everyone
Takodah, Takodia, Takodya, Takota

Tala (Native American) A stalking wolf
Talah, Talla

Talia (Hebrew / Greek) Morning dew from heaven / blooming
Taliah, Talea, Taleah, Taleya, Tallia, Talieya, Taleea, Taleia

Talihah (Arabic) One who seeks knowledge
Taliha, Talibah, Taliba, Talyha, Taleehah, Taleahah

Taline (Armenian) Of the monestary
Talene, Taleen, Taleene, Talyne, Talinia, Talinya, Taliniya

Talisa (American) Consecrated to God
Talisah, Talysa, Taleesa, Talissa, Talise, Taleese, Talisia, Talisya

Talisha (American) A damsel; an innocent
Talesha, Taleisha, Talysha, Taleesha, Tylesha, Taleysha, Taleshia, Talishia

Talitha (Arabic) A maiden; young girl
Talithah, Taletha, Taleetha, Talytha, Talithia, Talethia, Tiletha, Talith

Tamanna (Indian) One who is desired
Tamannah, Tamana, Tamanah, Tammana, Tammanna

Tamasha (African) Pageant winner
Tamasha, Tomosha, Tomasha, Tamashia, Tamashya

Tamesis (Celtic) In mythology, the goddess of water; source of the name for the river Thames
Tamesiss, Tamesys, Tamesyss

Tangia (American) The angel
Tangiah, Tangya, Tangiya, Tangeah

Tani (Japanese / Melanesian / Tonkinese) From the valley / a sweetheart / a young woman
Tanie, Tany, Taney, Tanee, Tanni, Tanye, Tannie, Tanny

Tania (Russian) Queen of the fairies
Tanya, Tannie, Tanny, Tanika

Tanner (English) One who tans hides
Taner, Tannar, Tannor, Tannis

Tansy (English / Greek) An aromatic yellow flower / having immortality
Tansey, Tansi, Tansie, Tansee, Tansye, Tansea, Tancy, Tanzy

Tanushri (Indian) One who is beautiful; attractive
Tanushrie, Tanushry, Tanushrey, Tanushree, Tanushrea

Tanvi (Indian) Slender and beautiful woman
Tanvie, Tanvy, Tanvey, Tanvee, Tanvye, Tannvi, Tanvea

Tapati (Indian) In mythology, the daughter of the sun god
Tapatie, Tapaty, Tapatey, Tapatee, Tapatye, Tapatea

Taphath (Hebrew) In the Bible, Solomon's daughter
Tafath, Taphathe, Tafathe

Tara (Gaelic / Indian) Of the tower; rocky hill / star; in mythology, an astral goddess
Tarah, Tarra, Tayra, Taraea, Tarai, Taralee, Tarali, Taraya

Tarachand (Indian) Silver star
Tarachande, Tarachanda,
Tarachandia, Tarachandea,
Tarachandiya, Tarachandya

Taree (Japanese) A bending
branch
Tarea, Tareya

Taregan (Native American)
Resembling a crane
Tareganne, Taregann

Tariana (American) From the
holy hillside
Tarianna, Taryana, Taryanna

Tarika (Indian) A starlet
Tarikah, Taryka, Tarykah,
Taricka, Tarickah

Tarisai (African) One to
behold; to look at
Tarysai

Tasanee (Thai) A beautiful
view
Tasane, Tasani, Tasanie,
Tasany, Tasaney, Tasanye,
Tasanea

Taskin (Arabic) One who
provides peace; satisfaction
Taskine, Taskeen, Taskeene,
Taskyne, Takseen, Taksin,
Taksyn

Tasnim (Arabic) From the
fountain of paradise
Tasnime, Tasneem, Tasneeme,
Tasnyme, Tasnym, Tasneam,
Tasneame

Tatum (English) Bringer of
joy; spirited
Tatom, Tatim, Tatem, Tatam,
Tatym

Tavi (Aramaic) One who is
well-behaved
Tavie, Tavee, Tavy, Tavey,
Tavea

Taylor (English) Cutter
of cloth; one who alters
garments
Tailor, Taylore, Taylar, Tayler,
Talour, Taylre, Tailore, Tailar

Teagan (Gaelic) One who is
attractive
Teegan

Tehya (Native American) One
who is precious
Tehyah, Tehiya, Tehiyah

Teigra (Greek) Resembling a
tiger
Teigre

Temperance (English) Having
self-restraint
Temperence, Temperince,
Temperancia, Temperanse,
Temperense, Temperinse

Tendai (African) Thankful to God
Tenday, Tendae, Tendaa, Tendaye

Tender (American) One who is sensitive; young and vulnerable
Tendere, Tendera, Tenderia, Tenderre, Tenderiya

Teranika (Gaelic) Victory of the earth
Teranikah, Teranieka, Teraneika, Teraneeka, Teranica, Teranicka, Teranicca, Teraneaka

Teresa (Greek) A harvester
Theresa, Theresah, Theresia, Therese, Thera, Tresa, Tressa, Tressam, Reese, Reza

Terra (Latin) From the earth; in mythology, an earth goddess
Terrah, Terah, Teralyn, Terran, Terena, Terenah, Terenna, Terrena

Terrian (Greek) One who is innocent
Terriane, Terrianne, Terriana, Terianna, Terian, Terianne

Tessa (Greek) Form of Teresa, meaning "a harvester"

Tetsu (Japanese) A strong woman
Tetsue

Tetty (English) Form of Elizabeth, meaning "my God is bountiful; God's promise"
Tettey, Tetti, Tettie, Tettee, Tettea

Thandiwe (African) The loving one
Thandywe, Thandiewe, Thandeewe, Thandie, Thandi, Thandee, Thandy, Thandey

Thara (Arabic) One who is wealthy; prosperous
Tharah, Tharra, Tharrah, Tharwat

Thea (Greek) A goddess; in mythology, the mother of the sun, moon, and dawn
Thia, Thya, Theia

Thelma (Greek) One who is ambitious and willful
Thelmah, Telma, Thelmai, Thelmia, Thelmalina

Thelred (English) One who is well-advised
Thelrede, Thelread, Thelredia, Thelredina, Thelreid, Thelreed, Thelryd

Thema (African) A queen
Themah, Theema, Thyma, Theyma, Theama

Theora (Greek) A watcher
Theorra, Theoria, Theoriya, Theorya

Theta (Greek) Eighth letter of the Greek alphabet
Thetta

Thistle (English) Resembling the prickly, flowered plant
Thistel, Thissle, Thissel

Thomasina (Hebrew) Feminine form of Thomas; a twin
Thomasine, Thomsina, Thomasin, Tomasina, Tomasine, Thomasa, Thomaseena, Thomaseana

Thorberta (Norse) Brilliance of Thor
Thorbiartr, Thorbertha

Thordia (Norse) Spirit of Thor
Thordiah, Thordis, Tordis, Thordissa, Tordissa, Thoridyss

Thuy (Vietnamese) One who is gentle and pure
Thuye, Thuyy, Thuyye

Thy (Vietnamese / Greek) A poet / one who is untamed
Thye

Tia (Spanish / Greek) An aunt / daughter born to royalty
Tiah, Tea, Teah, Tiana, Teea, Tya, Teeya, Tiia

Tiberia (Italian) Of the Tiber river
Tiberiah, Tiberiya, Tiberya, Tibeeria, Tibearia, Tibieria, Tibeiria

Tiegan (Aztec) A little princess in a big valley
Tiegann, Tieganne

Tierney (Gaelic) One who is regal; lordly
Tiernie, Tierni, Tiernee, Tierny, Tiernea

Tiffany (Greek) Lasting love
Tiffaney, Tiffani, Tiffanie, Tiffanee, Tifany, Tifaney, Tifanee, Tifani

Timothea (English) Feminine form of Timothy; honoring God
Timotheah, Timothia, Timothya, Timothiya

Tina (English) From the river; also shortened form of names ending in -tina
Tinah, Teena, Tena, Teyna, Tyna, Tinna, Teana

Ting (Chinese) Graceful and slim woman

Tirza (Hebrew) One who is pleasant; a delight
Tirzah

Tisa (African) The ninth-born child
Tisah, Tiza

Tita (Latin) Holding a title of honor
Titah, Teeta, Tyta, Teata

Tivona (Hebrew) Lover of nature
Tivonna, Tivone, Tivonia, Tivoniya

Toan (Vietnamese) Form of An-toan, meaning "safe and secure"
Toane, Toanne

Toinette (French) Form of Antoinette, meaning "praiseworthy"
Toinett, Toinete, Toinet, Toineta, Toinetta, Tola

Toki (Japanese / Korean) One who grasps opportunity; hopeful / resembling a rabbit
Tokie, Toky, Tokey, Tokye, Tokiko, Tokee, Tokea

Tola (Polish / Cambodian) Form of Toinette, meaning "praiseworthy" / born during October
Tolah, Tolla, Tollah

Topanga (Native American) From above or a high place
Topangah

Topaz (Latin) Resembling a yellow gemstone
Topazz, Topaza, Topazia, Topaziya, Topazya, Topazea

Tordis (Norse) A goddess
Tordiss, Tordisse, Tordys, Tordyss, Tordysse

Torny (Norse) New; just discovered
Torney, Tornie, Torni, Torne, Torn, Tornee, Tornea

Torunn (Norse) Thor's love
Torun, Torrun, Torrunn

Tory (American) Form of Victoria, meaning "victorious woman; winner; conqueror"
Torry, Torey, Tori, Torie, Torree, Tauri, Torye, Toya

Tosca (Latin) From the Tuscany region
Toscah, Toscka, Toska, Tosckah, Toskah

Tosha (English) Form of Natasha, meaning "born on Christmas"
Toshah, Toshiana, Tasha, Tashia, Tashi, Tassa

Tourmaline (Singhalese) A stone of mixed colors
Tourmalyne, Tourmalina, Tourmalinia

Tova (Hebrew) One who is well-behaved
Tovah, Tove, Tovi, Toba, Toibe, Tovva

Treasa (Irish) Having great strength
Treasah, Treesa, Treisa, Triesa, Treise, Treese, Toirease

Trinity (Latin) The holy three
Trinitey, Triniti, Trinitie, Trinitee, Trynity, Trynitey, Tryniti, Trynitie

Trisha (Latin) Form of Patricia, meaning "of noble descent"
Trishah, Trishia, Tricia, Trish, Trissa, Trisa

Trishna (Polish) In mythology, the goddess of the deceased, protector of graves
Trishnah, Trishnia, Trishniah, Trishnea, Trishneah, Trishniya, Trishniyah, Trishnya

Trisna (Indian) The one desired
Trisnah, Trisnia, Trisniah, Trisnea, Trisneah, Trisniya, Trisniyah, Trisnya

Trudy (German) Form of Gertrude, meaning "adored warrior"
Trudey, Trudi, Trudie, Trude, Trudye, Trudee, Truda, Trudia

Trupti (Indian) State of being satisfied
Truptie, Trupty, Truptey, Truptee, Trupte, Truptea

Tryamon (English) In Arthurian legend, a fairy princess
Tryamonn, Tryamonne, Tryamona, Tryamonna

Tryna (Greek) The third-born child
Trynah

Tsifira (Hebrew) One who is crowned
Tsifirah, Tsifyra, Tsiphyra, Tsiphira, Tsipheera, Tsifeera

Tuccia (Latin) A vestal virgin

Tula (Hindi) Balance; a sign of the zodiac
Tulah, Tulla, Tullah

Tullia (Irish) One who is peaceful
Tulliah, Tullea, Tulleah, Tullya, Tulia, Tulea, Tuleah, Tulya

Tusti (Hindi) One who brings happiness and peace
Tustie, Tusty, Tustey, Tustee, Tuste, Tustea

Tutilina (Latin) In mythology, the protector goddess of stored grain
Tutilinah, Tutileena, Tutileana, Tutilyna, Tutileina, Tutiliena, Tutilena, Tutylina

Tuuli (Finnish) Of the wind
Tuulie, Tuulee, Tuula, Tuuly, Tuuley, Tuulea

Tuyet (Vietnamese) Snow white woman
Tuyett, Tuyete, Tuyette, Tuyeta, Tuyetta

Tyler (English) Tiler of roofs

Tyme (English) The aromatic herb thyme
Time, Thyme, Thime

Tyne (English) Of the river
Tyna

Tyro (Greek) In mythology, a woman who bore twin sons to Poseidon

Tzidkiya (Hebrew) Righteousness of the Lord
Tzidkiyah, Tzidkiyahu

Tzigane (Hungarian) A gypsy
Tzigan, Tzigain, Tzigaine, Tzigayne

Uadjit (Egyptian) In mythology, a snake goddess
Ujadet, Uajit, Udjit, Ujadit

Ualani (Hawaiian) Of the heavenly rain
Ualanie, Ualany, Ualaney, Ualanee, Ualanea, Ualania, Ualana

Udavine (American) A thriving woman
Udavyne, Udavina, Udavyna, Udevine, Udevyne, Udevina, Udevyna

Udele (English) One who is wealthy; prosperous
Udelle, Udela, Udella, Udelah, Udellah, Uda, Udah

Uela (American) One who is devoted to God
Uelah, Uella, Uellah

Uganda (African) From the country in Africa
Ugandah, Ugaunda, Ugaundah, Ugawnda, Ugawndah, Ugonda, Ugondah

Ulalia (Greek) Form of Eulalia, meaning "well-spoken"
Ulaliah, Ulalya, Ulalyah

Ulan (African) Firstborn of twins
Ulann, Ulanne

Ulima (Arabic) One who is wise and astute
Ulimah, Ullima, Ulimma, Uleema, Uleama, Ulyma, Uleima, Uliema

Ulla (German) A willful woman
Ullah, Ullaa, Ullai, Ullae

Uma (Hindi) Mother; in mythology, the goddess of beauty and sunlight
Umah, Umma

Umberla (French) Feminine form of Umber; providing shade; of an earth color
Umberlah, Umberly, Umberley, Umberlee, Umberleigh, Umberli, Umberlea, Umberlie

Ummi (African) Born of my mother
Ummie, Ummy, Ummey, Ummee, Umi

Unity (American) Woman who upholds oneness; togetherness
Unitey, Unitie, Uniti, Unitee, Unitea, Unyty, Unytey, Unytie

Ura (Indian) Loved from the heart
Urah, Urra

Ural (Slavic) From the mountains
Urall, Urale, Uralle

Urbai (American) One who is gentle
Urbae, Urbay, Urbaye

Urbana (Latin) From the city; city dweller
Urbanah, Urbanna, Urbane, Urbania, Urbanya, Urbanne

Uriela (Hebrew) The angel of light
Uriella, Urielle, Uriel, Uriele, Uriell

Urta (Latin) Resembling the spiny plant
Urtah

Utah (Native American) People of the mountains; from the state of Utah

Uzoma (African) One who takes the right path
Uzomah, Uzomma, Uzommah

Uzzi (Hebrew / Arabic) God is my strength / a strong woman
Uzzie, Uzzy, Uzzey, Uzzee, Uzi, Uzie, Uzy, Uzey

V

Vala (German) The chosen one; singled out
Valah, Valla

Valda (Teutonic / German) Spirited in battle / famous ruler
Valdah, Valida, Velda, Vada, Vaida, Vayda, Vaeda

Valdis (Norse) In mythology, the goddess of the dead
Valdiss, Valdys, Valdyss

Valencia (Spanish) One who is powerful; strong; from the city of Valencia
Valenciah, Valyncia, Valencya, Valenzia, Valancia, Valenica, Valanca, Valecia

Valentina (Latin) One who is vigorous and healthy
Valentinah, Valentine, Valenteena, Valenteana, Valentena, Valentyna, Valantina, Valentyne

Valeria (Latin) Form of Valerie, meaning "strong and valiant"
Valara, Valera, Valaria, Valeriana, Veleria, Valora

Valerie (Latin) Feminine form of Valerius; strong and valiant
Valeri, Valeree, Valerey, Valery, Valarie, Valari, Vallery

Vandani (Hindi) One who is honorable and worthy
Vandany, Vandaney, Vandanie, Vandanee, Vandania, Vandanya

Vanessa (Greek) Resembling a butterfly
Vanessah, Vanesa, Vannesa, Vannessa, Vanassa, Vanasa, Vanessia, Vanysa, Yanessa

Vanity (English) Having excessive pride
Vanitey, Vanitee, Vaniti, Vanitie, Vanitty, Vanyti, Vanyty, Vanytie

Vanmra (Russian) A stranger; from a foreign place
Vanmrah

Varda (Hebrew) Resembling a rose
Vardah, Vardia, Vardina, Vardissa, Vardita, Vardysa, Vardyta, Vardit

Varuna (Hindi) Wife of the sea
*Varunah, Varuna, Varun,
Varunani, Varuni*

Vashti (Persian) A lovely
woman
*Vashtie, Vashty, Vashtey,
Vashtee*

Vasta (Persian) One who is
pretty
Vastah

Vasteen (American) A capable
woman
*Vasteene, Vastiene, Vastien,
Vastein, Vasteine, Vastean,
Vasteane*

Vasuda (Hindi) Of the earth
*Vasudah, Vasudhara,
Vasundhara, Vasudhra,
Vasundhra*

Vayu (Hindi) A vital life force;
the air
Vayyu

Vedette (French) From the
guard tower
*Vedete, Vedett, Vedet, Vedetta,
Vedeta*

Vedi (Sanskrit) Filled with
wisdom
*Vedie, Vedy, Vedey, Vedee,
Vedea, Vedeah*

Vega (Latin) A falling star
Vegah

Vellamo (Finnish) In mythology, the goddess of the sea
Velamo, Vellammo

Ventana (Spanish) As trans-
parent as a window
*Ventanah, Ventanna, Ventane,
Ventanne*

Venus (Greek) In mythology, the goddess of love and
beauty
*Venis, Venys, Vynys, Venusa,
Venusina, Venusia*

Veradis (Latin) One who is
genuine; truthful
*Veradise, Veradys, Veradisa,
Verdissa, Veradysa, Veradyssa,
Veradisia, Veraditia*

Verda (Latin) Springlike; one
who is young and fresh
*Verdah, Verdea, Virida, Verdy,
Verdey, Verde, Verdi, Verdie*

Verenase (Swedish) One who
is flourishing
*Verenese, Verennase, Vyrenase,
Vyrennase, Vyrenese, Verenace,
Vyrenace*

Veronica (Latin) Displaying
her true image
*Veronicah, Veronic, Veronicca,
Veronicka, Veronika, Veronicha,
Veronique, Veranique, Ronni*

Vesna (Slavic) Messenger; in mythology, the goddess of spring
Vesnah, Vezna, Vesnia, Vesnaa

Vespera (Latin) Evening star; born in the evening
Vesperah, Vespira, Vespeera, Vesperia, Vesper

Vevila (Gaelic) Woman with a melodious voice
Vevilah, Veveela, Vevyla, Vevilla, Vevylla, Vevylle, Vevyle, Vevillia

Vibhuti (Hindi) Of the sacred ash; a symbol
Vibuti, Vibhutie, Vibhutee

Victoria (Latin) Victorious woman; winner; conqueror
Victoriah, Victorea, Victoreah, Victorya, Victorria, Victoriya, Vyctoria, Victorine, Tory

Vidya (Indian) Having great wisdom
Vidyah

Viet (Vietnamese) A woman from Vietnam
Vyet, Viett, Vyett, Viette, Vyette

Vigilia (Latin) Wakefulness; watchfulness
Vigiliah, Vygilia, Vygylia, Vijilia, Vyjilia

Vignette (French) From the little vine
Vignete, Vignet, Vignetta, Vignett, Vigneta, Vygnette, Vygnete, Vygnet

Vilina (Hindi) One who is dedicated
Vilinah, Vileena, Vileana, Vylina, Vyleena, Vyleana, Vylyna, Vilinia

Villette (French) From the small village
Vilette, Villete, Vilete, Vilet, Vilett, Villet, Villett, Vylet

Vimala (Indian) Feminine form of Vamal; clean and pure
Vimalah, Vimalia, Vimalla

Vincentia (Latin) Feminine form of Vincent; conquerer; triumphant
Vincentiah, Vincenta, Vincensia, Vincenzia, Vyncentia, Vyncyntia, Vyncenzia, Vycenzya

Violet (French) Resembling the purplish-blue flower
Violett, Violette, Violete, Vyolet, Vyolett, Vyolette, Vyolete, Violeta

Virginia (Latin) One who is chaste; virginal; from the state of Virginia
Virginiah, Virginnia, Virgenya, Virgenia, Virgeenia, Virgeena, Virgena, Ginny

Virtue (Latin) Having moral excellence, chastity, and goodness
Virtu, Vyrtue, Vyrtu, Vertue, Vertu

Viveka (German) Little woman of the strong fortress
Vivekah, Vivecka, Vyveka, Viveca, Vyveca, Vivecca, Vivika, Vivieka

Vivian (Latin) Lively woman
Viv, Vivi, Vivienne, Bibiana

Vixen (American) A flirtatious woman
Vixin, Vixi, Vixie, Vixee, Vixea, Vixeah, Vixy, Vixey

Vlasta (Slavic) A friendly and likable woman
Vlastah, Vlastia, Vlastea, Vlastiah, Vlasteah

Voleta (Greek) The veiled one
Voletah, Voletta, Volita, Volitta, Volyta, Volytta, Volet, Volett

Volva (Scandinavian) In mythology, a female shaman
Volvah, Volvya, Volvaa, Volvae, Volvai, Volvay, Volvia

Vondila (African) Woman who lost a child
Vondilah, Vondilla, Vondilya, Vondilia, Vondyla, Vondylya

Vonna (French) Form of Yvonne, meaning "young archer"
Vonnah, Vona, Vonah, Vonnia, Vonnya, Vonia, Vonya, Vonny

Vonshae (American) One who is confident
Vonshay, Vonshaye, Vonshai

Vor (Norse) In mythology, an omniscient goddess
Vore, Vorr, Vorre

Vulpine (English) A cunning woman; like a fox
Vulpyne, Vulpina, Vulpyna

Vyomini (Indian) A gift of the divine
Vyominie, Vyominy, Vyominey, Vyominee, Vyomyni, Vyomyny, Viomini, Viomyni

W

Wafa (Arabic) One who is faithful; devoted
Wafah, Wafaa, Waffa, Wapha, Waffah, Waphah

Wainani (Hawaiian) Of the
beautiful waters
*Wainanie, Wainany, Wainaney,
Wainanee, Wainanea,
Wainaneah*

Wajihah (Arabic) One who is
distinguished; eminent
*Wajiha, Wajeeha, Wajyha,
Wajeehah, Wajyhah, Wajieha,
Wajiehah, Wajeiha*

Wakanda (Native American)
One who possesses magical
powers
*Wakandah, Wakenda,
Wakinda, Wakynda*

Walda (German) One who has
fame and power
*Waldah, Wallda, Walida,
Waldine, Waldina, Waldyne,
Waldyna, Welda*

Walker (English) Walker of the
forests
Wallker, Walkher

Walta (African) One who acts
as a shield
Waltah

Wanetta (English) A pale-
skinned woman
*Wanettah, Wanette, Wannette,
Wannetta, Wonetta, Wonette,
Wonitta, Wonitte*

Wangari (African) Resembling
the leopard
*Wangarie, Wangarri, Wangary,
Wangarey, Wangaria,
Wangaree*

Wanyika (African) Of the bush
*Wanyikka, Wanyicka,
Wanyicca, Wanyica*

Waqi (Arabic) Falling;
swooping
Waqqi

Warma (American) A caring
woman
*Warm, Warme, Warmia,
Warmiah, Warmea, Warmeah*

Warna (German) One who
defends her loved ones
Warnah

Washi (Japanese) Resembling
an eagle
*Washie, Washy, Washey,
Washee, Washea, Washeah*

Waynette (English) One who
makes wagons
*Waynett, Waynet, Waynete,
Wayneta, Waynetta*

Wednesday (American) Born
on a Wednesday
*Wensday, Winsday,
Windnesday, Wednesdae,
Wensdae, Winsdae,
Windnesdae, Wednesdai*

Welcome (English) A welcome guest
Welcom, Welcomme

Wendy (Welsh) Form of Gwendolyn, meaning "one who is fair; of the white ring"
Wendi, Wendie, Wendee, Wendey, Wenda, Wendia, Wendea, Wendya

Wesley (English) From the western meadow
Wesly, Weslie, Wesli, Weslee, Weslia, Wesleigh, Weslea, Weslei

Whitley (English) From the white meadow
Whitly, Whitlie, Whitli, Whitlee, Whitleigh, Whitlea, Whitlia, Whitlya

Whitney (English) From the white island
Whitny, Whitnie, Whitni, Whitnee, Whittney, Whitneigh, Whytny, Whytney

Wicapi (Native American) A holy star

Wijida (Arabic) An excited seeker
Wijidah, Weejida, Weejidah, Wijeeda, Wijeedah, Wijyda, Wijydah, Wijieda

Wileen (Teutonic) A firm defender
Wiline, Wilean, Wileane, Wilyn, Wileene, Wilene, Wyleen, Wyline

Wilhelmina (German) Feminine form of Wilhelm; determined protector
Wilhelminah, Wylhelmina, Wylhelmyna, Willemina, Wilhelmine, Wilhemina, Wilhemine, Helma, Ilma

Willa (English) Feminine version of William, meaning "protector"
Willah, Wylla

Willow (English) One who is hoped for; desired
Willo, Willough

Winetta (American) One who is peaceful
Wineta, Wynetta, Wyneta, Winet, Winett, Winette, Wynet, Wynett

Winnielle (African) A victorious woman
Winniell, Winniele, Winniel, Winniella

Winola (German) Gracious and charming friend
Winolah, Wynola, Winolla, Wynolla, Wynolah, Winollah, Wynollah

Winta (African) One who is desired
Wintah, Whinta, Wynta, Whynta, Whintah, Wyntah, Whyntah

Woody (American) A woman of the forest
Woodey, Woodi, Woodie, Woodee, Woodea, Woodeah, Woods

Wren (English) Resembling a small songbird
Wrenn, Wrene, Wrena, Wrenie, Wrenee, Wreney, Wrenny, Wrenna

Wynda (Scottish) From the narrow passage
Wyndah, Winda, Windah

Xalvadora (Spanish) A savior
Xalvadorah, Xalbadora, Xalbadorah, Xalvadoria, Xalbadoria

Xanadu (African) From the exotic paradise

Xantara (American) Protector of the Earth
Xantarah, Xanterra, Xantera, Xantarra, Xantarrah, Xanterah, Xanterrah

Xaquelina (Galician) Form of Jacqueline, meaning "the supplanter"
Xaqueline, Xaqueleena, Xaquelyna, Xaquelayna, Xaqueleana

Xerena (Latin) Form of Serena, meaning "having a peaceful disposition"
Xerenah, Xerene, Xeren, Xereena, Xeryna, Xereene, Xerenna

Xhosa (African) Leader of a nation
Xosa, Xhose, Xhosia, Xhosah, Xosah

Xiang (Chinese) Having a nice fragrance
Xyang, Xeang, Xhiang, Xhyang, Xheang

Xiao Hong (Chinese) Of the morning rainbow

Xin Qian (Chinese) Happy and beautiful woman

Xinavane (African) A mother; to propagate
Xinavana, Xinavania, Xinavain, Xinavaine, Xinavaen, Xinavaene

Xirena (Greek) Form of Sirena, meaning "enchantress"
Xirenah, Xireena, Xirina, Xirene, Xyrena, Xyreena, Xyrina, Xyryna

Xi-Wang (Chinese) One with hope

Xochiquetzal (Aztec) Resembling a flowery feather; in mythology, the goddess of love, flowers, and the earth

Xola (African) Stay in peace
Xolah, Xolia, Xolla, Xollah

Xue (Chinese) Woman of snow

Yachne (Hebrew) One who is gracious and hospitable
Yachnee, Yachney, Yachnie, Yachni, Yachnea, Yachneah

Yadra (Spanish) Form of Madre, meaning "mother"
Yadre, Yadrah

Yaffa (Hebrew) A beautiful woman
Yaffah, Yaffit, Yafit, Yafeal

Yakini (African) An honest woman
Yakinie, Yakiney, Yakiny, Yackini, Yackinie, Yackiney, Yackiny, Yakinee

Yalena (Greek) Form of Helen, meaning "the shining light"
Yalenah, Yalina, Yaleena, Yalyna, Yalana, Yaleana, Yalane, Yaleene

Yama (Japanese) From the mountain
Yamma, Yamah, Yammah

Yamin (Hebrew) Right hand
Yamine, Yamyn, Yamyne, Yameen, Yameene, Yamein, Yameine, Yamien

Yana (Hebrew) He answers
Yanna, Yaan, Yanah, Yannah

Yanessa (American) Form of Vanessa, meaning "resembling a butterfly"
Yanessah, Yanesa, Yannesa, Yannessa, Yanassa, Yanasa, Yanessia, Yanysa

Yanka (Slavic) God is good
Yancka, Yancca, Yankka

Yara (Brazilian) In mythology, the goddess of the river; a mermaid
Yarah, Yarrah, Yarra

Yareli (American) The Lord is my light
Yarelie, Yareley, Yarelee, Yarely, Yaresly, Yarelea, Yareleah

Yaretzi (Spanish) Always beloved
Yaretzie, Yaretza, Yarezita

Yashira (Japanese) Blessed with God's grace
Yashirah, Yasheera, Yashyra, Yashara, Yashiera, Yashierah, Yasheira, Yasheirah

Yashona (Hindi) A wealthy woman
Yashonah, Yashawna, Yashauna, Yaseana, Yashawnah, Yashaunah, Yaseanah

Yasmine (Persian) Resembling the jasmine flower
Yasmin, Yasmene, Yasmeen, Yasmeene, Yasmen, Yasemin, Yasemeen, Yasmyn

Yatima (African) An orphan
Yatimah, Yateema, Yatyma, Yateemah, Yatymah, Yatiema, Yatiemah, Yateima

Yedidah (Hebrew) A beloved friend
Yedida, Yedyda, Yedydah, Yedeeda, Yedeedah

Yeira (Hebrew) One who is illuminated
Yeirah, Yaira, Yeyra, Yairah, Yeyrah

Yenge (African) A hardworking woman
Yenga, Yengeh, Yengah

Yeshi (African) For a thousand
Yeshie, Yeshey, Yeshy, Yeshee, Yeshea, Yesheah

Yessica (Hebrew) Form of Jessica, meaning "the Lord sees all"
Yesica, Yessika, Yesika, Yesicka, Yessicka, Yesyka, Yesiko

Yetta (English) Form of Henrietta, meaning "ruler of the house"
Yettah, Yeta, Yette, Yitta, Yettie, Yetty

Yi Min (Chinese) An intelligent woman

Yi Ze (Chinese) Happy and shiny as a pearl

Yihana (African) One deserving congratulations
Yihanah, Yhana, Yihanna, Yihannah, Yhanah, Yhanna, Yhannah

Yinah (Spanish) A victorious woman
Yina, Yinna, Yinnah

Yitta (Hebrew) One who emanates light
Yittah, Yita, Yitah

Ynes (French) Form of Agnes, meaning "pure; chaste"
Ynez, Ynesita

Yogi (Hindi) One who practices yoga
Yogini, Yoginie, Yogie, Yogy, Yogey, Yogee, Yogea, Yogeah

Yohance (African) A gift from God
Yohanse

Yoki (Native American) Of the rain
Yokie, Yokee, Yoky, Yokey, Yokea, Yokeah

Yolanda (Greek) Resembling the violet flower
Yola, Yolana, Yolandah, Colanda

Yomaris (Spanish) I am the sun
Yomariss, Yomarise, Yomarris

Yon (Korean) Resembling a lotus blossom

Yoruba (African) Woman from Nigeria
Yorubah, Yorubba, Yorubbah

Yoshi (Japanese) One who is respectful and good
Yoshie, Yoshy, Yoshey, Yoshee, Yoshiyo, Yoshiko, Yoshino, Yoshea

Ysabel (Spanish) Form of Isabel, meaning "my God is bountiful; God's promise"
Ysabelle, Ysabela, Ysabele, Ysabell, Ysabella, Ysbel, Ysibel, Ysibela

Ysbail (Welsh) A spoiled girl
Ysbale, Ysbayle, Ysbaile, Ysbayl, Ysbael, Ysbaele

Yue (Chinese) Of the moonlight

Yuette (American) A capable woman
Yuett, Yuete, Yuet, Yueta, Yuetta

Yulan (Spanish) A splendid woman
Yulann

Yuna (African) A gorgeous woman
Yunah, Yunna, Yunnah

Yuta (Hebrew / Japanese) One who is awarded praise / one who is superior
Yutah, Yoota, Yootah

Yvonne (French) Young archer
Yvone, Vonne, Vonna

Zabrina (American) Form of Sabrina, meaning "a legendary princess"
Zabreena, Zabrinah, Zabrinna, Zabryna, Zabryne, Zabrynya, Zabreana, Zabreane

Zachah (Hebrew) Feminine form of Zachary; God is remembered
Zacha, Zachie, Zachi, Zachee, Zachea, Zacheah

Zafara (Hebrew) One who sings
Zaphara, Zafarra, Zapharra, Zafarah, Zafarrah, Zapharah, Zapharrah

Zagir (Armenian) Resembling a flower
Zagiri, Zagirie, Zagiree, Zagirea, Zagireah, Zagiry, Zagirey, Zagira

Zahiya (Arabic) A brilliant woman; radiant
Zahiyah, Zehiya, Zehiyah, Zeheeya, Zaheeya, Zeheeyah, Zaheeyah, Zaheiya

Zahra (Arabic / Swahili) White-skinned / flowerlike
Zahrah, Zahraa, Zahre, Zahreh, Zahara, Zaharra, Zahera, Zahira

Zainab (Arabic) A fragrant flowering plant
Zaynab, Zaenab

Zainabu (Swahili) One who is known for her beauty
Zaynabu, Zaenabu

Zalina (French) Form of Selene, meaning "of the moon"; in mythology Selene was the Greek goddess of the moon
Zalinah, Zaleana, Zaleena, Zalena, Zalyna, Zaleen, Zaleene, Zalene

Zama (Latin) One from the town of Zama
Zamah, Zamma, Zammah

Zambda (Hebrew) One who meditates
Zambdah

Zamella (Zulu) One who strives to succeed
Zamellah, Zamy, Zamie, Zami, Zamey, Zamee, Zamea, Zameah

Zamilla (Greek) Having the strength of the sea
Zamillah, Zamila, Zamilah, Zamylla, Zamyllah, Zamyla, Zamylah

Zamora (Spanish) From the city of Zamora
Zamorah, Zamorrah, Zamorra

Zana (Romanian / Hebrew) In mythology, the three graces / shortened form of Susanna, meaning "lily"
Zanna, Zanah, Zannah

Zane (Scandinavian) One who is bold
Zain, Zaine, Zayn, Zayne, Zaen, Zaene

Zanta (Swahili) A beautiful young woman
Zantah

Zarahlinda (Hebrew) Of the beautiful dawn
Zaralinda, Zaralynda, Zarahlindah, Zaralyndah, Zarahlynda, Zarahlyndah, Zaralenda, Zarahlenda

Zariah (Russian / Slavic) Born at sunrise
Zarya, Zariah, Zaryah

Zarifa (Arabic) One who is successful; moves with grace
Zarifah, Zaryfa, Zaryfah, Zareefa, Zareefah, Zariefa, Zariefah, Zareifa

Zarna (Hindi) Resembling a spring of water
Zarnah, Zarnia, Zarniah

Zarqa (Arabic) Having bluish-green eyes; from the city of Zarqa
Zarqaa

Zaylee (English) A heavenly woman
Zayleigh, Zayli, Zaylie, Zaylea, Zayleah, Zayley, Zayly, Zalee

Zaypana (Tibetan) A beautiful woman
Zaypanah, Zaypo, Zaypanna, Zaypannah

Zaza (Hebrew / Arabic) Belonging to all / one who is flowery
Zazah, Zazu, Zazza, Zazzah, Zazzu

Zdenka (Slovene) Feminine form of Zdenek, meaning "from Sidon"
Zdena, Zdenuska, Zdenicka, Zdenika, Zdenyka, Zdeninka, Zdenynka

Zebba (Persian) A known beauty
Zebbah, Zebara, Zebarah, Zebarra, Zebarrah

Zelia (Greek / Spanish) Having great zeal / of the sunshine
Zeliah, Zelya, Zelie, Zele, Zelina, Zelinia

Zenaida (Greek) White-winged dove; in mythology, a daughter of Zeus
Zenaidah, Zenayda, Zenaide, Zenayde, Zinaida, Zenina, Zenna, Zenaydah

Zenechka (Russian) Form of Eugenia, meaning "a well-born woman"

Zenobia (Greek) Child of Zeus
Sinobia

Zephyr (Greek) Of the west wind
Zephyra, Zephira, Zephria, Zephra, Zephyer, Zefiryn, Zefiryna, Zefyrin

Zera (Hebrew) A sower of seeds
Zerah, Zeria, Zeriah, Zera'im, Zerra, Zerrah

Zeraldina (Polish) One who rules with the spear
Zeraldinah, Zeraldeena, Zeraldeenah, Zeraldiena, Zeraldienah, Zeraldeina, Zeraldeinah, Zeraldyna

Zerdali (Turkish) Resembling the wild apricot
Zerdalie, Zerdaly, Zerdaley, Zerdalya, Zerdalia, Zerdalee, Zerdalea

Zesta (American) One with energy and gusto
Zestah, Zestie, Zestee, Zesti, Zesty, Zestey, Zestea, Zesteah

Zetta (Portuguese) Resembling the rose
Zettah

Zhen (Chinese) One who is precious and chaste
Zen, Zhena, Zenn, Zhenni

Zhi (Chinese) A woman of high moral character

Zhong (Chinese) An honorable woman

Zi (Chinese) A flourishing young woman

Zia (Arabic) One who emanates light; splendor
Ziah, Zea, Zeah, Zya, Zyah

Zilias (Hebrew) A shady woman; a shadow
Zilyas, Zylias, Zylyas

Zillah (Hebrew) The shadowed one
Zilla, Zila, Zyla, Zylla, Zilah, Zylah, Zyllah

Zilpah (Hebrew) One who is frail but dignified; in the Bible, a concubine of Jacob
Zilpa, Zylpa, Zilpha, Zylpha, Zylpah, Zilphah, Zylphah

Zimbab (African) Woman from Zimbabwe
Zymbab, Zimbob, Zymbob

Zinat (Arabic) A decoration; graceful beauty
Zeenat, Zynat, Zienat, Zeinat, Zeanat

Zinchita (Incan) One who is dearly loved
Zinchitah, Zinchyta, Zinchytah, Zincheeta, Zincheetah, Zinchieta, Zinchietah, Zincheita

Zintkala Kinyan (Native American) Resembling a flying bird
Zintkalah Kinyan

Ziona (Hebrew) One who symbolizes goodness
Zionah, Zyona, Zyonah

Zipporah (Hebrew) A beauty; little bird; in the Bible, the wife of Moses
Zippora, Ziporah, Zipora, Zypora, Zyppora, Ziproh, Zipporia

Zira (African) The pathway
Zirah, Zirra, Zirrah, Zyra, Zyrah, Zyrra, Zyrrah

Zisel (Hebrew) One who is sweet
Zissel, Zisal, Zysel, Zysal, Zyssel, Zissal, Zyssal

Zita (Latin / Spanish) Patron of housewives and servants / little rose
Zitah, Zeeta, Zyta, Zeetah

Ziwa (Swahili) Woman of the lake
Ziwah, Zywa, Zywah

Zizi (Hungarian) Dedicated to God
Zeezee, Zyzy, Ziezie, Zeazea, Zeyzey

Zoa (Greek) One who is full of life; vibrant

Zoe (Greek) A life-giving woman; alive
Zoee, Zowey, Zowie, Zowe, Zoelie, Zoeline, Zoelle, Zoey

Zofia (Slavic) Form of Sophia, meaning "wisdom"
Zofiah, Zophia, Zophiah, Zophya, Zofie, Zofee, Zofey

Zora (Slavic) Born at dawn; aurora
Zorah, Zorna, Zorra, Zorya, Zorane, Zory, Zorrah, Zorey

Zoria (Basque) One who is lucky
Zoriah

Zoriona (Basque) One who is happy

Zubeda (Swahili) The best one
Zubedah

Zudora (Arabic) A laborer; hardworking woman
Zudorah, Zudorra

Zula (African) One who is brilliant; from the town of Zula
Zul, Zulay, Zulae, Zulai, Zulah, Zulla, Zullah

Zuni (Native American) One who is creative
Zunie, Zuny, Zuney, Zunee, Zunea, Zuneah

Zurafa (Arabic) A lovely woman
Zurafah, Zirafa, Zirafah, Ziraf, Zurufa, Zurufah

Zuri (Swahili / French) A beauty / lovely and white
Zurie, Zurey, Zuria, Zuriaa, Zury, Zuree, Zurya, Zurisha

Zuwena (African) One who is pleasant and good
Zuwenah, Zwena, Zwenah, Zuwenna, Zuwennah, Zuwyna, Zuwynah

Zuyana (Sioux) One who has a brave heart
Zuyanah, Zuyanna

Zuzena (Basque) One who is correct
Zuzenah, Zuzenna

Zwi (Scandinavian) Resembling a gazelle
Zui, Zwie, Zwee, Zwey

Boys

Aabha (Indian) One who shines
Abha, Abbha

Aabharan (Hindu) One who is treasured; jewel
Abharan, Abharen, Aabharen, Aabharon

Aaden (Irish) Form of Aidan, meaning "a fiery young man"
Adan, Aden

Aage (Norse) Representative of ancestors
Age, Ake, Aake

Aarif (Arabic) A learned man
Arif, Aareef, Areef, Aareaf, Areaf, Aareif, Areif, Aarief

Aaron (Hebrew) One who is exalted; from the mountain of strength
Aaran, Aaren, Aarin, Aaro, Aaronas, Aaronn, Aarron, Aaryn, Eron, Aron, Eran

Abdi (Hebrew) My servant
Abdie, Abdy, Abdey, Abdee

Abdul (Arabic) A servant of God
Abdal, Abdall, Abdalla, Abdallah, Abdel, Abdell, Abdella, Abdellah

Abedi (African) One who worships God
Abedie, Abedy, Abedey, Abedee, Abedea

Abednago (Aramaic) Servant of the god of wisdom, Nabu
Abednego

Abejundio (Spanish) Resembling a bee
Abejundo, Abejundeo, Abedjundiyo, Abedjundeyo

Abel (Hebrew) The life force, breath
Abele, Abell, Abelson, Able, Avel, Avele

Abraham (Hebrew) Father of a multitude; father of nations
Abarran, Avraham, Aberham, Abrahamo, Abrahan, Abrahim, Abram, Abrami, Ibrahim

Abram (Hebrew) Form of Abraham, meaning "father of nations"

Absalom (Hebrew) The father of peace
Absalon, Abshalom, Absolem, Absolom, Absolon, Avshalom, Avsholom

Abu (African) A father
Abue, Aboo, Abou

Abundio (Spanish) A man of
plenty
*Abbondio, Abondio, Aboundio,
Abundo, Abundeo, Aboundeo*

Adael (Hebrew) God witnesses
Adaele, Adayel, Adayele

Adam (Hebrew) Of the earth
*Ad, Adamo, Adams, Adan,
Adao, Addam, Addams, Addem*

Addy (Teutonic) One who is
awe-inspiring
*Addey, Addi, Addie, Addee,
Addea, Adi, Ady, Adie*

Adelpho (Greek) A brotherly
man
*Aldelfo, Adelfus, Adelfio,
Adelphe*

Adil (Arabic) A righteous man;
one who is fair and just
*Adyl, Adiel, Adeil, Adeel, Adeal,
Adyeel*

Aditya (Hindi) Of the sun
*Adithya, Adithyan, Adityah,
Aditeya, Aditeyah*

Adonis (Greek) In mythology,
a handsome young man loved
by Aphrodite
Addonia, Adohnes, Adonys

Adrian (Latin) A man from
Hadria
*Adrien, Adrain, Adrean,
Adreean, Adreyan, Adreeyan,
Adriaan*

Adriel (Hebrew) From God's
flock
*Adriell, Adriele, Adryel, Adryell,
Adryele*

Afif (Arabic) One who is
chaste; pure
*Afeef, Afief, Afeif, Affeef, Affif,
Afyf, Afeaf*

Agamemnon (Greek) One who
works slowly; in mythology,
the leader of the Greeks at Troy
Agamemno, Agamenon

Ahmad (Arabic) One who
always thanks God; a name of
Muhammed
Ahmed

Aidan (Irish) A fiery young man
*Aiden, Aedan, Aeden, Aidano,
Aidyn, Ayden, Aydin, Aydan*

Aiken (English) Constructed of
oak; sturdy
*Aikin, Aicken, Aickin, Ayken,
Aykin, Aycken, Ayckin*

Ainsworth (English) From
Ann's estate
*Answorth, Annsworth,
Ainsworthe, Answorthe,
Annsworthe*

Ajax (Greek) In mythology, a hero of the Trojan war
Aias, Aiastes, Ajaxx, Ajaxe

Ajit (Indian) One who is invincible
Ajeet, Ajeat, Ajeit, Ajiet, Ajyt

Akiko (Japanese) Surrounded by bright light
Akyko

Akin (African) A brave man; a hero
Akeen, Akean, Akein, Akien, Akyn

Akiva (Hebrew) One who protects or provides shelter
Akyva, Akeeva, Akeava, Akieva, Akeiva, Akeyva

Akmal (Arabic) A perfect man
Aqmal, Akmall, Aqmall, Acmal, Acmall, Ackmal, Ackmall

Alaire (French) Filled with joy
Alair, Alaer, Alaere, Alare, Alayr, Alayre

Alamar (Arabic) Covered with gold
Alamarr, Alemar, Alemarr, Alomar, Alomarr

Alan (German / Gaelic) One who is precious / resembling a little rock
Alain, Alann, Allan, Alson, Allin, Allen, Allyn

Alard (German) Of noble strength
Aliard, Allard, Alliard

Albert (German) One who is noble and bright
Alberto, Albertus, Alburt, Albirt, Aubert, Albyrt, Albertos, Albertino

Alden (English) An old friend
Aldan, Aldin, Aldyn, Aldon, Aldun

Aldo (German) Old or wise one; elder
Aldous, Aldis, Aldus, Alldo, Aldys

Aldred (English) An old advisor
Alldred, Aldraed, Alldraed, Aldread, Alldread

Alejandro (Spanish) Form of Alexander, meaning "a helper and defender of mankind"
Alejandrino, Alejo

Alex (English) Form of Alexander, meaning "a helper and defender of mankind"
Aleks, Alecks, Alecs, Allex, Alleks, Allecks, Alexis

Alexander (Greek) A helper and defender of mankind
Alex, Alec, Alejandro, Alaxander, Aleksandar, Aleksander, Aleksandr, Alessandro, Alexzander, Zander

Alfonso (Italian) Prepared for battle; eager and ready
Alphonso, Alphonse, Affonso, Alfons, Alfonse, Alfonsin, Alfonsino, Alfonz, Alfonzo

Ali (Arabic) The great one; one who is exalted
Alie, Aly, Aley, Alee

Alijah (American) Form of Elijah, meaning "Jehovah is my god"

Alon (Hebrew) Of the oak tree
Allona, Allon, Alonn

Alonzo (Spanish) Form of Alfonso, meaning "prepared for battle; eager and ready"
Alonso, Alanso, Alanzo, Allonso, Allonzo, Allohnso, Allohnzo, Alohnso

Aloysius (German) A famous warrior
Ahlois, Aloess, Alois, Aloisio, Aloisius, Aloisio, Aloj, Alojzy

Alpha (Greek) The first-born child; the first letter of the Greek alphabet
Alphah, Alfa, Alfah

Alter (Hebrew) One who is old
Allter, Altar, Alltar

Alton (English) From the old town
Aldon, Aldun, Altun, Alten, Allton, Alltun, Allten

Alvin (English) Friend of the elves
Alven, Alvan, Alvyn

Amani (African / Arabic) One who is peaceful / one with wishes and dreams
Amanie, Amany, Amaney, Amanee, Amanye, Amanea, Amaneah

Amari (African) Having great strength; a builder
Amare, Amarie, Amaree, Amarea, Amary, Amarey

Amil (Hindi) One who is invaluable
Ameel, Ameal, Ameil, Amiel, Amyl

Amit (Hindi) Without limit; endless
Ameet, Ameat, Ameit, Amiet, Amyt

Amory (German) Ruler and lover of one's home
Aimory, Amery, Amorey, Amry, Amori, Amorie, Amoree, Amorea

Amos (Hebrew) To carry; hardworking
Amoss, Aymoss, Aymos

Andino (Italian) Form of Andrew, meaning "one who is manly; a warrior"
Andyno, Andeeno, Andeano, Andieno, Andeino

Andre (French) Form of Andrew, meaning "manly, a warrior"
Andreas, Andrei, Andrej, Andres, Andrey

Andrew (Greek) One who is manly; a warrior
Andy, Aindrea, Andreas, Andie, Andonia, Andor, Andresj, Anderson, Anders

Andrik (Slavic) Form of Andrew, meaning "one who is manly; a warrior"
Andric, Andrick, Andryk, Andryck, Andryc

Angel (Greek) A messenger of God
Andjelko, Ange, Angelino, Angell, Angelmo, Angelo, Angie, Angy

Angus (Scottish) One force; one strength; one choice
Aengus, Anngus, Aonghus

Ankur (Indian) One who is blossoming; a sapling

Annan (Celtic) From the brook
Anan

Ansley (English) From the noble's pastureland
Ansly, Anslie, Ansli, Anslee, Ansleigh, Anslea, Ansleah, Anslye

Anthony (Latin) A flourishing man; of an ancient Roman family
Antal, Antony, Anthoney, Anntoin, Antin, Anton, Antone, Antonello, Antonio

Antoine (French) Form of Anthony, meaning "a flourishing man; of an ancient Roman family"
Antione, Antjuan, Antuan, Antuwain, Antuwaine, Antuwayne, Antuwon, Antwahn

Antonio (Italian) Form of Anthony, meaning "a flourishing man, from an ancient Roman family"
Antonin, Antonino, Antonius, Antonyo

Apollo (Greek) In mythology, the god of archery, music, and poetry

Ara (Armenian / Latin) A legendary king / of the altar; the name of a constellation
Araa, Aira, Arah, Arae, Ahraya

Arcadio (Greek) From an ideal country paradise
Alcadio, Alcado, Alcedio, Arcadios, Arcadius, Arkadi, Arkadios, Arkadius

Arcelio (Spanish) From the altar of heaven
Arcelios, Arcelius, Aricelio, Aricelios, Aricelius

Archard (German) A powerful holy man
Archerd, Archird, Archyrd

Archelaus (Greek) The ruler of the people
Archelaios, Arkelaos, Arkelaus, Arkelaios, Archelaos

Archer (Latin) A skilled bowman

Ardell (Latin) One who is eager
Ardel, Ardelle, Ardele

Arden (Latin / English) One who is passionate and enthusiastic / from the valley of the eagles
Ardan, Arrden, Arrdan, Ardin, Arrdin, Ard, Ardyn, Arrdyn

Arduino (German) A valued friend
Ardwino, Arrduino, Ardueno

Ari (Hebrew) Resembling a lion or an eagle
Aree, Arie, Aristide, Aristides, Arri, Ary, Arye, Arrie

Ariel (Hebrew) A lion of God
Arielle, Ariele, Ariell, Arriel, Ahriel, Airial, Arieal, Arial

Aries (Latin) Resembling a ram; the first sign of the zodiac; a constellation
Arese, Ariese

Arion (Greek) A poet or musician
Arian, Arien, Aryon

Aristotle (Greek) Of high quality
Aristotelis, Aristotellis

Arius (Greek) Enduring life; everlasting; immortal
Areos, Areus, Arios

Arley (English) From the hare's meadow
Arlea, Arleigh, Arlie, Arly, Arleah, Arli, Arlee

Armani (Persian) One who is desired

Arnold (German) The eagle ruler
Arnaldo, Arnaud, Arnauld, Arnault, Arnd, Arndt, Arnel, Arnell

Arthur (Celtic) As strong as a bear; a hero
Aart, Arrt, Art, Artair, Arte, Arther, Arthor, Arthuro

Arvin (English) A friend to everyone
Arvinn, Arvinne, Arven, Arvenn, Arvenne, Arvyn, Arvynn, Arvynne

Asa (Hebrew) One who heals others
Asah

Asaph (Hebrew) One who gathers or collects
Asaf, Asaphe, Asafe, Asiph, Asiphe, Asif, Asife

Ash (English) From the ash tree
Ashe

Asher (Hebrew) Filled with happiness
Ashar, Ashor, Ashir, Ashyr, Ashur

Ashley (English) From the meadow of ash trees
Ashely, Asheley, Ashelie, Ashlan, Ashleigh, Ashlen, Ashli, Ashlie

Ashton (English) From the ash-tree town
Asheton, Ashtun, Ashetun, Ashtin, Ashetin, Ashtyn, Ashetyn, Aston

Aslan (Turkish) Resembling a lion
Aslen, Azlan, Azlen

Athens (Greek) From the capital of Greece
Athenios, Athenius, Atheneos, Atheneus

Atticus (Latin) A man from Athens
Attikus, Attickus, Aticus, Atickus, Atikus

Atwell (English) One who lives at the spring
Attwell, Atwel, Attwel

Aubrey (English) One who rules with elf-wisdom
Aubary, Aube, Aubery, Aubry, Aubury, Aubrian, Aubrien, Aubrion

Auburn (Latin) Having a reddish-brown color
Aubirn, Auburne, Aubyrn, Abern, Abirn, Aburn, Abyrn, Aubern

Audley (English) From the old meadow
Audly, Audleigh, Audlee, Audlea, Audleah, Audli, Audlie

August (Irish) One who is venerable; majestic
Austin, Augustine, Agoston, Aguistin, Agustin, Augustin, Augustyn, Avgustin, Augusteen, Agosteen

Austin (English) Form of August, meaning "one who is venerable; majestic"
Austen, Austyn, Austan, Auston, Austun

Avery (English) One who is a wise ruler; of the nobility
Avrie, Averey, Averie, Averi, Averee

Aviram (Hebrew) My Father is mighty
Avyram, Avirem, Avyrem

Axel (German / Latin / Hebrew) Source of life; small oak / ax / peace
Aksel, Ax, Axe, Axell, Axil, Axill, Axl

Aya (Hebrew) Resembling a bird
Ayah

Ayden (Irish) Form of Aiden, meaning "a fiery young man"

Ayo (African) Filled with happiness
Ayoe, Ayow, Ayowe

Azamat (Arabic) A proud man; one who is majestic

Azi (African) One who is youthful
Azie, Azy, Azey, Azee, Azea

Azmer (Islamic) Resembling a lion
Azmar, Azmir, Azmyr, Azmor, Azmur

B

Baakir (African) The eldest child
Baakeer, Baakyr, Baakear, Baakier, Baakeir

Bachir (Hebrew) The oldest son
Bacheer, Bachear, Bachier, Bacheir, Bachyr

Baha (Arabic) A glorious and splendid man
Bahah

Bailintin (Irish) A valiant man
Bailinten, Bailentin, Bailenten, Bailintyn, Bailentyn

Bain (Irish) A fair-haired man
Baine, Bayn, Bayne, Baen, Baene, Bane, Baines, Baynes

Bakari (Swahili) One who is promised
Bakarie, Bakary, Bakarey, Bakaree, Bakarea

Bakhit (Arabic) A lucky man
Bakheet, Bakheat, Bakheit, Bakhiet, Bakhyt, Bakht

Bala (Hindi) One who is youthful
Balu, Balue, Balou

Balark (Hindi) Born with the rising sun

Balasi (Basque) One who is flat-footed
Balasie, Balasy, Balasey, Balasee, Balasea

Baldwin (German) A brave friend
Baldwine, Baldwinn, Baldwinne, Baldwen, Baldwenn, Baldwenne, Baldwyn, Baldwynn

Balint (Latin) A healthy and strong man
Balent, Balin, Balen, Balynt, Balyn

Balloch (Scottish) From the grazing land

Bancroft (English) From the bean field
Bancrofte, Banfield, Banfeld, Bankroft, Bankrofte

Bandana (Spanish) A brightly colored headwrap
Bandanah, Bandanna, Bandannah

Bandy (American) A fiesty man
Bandey, Bandi, Bandie, Bandee, Bandea

Bansi (Indian) One who plays the flute
Bansie, Bansy, Bansey, Bansee, Bansea

Bao (Vietnamese / Chinese) To order / one who is prized

Baqir (Arabic) A learned man
Baqeer, Baqear, Baqier, Baqeir, Baqyr, Baqer

Barak (Hebrew) Of the lightning flash
Barrak, Barac, Barrac, Barack, Barrack

Baram (Hebrew) The son of the nation
Barem, Barum, Barom, Barim, Barym

Bard (English) A minstrel; a poet
Barde, Bardo

Barden (English) From the barley valley; from the boar's valley
Bardon, Bardun, Bardin, Bardyn, Bardan, Bardene

Bardol (Basque) A farmer
Bardo, Bartol

Bardrick (Teutonic) An ax ruler
Bardric, Bardrik, Bardryck, Bardryk, Bardryc, Bardarick, Bardaric, Bardarik

Barek (Arabic) One who is noble
Barec, Bareck

Barend (German) The hard bear
Barende, Barind, Barinde, Barynd, Barynde

Barnett (English) Of honorable birth
Barnet, Baronet, Baronett

Baron (English) A title of nobility
Barron

Barr (English) A lawyer
Barre, Bar

Barra (Gaelic) A fair-haired man

Barrett (German / English) Having the strength of a bear / one who argues
Baret, Barrat, Barratt, Barret, Barrette

Barry (Gaelic) A fair-haired man
Barrey, Barri, Barrie, Barree, Barrea, Barrington, Barryngton, Barringtun

Bartholomew (Aramaic) The son of the farmer
Bart, Bartel, Barth, Barthelemy, Bartho, Barthold, Bartholoma, Bartholomaus, Bartlett, Bartol

Bartlett (French) Form of Bartholomew, meaning "the son of the farmer"
Bartlet, Bartlitt, Bartlit, Bartlytt, Bartlyt

Bartley (English) From the meadow of birch trees
Bartly, Bartli, Bartlie, Bartlee, Bartlea, Bartleah, Bartleigh

Bartoli (Spanish) Form of Bartholomew, meaning "the son of the farmer"
Bartolie, Bartoly, Bartoley, Bartolee, Bartoleigh, Bartolea, Bartolo, Bartolio

Barton (English) From the barley town
Bartun, Barten, Bartan, Bartin, Bartyn

Barwolf (English) The ax-wolf
Barrwolf, Barwulf, Barrwulf

Basant (Arabic) One who smiles often
Basante

Bassett (English) A little person
Baset, Basset, Basett

Baurice (American) Form of Maurice, meaning "a dark-skinned man; Moorish"
Baurell, Baureo, Bauricio, Baurids, Baurie, Baurin

Bay (Vietnamese / English) The seventh-born child; born during the month of July / from the bay
Baye, Bae, Bai

Beamer (English) One who plays the trumpet
Beamor, Beamir, Beamyr, Beamur, Beamar, Beemer, Beemar, Beemir

Beau (French) A handsome man, an admirer
Bo

Becher (Hebrew) The firstborn son

Beckett (English) From the small stream; from the brook
Becket

Bedar (Arabic) One who is attentive
Beder, Bedor, Bedur, Bedyr, Bedir

Bela (Slavic) A white-skinned man
Belah, Bella, Bellah

Belden (English) From the beautiful valley
Beldan, Beldon, Beldun, Beldin, Beldyn, Bellden, Belldan, Belldon, Belldun, Belldin, Belldyn

Belen (Greek) Of an arrow
Belin, Belyn, Belan, Belon, Belun

Belindo (English) A handsome and tender man
Belyndo, Belindio, Belyndio, Belindeo, Belyndeo, Belindiyo, Belyndiyo, Belindeyo

Bellarmine (Italian) One who is handsomely armed
Bellarmin, Bellarmeen, Bellarmeene, Bellarmean, Bellarmeane, Bellarmyn, Bellarmyne

Belton (English) From the beautiful town
Bellton, Beltun, Belltun, Belten, Bellten

Belvin (American) Form of Melvin, meaning "a friend who offers counsel"
Belven, Belvyn, Belvon, Belvun, Belvan

Bem (African) A peaceful man

Ben (English) Form of Benjamin, meaning "son of the south; son of the right hand"
Benn, Benni, Bennie, Bennee, Benney, Benny, Bennea, Benno

Benjamin (Hebrew) Son of the south; son of the right hand
Ben, Benejamen, Beniamino, Benjaman, Benjamen, Benjamino, Benjamon, Benjiman, Benjimen

Bennett (English) Form of Benedict, meaning "one who is blessed"
Benett, Bennet, Benet

Bentley (English) From the meadow of bent grass
Bently, Bentleigh, Bentlee, Bentlie

Berdy (German) Having a brilliant mind
Berdey, Berdee, Berdea, Berdi, Berdie

Berkeley (English) From the meadow of birch trees
Berkely, Berkeli, Berkelie, Berkelea, Berkeleah, Berkelee, Berkeleigh, Berkley

Bernard (German) As strong and brave as a bear
Barnard, Barnardo, Barnhard, Barnhardo, Bearnard, Bernardo, Bernarr, Bernd

Berry (English) Resembling a berry fruit
Berrey, Berri, Berrie, Berree, Berrea

Bert (English) One who is illustrious
Berte, Berti, Bertie, Bertee, Bertea, Berty, Bertey

Bethel (Hebrew) The house of God
Bethell, Bethele, Bethelle, Betuel, Betuell, Betuele, Betuelle

Bevis (Teutonic) An archer
Beviss, Bevys, Bevyss, Beavis, Beaviss, Beavys, Beavyss

Biagio (Italian) One who has a stutter
Biaggio

Birney (English) From the island with the brook
Birny, Birnee, Birnea, Birni, Birnie

Black (English) A dark-skinned man
Blak, Blac, Blacke

Blackwell (English) From the dark spring
Blackwel, Blackwelle, Blackwele

Blade (English) One who wields a sword or knife
Blayd, Blayde, Blaid, Blaide, Blaed, Blaede

Blaine (Scottish / Irish) A saint's servant / a thin man
Blayne, Blane, Blain, Blayn, Blaen, Blaene, Blainy, Blainey

Blaise (Latin / American) One with a lisp or a stutter / a fiery man
Blaze, Blaize, Blaiz, Blayze, Blayz, Blaez, Blaeze

Blake (English) A dark, handsome man
Blayk, Blayke, Blaik, Blaike, Blaek, Blaeke

Bliss (English) Filled with happiness
Blis, Blyss, Blys

Blondell (English) A fair-haired boy
Blondel, Blondele, Blondelle

Boaz (Hebrew) One who is swift
Boaze, Boas, Boase

Bob (English) Form of Robert, meaning "one who is bright with fame"
Bobbi, Bobbie, Bobby, Bobbey, Bobbee, Bobbea

Bodhi (Buddhist) To become aware
Bode, Bodie

Bogart (French) One who is strong with the bow
Bogaard, Bogaart, Bogaerd, Bogey, Bogie, Bogi, Bogy, Bogee

Bonaventure (Latin) One who undertakes a blessed venture
Bonaventura, Buenaventure, Buenaventura, Bueaventure, Bueaventura

Booker (English) One who binds books; a scribe
Bookar, Bookir, Bookyr, Bookur, Bookor

Bosley (English) From the meadow near the forest
Bosly, Boslee, Boslea, Bosleah, Bosleigh, Bosli, Boslie, Bozley

Boston (English) From the town near the forest; from the city of Boston
Bostun, Bostin, Bostyn, Bosten, Bostan

Boyce (French) One who lives near the forest
Boice, Boyse, Boise

Boyd (Celtic) A blond-haired man
Boyde, Boid, Boide, Boyden, Boydan, Boydin, Boydyn, Boydon

Bracken (English) Resembling the large fern
Braken, Brackan, Brakan, Brackin, Brakin, Brackyn

Braddock (English) From the broadly spread oak
Bradock, Braddoc, Bradoc, Braddok, Bradok

Braden (Gaelic / English)
Resembling salmon / from
the wide valley
*Bradan, Bradon, Bradin,
Bradyn, Braeden, Brayden*

Bradford (English) From the
wide ford
Bradforde, Bradferd, Bradferde

Bradley (English) From the
wide meadow
*Bradly, Bradlea, Bradleah,
Bradlee, Bradleigh, Bradli*

Brady (Irish) The son of a
large-chested man
*Bradey, Bradee, Bradea, Bradi,
Bradie, Braidy, Braidey, Braidee*

Bramley (English) From the
wild gorse meadow; from the
raven's meadow
Bramly, Bramlee, Bramlea

Brandon (English) From the
broom or gorse hill
*Brandun, Brandin, Brandyn,
Brandan, Branden, Brannon,
Brannun, Brannen*

Branson (English) The son of
Brand or Brandon
*Bransun, Bransen, Bransan,
Bransin, Bransyn*

Brant (English) Steep, tall

Brantley (English) Form of
Brant, meaning "steep, tall"
Brantly

Braxton (English) From
Brock's town
*Braxtun, Braxten, Braxtan,
Braxtyn*

Brayden (Gaelic / English)
Form of Braden, meaning
"resembling salmon / from
the wide valley"
*Braydon, Braydan, Braydin,
Braydyn*

Braylen (American)
Combination of Brayden and
Lynn
Braylon

Brendan (Irish) Born to
royalty; a prince
*Brendano, Brenden, Brendin,
Brendon, Brendyn, Brendun*

Brennan (Gaelic) A sorrowful
man; a teardrop
*Brenan, Brenn, Brennen,
Brennin, Brennon, Brenin,
Brennun, Brennyn*

Brent (English) From the hill
*Brendt, Brennt, Brentan,
Brenten, Brentin, Brenton,
Brentun, Brentyn*

Brett (Latin) A man from
Britain or Brittany
*Bret, Breton, Brette, Bretton,
Brit, Briton, Britt, Brittain*

Brewster (English) One who
brews
Brewer, Brewstere

Brian (Gaelic / Celtic) Of noble birth / having great strength
Briano, Briant, Brien, Brion, Bryan, Bryant, Bryen, Bryent

Briar (English) Resembling a thorny plant
Brier, Bryar, Bryer

Brock (English) Resembling a badger
Broc

Broderick (English) From the wide ridge
Broderik, Broderic, Brodrick, Brodryk, Brodyrc, Brodrik, Broderyc, Brodrig

Brody (Gaelic / Irish) From the ditch
Brodie, Brodey, Brodi, Brodee

Brogan (Gaelic) One who is sturdy
Broggan, Brogen, Broggen, Brogon, Broggon, Brogun, Broggun, Brogin, Broggin, Brogyn

Brooks (English) From the running stream
Brookes

Bruce (Scottish) A man from Brieuse; one who is well-born; from an influential family
Brouce, Brooce, Bruci, Brucie, Brucey, Brucy

Bruno (German) A brown-haired man
Brunoh, Brunoe, Brunow, Brunowe, Bruin, Bruine, Brunon, Brunun

Bryce (Scottish / Anglo-Saxon) One who is speckled / the son of a nobleman
Brice, Bricio, Brizio, Brycio

Bryson (Welsh) The son of Brice
Brisen, Brysin, Brysun, Brysyn, Brycen

Bud (English) One who is brotherly
Budd, Buddi, Buddie, Buddee, Buddey, Buddy

Budha (Hindi) Another name for the planet Mercury
Budhan, Budhwar

Burbank (English) From the riverbank of burrs
Burrbank, Burhbank

Burgess (German) A free citizen of the town
Burges, Burgiss, Burgis, Burgyss, Burgys, Burgeis

Burne (English) Resembling a bear; from the brook; the brown-haired one
Burn, Beirne, Burnis, Byrn, Byrne, Burns, Byrnes

Burnet (French) Having brown hair
Burnett, Burnete, Burnette, Bernet, Bernett, Bernete, Bernette

Burton (English) From the fortified town
Burtun, Burten, Burtin, Burtyn, Burtan

Butler (English) The keeper of the bottles (wine, liquor)
Buttler, Butlar, Butlor, Butlir, Buttlir, Butlyr

Byron (English) One who lives near the cow sheds
Byrom, Beyren, Beyron, Biren, Biron, Buiron, Byram, Byran

Cable (French) One who makes rope
Cabel, Caibel, Caible, Caybel, Cayble, Caebel, Caeble, Cabe

Caddis (English) Resembling a worsted fabric
Caddys, Caddiss, Caddice

Cade (English / French) One who is round / of the cask
Caid, Caide, Cayd, Cayde, Caed, Caede

Cadell (Welsh) Having the spirit of battle
Cadel, Caddell, Caddel

Caden (Welsh) Spirit of Battle
Caiden, Cayden

Cadmus (Greek) A man from the east; in mythology, the man who founded Thebes
Cadmar, Cadmo, Cadmos, Cadmuss

Cadogan (Welsh) Having glory and honor during battle
Cadogawn, Cadwgan, Cadwgawn, Cadogaun

Caesar (Latin) An emperor
Caezar, Casar, Cezar, Chezare, Caesarius, Ceasar, Ceazer

Cain (Hebrew) One who wields a spear; something acquired; in the Bible, Adam and Eve's first son who killed his brother Abel
Cayn, Caen, Cane, Caine, Cayne, Caene

Caird (Scottish) A traveling metal worker
Cairde, Cayrd, Cayrde, Caerd, Caerde

Cairn (Gaelic) From the mound of rocks
Cairne, Cairns, Caern, Caerne, Caernes

Caith (Irish) Of the battlefield
Caithe, Cayth, Caythe, Cathe, Caeth, Caethe

Calbert (English) A cowboy
Calberte, Calburt, Calburte, Calbirt, Calbirte, Calbyrt, Calbyrte

Cale (English) Form of Charles, meaning "one who is manly and strong / a free man"
Cail, Caile, Cayl, Cayle, Cael, Caele

Caleb (Hebrew) Resembling a dog
Cayleb, Caileb, Caeleb, Calob, Cailob, Caylob, Caelob, Kaleb

Calian (Native American) A warrior of life
Calien, Calyan, Calyen

Callum (Gaelic) Resembling a dove
Calum

Calvin (French) The little bald one
Cal, Calvyn, Calvon, Calven, Calvan, Calvun, Calvino

Camara (African) One who teaches others

Camden (Gaelic) From the winding valley
Camdene, Camdin, Camdyn, Camdan, Camdon, Camdun

Cameo (English) A small, perfect child
Cammeo

Cameron (Scottish) Having a crooked nose
Cameren, Cameran, Camerin, Cameryn, Camerun, Camron, Camren, Camran, Tameron

Campbell (Scottish) Having a crooked mouth
Campbel, Cambell, Cambel, Camp, Campe, Cambeul, Cambeull, Campbeul

Cannon (French) An official of the church
Canon, Cannun, Canun, Cannin, Canin

Canyon (Spanish / English) From the footpath / from the deep ravine
Caniyon, Canyun, Caniyun

Capricorn (Latin) The tenth sign of the zodiac; the goat

Cargan (Gaelic) From the small rock
Cargen, Cargon, Cargun, Cargin, Cargyn

Carl (German) Form of Karl, meaning "a free man"
Carel, Carlan, Carle, Carlens, Carlitis, Carlin, Carlo, Carlos

Carlos (Spanish) Form of Karl, meaning "a free man"
Carolos, Carolo, Carlito

Carlsen (Scandinavian) The son of Carl
Carlssen, Carlson, Carlsson, Carlsun, Carllsun, Carlsin, Carllsin, Carlsyn

Carlton (English) From the free man's town
Carltun, Carltown, Carston, Carstun, Carstown, Carleton, Carletun, Carlten

Carmichael (Scottish) A follower of Michael

Carmine (Latin / Aramaic) A beautiful song / the color crimson
Carman, Carmen, Carmin, Carmino, Carmyne, Carmon, Carmun, Carmyn

Carson (Scottish) The son of a marsh dweller
Carsen, Carsun, Carsan, Carsin, Carsyn

Carter (English) One who transports goods; one who drives a cart
Cartar, Cartir, Cartyr, Cartor, Cartur, Cartere, Cartier, Cartrell

Cartland (English) From Carter's land
Carteland, Cartlan, Cartlend, Cartelend, Cartlen

Cary (Celtic / Welsh / Gaelic) From the river / from the fort on the hill / having dark features
Carey, Cari, Carie, Caree, Carea, Carry, Carrey, Carri

Case (French) Refers to a chest or box
Cace

Cash (Latin) money

Cason (Greek) A seer
Casen, Kaysen

Cassander (Spanish) A brother of heroes
Casander, Casandro, Cassandro, Casandero

Cassius (Latin) One who is empty; hollow; vain
Cassios, Cassio, Cach, Cache, Cashus, Cashos, Cassian, Cassien

Castel (Spanish) From the castle
Castell, Castal, Castall, Castol, Castoll, Castul, Castull, Castil

Castor (Greek) Resembling a beaver; in mythology, one of the Dioscuri
Castur, Caster, Castar, Castir, Castyr, Castorio, Castoreo, Castoro

Cathmore (Irish) A renowned
fighter
Cathmor, Cathemore

Cato (Latin) One who is
all-knowing
Cayto, Caito, Caeto

Caton (Spanish) One who is
knowledgable
*Caten, Catun, Catan, Catin,
Catyn*

Cavell (Teutonic) One who is
bold
Cavel, Cavele, Cavelle

Celesto (Latin) From heaven
*Célestine, Celestino, Celindo,
Celestyne, Celestyno*

Cephas (Hebrew) As solid as
a rock

Cesar (Spanish) Form of
Caesar, meaning "emperor"
Cesare, Cesaro, Cesario

Chad (English) One who is
warlike
*Chaddie, Chadd, Chadric,
Chadrick, Chadrik, Chadryck,
Chadryc, Chadryk*

Chadwick (English) From
Chad's dairy farm
*Chadwik, Chadwic, Chadwyck,
Chadwyk, Chadwyc*

Chai (Hebrew) A giver of life
*Chaika, Chaim, Cahyim,
Cahyyam*

Chalkley (English) From the
chalk meadow
*Chalkly, Chalkleigh, Chalklee,
Chalkleah, Chalkli, Chalklie,
Chalklea*

Champion (English) A warrior;
the victor
*Champeon, Champiun,
Champeun, Champ*

Chan (Spanish / Sanskrit)
Form of John, meaning "God
is gracious" / a shining man
Chayo, Chano, Chawn, Chaun

Chanan (Hebrew) God is com-
passionate
*Chanen, Chanin, Chanyn,
Chanun, Chanon*

Chance (English) Having good
fortune

Chandler (English) One who
makes candles
Chandlar, Chandlor

Chaniel (Hebrew) The grace
of God
Chanyel, Chaniell, Chanyell

Channing (French / English)
An official of the church /
resembling a young wolf
Channyng, Canning, Cannyng

Chao (Chinese) The great one

Chappel (English) One who works in the chapel
Capel, Capell, Capello, Cappel, Chappell

Charles (English / German) One who is manly and strong / a free man
Charls, Chas, Charli, Charlie, Charley, Charly, Charlee, Charleigh, Cale, Chuck, Chick

Charleson (English) The son of Charles
Charlesen, Charlesin, Charlesyn, Charlesan, Charlesun

Charlton (English) From the free man's town
Charleton, Charltun, Charletun, Charleston, Charlestun

Charro (Spanish) A cowboy
Charo

Chase (English) A huntsman
Chace, Chasen, Chayce, Chayse, Chaise, Chaice, Chaece, Chaese

Chatwin (English) A warring friend
Chatwine, Chatwinn, Chatwinne, Chatwen, Chatwenn, Chatwenne, Chatwyn, Chatwynn

Chaviv (Hebrew) One who is dearly loved
Chaveev, Chaveav, Chaviev, Chaveiv, Chavyv, Chavivi, Chavivie, Chavivy

Chay (Gaelic) From the fairy place
Chaye, Chae

Chelsey (English) From the landing place for chalk
Chelsee, Chelseigh, Chelsea, Chelsi, Chelsie, Chelsy, Chelcey, Chelcy

Cheslav (Russian) From the fortified camp
Cheslaw

Chester (Latin) From the camp of the soldiers
Chet, Chess, Cheston, Chestar, Chestor, Chestur, Chestir, Chestyr

Chien (Vietnamese) A combative man

Chiron (Greek) A wise tutor
Chyron, Chirun, Chyrun

Chogan (Native American) Resembling a blackbird
Chogen, Chogon, Chogun, Chogin, Chogyn

Choni (Hebrew) A gracious man
Chonie, Chony, Choney, Chonee, Chonea

Christian (Greek) A follower of Christ
Chrestien, Chretien, Chris, Christan, Christer, Christiano, Cristian

Christopher (Greek) One who bears Christ inside
Chris, Kit, Christof, Christofer, Christoffer, Christoforo, Christoforus, Christoph, Christophe, Cristopher, Cristofer

Chuck (English) Form of Charles, meaning "one who is manly and strong / a free man"
Chucke, Chucki, Chuckie, Chucky, Chuckey, Chuckee, Chuckea

Chul (Korean) One who stands firm

Chun (Chinese) Born during the spring

Cid (Spanish) A lord
Cyd

Cillian (Gaelic) One who suffers strife

Ciqala (Native American) The little one

Cirrus (Latin) A lock of hair; resembling the cloud
Cyrrus

Clair (Latin) One who is bright
Clare, Clayr, Claer, Clairo, Claro, Claero

Clancy (Celtic) Son of the red-haired warrior
Clancey, Clanci, Clancie, Clancee, Clancea, Clansey, Clansy, Clansi

Clark (English) A cleric; a clerk
Clarke, Clerk, Clerke, Clerc

Claude (English) One who is lame
Claud, Claudan, Claudell, Claidianus, Claudicio, Claudien, Claudino, Claudio

Clay (English) Of the earth's clay

Clayton (English) From the town settled on clay
Claytun, Clayten, Claytin, Claytyn, Claytan, Cleyton, Cleytun, Cleytan

Cleon (Greek) A well-known man
Cleone, Clion, Clione, Clyon, Clyone

Clifford (English) From the ford near the cliff
Cliff, Clyfford, Cliford, Clyford

Cliffton (English) From the town near the cliff
Cliff, Cliffe, Clyff, Clyffe, Clifft, Clift, Clyfft, Clyft

Clinton (English) From the town on the hill
Clynton, Clintun, Clyntun, Clint, Clynt, Clinte, Clynte

Clive (English) One who lives near the cliff
Clyve, Cleve

Cluny (Irish) From the meadow
Cluney, Cluni, Clunie, Clunee, Clunea, Cluneah

Clyde (Scottish) From the river Clyde
Clide

Clide Cobden (English) From the cottage in the valley
Cobdenn, Cobdale, Cobdail, Cobdaile, Cobdell, Cobdel, Cobdayl, Cobdayle

Coby (English) Form of Jacob, meaning "he who supplants"
Cobey

Cody (Irish / English) One who is helpful; a wealthy man / acting as a cushion
Codi, Codie, Codey, Codee, Codeah, Codea, Codier, Codyr

Colbert (French) A famous and bright man
Colvert, Culbert, Colburt, Colbirt, Colbyrt, Colbart, Culburt, Culbirt

Colby (English) From the coal town
Colbey, Colbi, Colbie, Colbee, Collby, Coalby, Colbea, Colbeah

Cole (English) Having dark features; having coal-black hair
Coley, Coli, Coly, Colie, Colee, Coleigh, Colea, Colson

Coleridge (English) From the dark ridge
Colerige, Colridge, Colrige

Colgate (English) From the dark gate
Colegate, Colgait, Colegait, Colgayt, Colegayt, Colgaet

Colin (Scottish) A young man; a form of Nicholas, meaning "of the victorious people"
Cailean, Colan, Colyn, Colon, Colen, Collin, Collan

Colt (English) A young horse; from the coal town
Colte

Colter (English) A horse herdsman
Coltere, Coltar, Coltor, Coltir, Coltyr, Coulter, Coultar, Coultir

Colton (English) From the coal town
Colten, Coltun, Coltan, Coltin, Coltyn, Coltrain

Comanche (Native American)
A tribal name
*Comanchi, Comanchie,
Comanchee, Comanchea,
Comanchy, Comanchey*

Comus (Latin) In mythology,
the god of mirth and revelry
Comas, Comis, Comys

Conan (English / Gaelic)
Resembling a wolf / one who
is high and mighty
Conant

Condon (Celtic) A dark,
wise man
*Condun, Condan, Conden,
Condin, Condyn*

Cong (Chinese) A clever man

Conn (Irish) The chief
Con

Connecticut (Native American)
From the place beside the
long river / from the state of
Connecticut

Connery (Scottish) A daring
man
*Connary, Connerie, Conneri,
Connerey, Connarie, Connari,
Connarey, Conary*

Connor (Gaelic) A wolf lover
*Conor, Conner, Coner, Connar,
Conar, Connur, Conur, Connir,
Conir*

Conroy (Irish) A wise adviser
Conroye, Conroi

Constantine (Latin) One who
is steadfast; firm
Dinos

Consuelo (Spanish) One who
offers consolation
*Consuel, Consuelio, Consueleo,
Consueliyo, Consueleyo*

Conway (Gaelic) The hound
of the plain; from the sacred
river
*Conwaye, Conwai, Conwae,
Conwy*

Cook (English) One who
prepares meals for others
Cooke

Cooney (Irish) A handsome
man
*Coony, Cooni, Coonie, Coonee,
Coonea*

Cooper (English) One who
makes barrels
*Coop, Coopar, Coopir, Coopyr,
Coopor, Coopur, Coopersmith,
Cupere*

Corbett (French) Resembling a
young raven
*Corbet, Corbete, Corbette,
Corbit, Corbitt, Corbite,
Corbitte*

Corcoran (Gaelic) Having a ruddy complexion
Cochran

Cordero (Spanish) Resembling a lamb
Corderio, Corderiyo, Cordereo, Cordereyo

Corey (Irish) From the hollow; of the churning waters
Cory, Cori, Corie, Coree, Corea, Correy, Corry, Corri

Coriander (Greek) A romantic man; resembling the spice
Coryander, Coriender, Coryender

Corlan (Irish) One who wields a spear
Corlen, Corlin, Corlyn, Corlon, Corlun

Corrado (German) A bold counselor
Corrade, Corradeo, Corradio

Corridon (Irish) One who wields a spear
Corridan, Corridun, Corriden, Corridin, Corridyn

Cortez (Spanish) A courteous man
Cortes

Cosmo (Greek) The order of the universe
Cosimo, Cosmé, Cosmos, Cosmas, Cozmo, Cozmos, Cozmas

Courtney (English) A courteous man; courtly
Cordney, Cordni, Cortenay, Corteney, Cortni, Cortnee, Cortneigh, Cortney

Covert (English) One who provides shelter
Couvert

Covey (English) A brood of birds
Covy, Covi, Covie, Covee, Covea, Covvey, Covvy, Covvi

Covington (English) From the town near the cave
Covyngton, Covingtun, Covyngtun

Cox (English) A coxswain
Coxe, Coxi, Coxie, Coxey, Coxy, Coxee, Coxea

Coyle (Irish) A leader during battle
Coyl, Coil, Coile

Craig (Gaelic) From the rocks; from the crag
Crayg, Craeg, Craige, Crayge, Craege, Crage, Crag

Crandell (English) From the valley of cranes
Crandel, Crandale, Crandail, Crandaile, Crandayl, Crandayle, Crandael, Crandaele

Crawford (English) From the crow's ford
Crawforde, Crawferd, Crawferde, Crawfurd, Crawfurde

Creed (Latin) A guiding principle; a belief
Creede, Cread, Creade, Creedon, Creadon, Creedun, Creadun, Creedin

Creek (English) From the small stream
Creeke, Creak, Creake, Creik, Creike

Creighton (Scottish) From the border town
Creightun, Crayton, Craytun, Craiton, Craitun, Craeton, Craetun, Crichton

Crescent (French) One who creates; increasing; growing
Creissant, Crescence, Cressant, Cressent, Crescant

Cruz (Spanish) Of the cross

Cuarto (Spanish) The fourth-born child
Cuartio, Cuartiyo, Cuarteo

Cullen (Gaelic) A good-looking young man
Cullin, Cullyn, Cullan, Cullon, Cullun

Cunningham (Gaelic) Descendant of the chief
Conyngham, Cuningham, Cunnyngham, Cunyngham

Curcio (French) One who is courteous
Curceo

Cuthbert (English) One who is bright and famous
Cuthbeorht, Cuthburt, Cuthbirt, Cuthbyrt

Cyneley (English) From the royal meadow
Cynely, Cyneli, Cynelie, Cynelee, Cynelea, Cyneleah, Cyneleigh

Czar (Russian) An emperor

Dacey (Gaelic / Latin) A man from the south / a man from Dacia
Dacy, Dacee, Dacea, Daci, Dacie, Daicey, Daicy

Daedalus (Greek) A craftsman
Daldalos, Dedalus

Dag (Scandinavian) Born during the daylight
Dagney, Dagny, Dagnee, Dagnea, Dagni, Dagnie, Daeg, Dagget

Daijon (American) A gift of hope
Dayjon, Daejon, Dajon

Dainan (Australian) A kindhearted man
Dainen, Dainon, Dainun, Dainyn, Dainin, Daynan, Daynen, Daynon

Daire (Irish) A wealthy man
Dair, Daere, Daer, Dayr, Dayre, Dare, Dari, Darie

Daivat (Hindi) A powerful man

Dakarai (African) Filled with happiness

Dakota (Native American) A friend to all
Daccota, Dakoda, Dakodah, Dakotah, Dakoeta, Dekota, Dekohta, Dekowta

Dallan (Irish) One who is blind
Dalan, Dallen, Dalen, Dalin, Dallin, Dallyn, Dalyn, Dallon, Dalon, Dallun, Dalun

Dallas (Scottish) From the dales
Dalles, Dallis, Dallys, Dallos

Dalton (English) from the town in the valley
Daltun, Dalten, Daltan, Daltin, Daltyn, Daleten, Dalte, Daulten

Damario (Greek / Spanish) Resembling a calf / one who is gentle
Damarios, Damarius, Damaro, Damero, Damerio, Damereo, Damareo, Damerios

Damian (Greek) One who tames or subdues others
Daemon, Daimen, Daimon, Daman, Damen, Dameon, Damiano, Damianos, Damon

Dane (English) A man from Denmark
Dain, Daine, Dayn, Dayne

Danely (Scandinavian) A man from Denmark
Daneley, Daneli, Danelie, Danelee, Daneleigh, Danelea, Daineley, Dainely

Daniachew (African) A mediator

Daniel (Hebrew) God is my judge
Dan, Danal, Daneal, Danek, Danell, Danial, Daniele, Danil, Danilo

Danso (African) A reliable man
Dansoe, Dansow, Dansowe

Dante (Latin) An enduring man; everlasting
Dantae, Dantay, Dantel, Daunte, Dontae, Dontay, Donte, Dontae

Daoud (Arabian) Form of David, meaning "the beloved one"
Daoude, Dawud, Doud, Daud, Da'ud

Daphnis (Greek) In mythology, the son of Hermes
Daphnys

Dar (Hebrew) Resembling a pearl
Darr

Darcel (French) Having dark features
Darcell, Darcele, Darcelle, Darcio, Darceo

Darek (English) Form of Derek, meaning "the ruler of the tribe"
Darrek, Darec, Darrec, Darreck, Dareck

Darion (Greek) A gift
Darian, Darien, Dariun, Darrion, Darrian, Darrien, Daryon, Daryan

Darius (Greek) A kingly man; one who is wealthy
Darias, Dariess, Dario, Darious, Darrius, Derrius, Derrious, Derrias

Darlen (American) A sweet man; a darling
Darlon, Darlun, Darlan, Darlin, Darlyn

Darnell (English) From the hidden place
Darnall, Darneil, Darnel, Darnele, Darnelle

Darold (English) Form of Harold, meaning "the ruler of an army"
Darrold, Derald, Derrald, Derold, Derrold

Darren (Gaelic / English) A great man / a gift from God
Darran, Darrin, Darryn, Darron, Darrun, Daren, Darin, Daran

Dash (American) A charming man

Darvell (French) From the eagle town
Darvel, Darvele, Darvelle

Dasras (Indian) A handsome man

Dasya (Indian) A servant

David (Hebrew) The beloved one
Dave, Davey, Davi, Davidde, Davide, Davie, Daviel, Davin, Daoud

Davis (English) The son of David
Davies, Daviss, Davys, Davyss

Davu (African) Of the beginning
Davue, Davoo, Davou, Davugh

Dawson (English) The son of David
Dawsan, Dawsen, Dawsin, Dawsun

Dax (French) From the French town Dax
Daxton

Dayton (English) From the sunny town

Deacon (Greek) The dusty one; a servant
Deecon, Deakon, Deekon, Deacun, Deecun, Deakun, Deekun, Deacan

Dean (English) From the valley; a church official
Deane, Deen, Deene, Dene, Deans, Deens, Deani, Deanie

DeAndre (American) A manly man
D'André, DeAndrae, DeAndray, Diandray, Diondrae, Diondray

Dearon (American) One who is much loved
Dearan, Dearen, Dearin, Dearyn, Dearun

Decker (German / Hebrew) One who prays / a piercing man
Deker, Decer, Dekker, Deccer, Deck, Decke

Declan (Irish) The name of a saint

Dedrick (English) Form of Dietrich, meaning "the ruler of the tribe"
Dedryck, Dedrik, Dedryk, Dedric, Dedryc

Deegan (Irish) A black-haired man
Deagan, Degan, Deegen, Deagen, Degen, Deegon, Deagon, Degon

Deinorus (American) A lively man
Denorius, Denorus, Denorios, Deinorius, Deinorios

Dejuan (American) A talkative man
Dejuane, Dewon, Dewonn, Dewan, Dewann, Dwon, Dwonn, Dajuan

Delaney (Irish / French) The dark challenger / from the elder-tree grove
Delany, Delanee, Delanea, Delani, Delanie, Delainey, Delainy, Delaini

Delaware (English) From the state of Delaware
Delawair, Delaweir, Delwayr, Delawayre, Delawaire, Delawaer, Delawaere

Delius (Greek) A man from Delos
Delios, Delos, Delus, Delo

Dell (English) From the small valley
Delle, Del

Delmon (English) A man of the mountain
Delmun, Delmen, Delmin, Delmyn, Delmont, Delmonte, Delmond, Delmonde

Delsi (American) An easy-going guy
Delsie, Delsy, Delsey, Delsee, Delsea, Delci, Delcie, Delcee

Delvin (English) A godly friend
Delvinn, Delvinne, Delvyn, Delvynn, Delvynne, Delven, Delvenn, Delvenne

Demarcus (American) The son of Marcus
DeMarcus, DaMarkiss, DeMarco, Demarkess, DeMarko, Demarkus, DeMarques, DeMarquez

Dembe (African) A peaceful man
Dembi, Dembie, Dembee, Dembea, Dembey, Demby

Denali (American) From the national park
Denalie, Denaly, Denaley, Denalee, Denalea, Denaleigh

Denley (English) From the meadow near the valley
Denly, Denlea, Denleah, Denlee, Denleigh, Denli, Denlie

Denman (English) One who lives in the valley
Denmann, Denmin, Denmyn, Denmen, Denmon, Denmun

Dennis (French) A follower of Dionysus
Den, Denies, Denis, Dennes, Dennet, Denney, Dennie, Denys, Dennys

Dennison (English) The son of Dennis
Denison, Dennisun, Denisun, Dennisen, Denisen, Dennisan, Denisan

Deo (Greek) A godly man

Deonte (French) An outgoing man
Deontay, Deontaye, Deontae, Dionte, Diontay, Diontaye, Diontae

Deotis (American) A learned man; a scholar
Deotiss, Deotys, Deotyss, Deotus, Deotuss

Derek (English) The ruler of the tribe
Dereck, Deric, Derick, Derik, Deriq, Derk, Derreck, Derrek, Derrick

Dervin (English) A gifted friend
Dervinn, Dervinne, Dervyn, Dervynn, Dervynne, Dervon, Dervan, Dervun

Deshan (Hindi) Of the nation
Deshal, Deshad

Desiderio (Latin) One who is desired; hoped for
Derito, Desi, Desideratus, Desiderios, Desiderius, Desiderus, Dezi, Diderot

Desmond (Gaelic) A man from South Munster
Desmonde, Desmund, Desmunde, Dezmond, Dezmonde, Dezmund, Dezmunde, Desmee

Desperado (Spanish) A renegade

Destin (French) Recognizing one's certain fortune; fate
Destyn, Deston, Destun, Desten, Destan

Destrey (American) A cowboy
Destry, Destree, Destrea, Destri, Destrie

Devanshi (Hindi) A divine messenger
Devanshie, Devanshy, Devanshey, Devanshee

Devante (Spanish) One who fights wrongdoing

Devlin (Gaelic) Having fierce bravery; a misfortunate man
Devlyn, Devlon, Devlen, Devlan, Devlun

Devon (English) From the beautiful farmland; of the divine
Devan, Deven, Devenn, Devin, Devonn, Devone, Deveon, Devonne

Dewitt (Flemish) A blond-haired man
DeWitt, Dewytt, DeWytt, Dewit, DeWit, Dewyt, DeWyt

Dexter (Latin) A right-handed man; one who is skillful
Dextor, Dextar, Dextur, Dextir, Dextyr, Dexton, Dextun, Dexten

Dhyanesh (Indian) One who meditates
Dhianesh, Dhyaneshe, Dhianeshe

Dichali (Native American) One who talks a lot
Dichalie, Dichaly, Dichaley, Dichalee, Dichalea, Dichaleigh

Diego (Spanish) Form of James, meaning "he who supplants"
Dyego, Dago

Diesel (American) Having great strength
Deisel, Diezel, Deizel, Dezsel

Dietrich (German) The ruler of the tribe
Dedrick

Digby (Norse) From the town near the ditch
Digbey, Digbee, Digbea, Digbi, Digbie

Diji (African) A farmer
Dijie, Dijee, Dijea, Dijy, Dijey

Dillon (Gaelic) Resembling a lion; a faithful man
Dillun, Dillen, Dillan, Dillin, Dillyn, Dilon, Dilan, Dilin

Dino (Italian) One who wields a little sword
Dyno, Dinoh, Dynoh, Deano, Deanoh, Deeno, Deenoh, Deino

Dinos (Greek) Form of Constantine, meaning "one who is steadfast; firm"
Dynos, Deanos, Deenos, Deinos, Dinose, Dinoz

Dins (American) One who climbs to the top
Dinz, Dyns, Dynz

Dionysus (Greek) The god of wine and revelry
Dion, Deion, Deon, Deonn, Deonys, Deyon, Diandre

Dior (French) The golden one
D'Or, Diorr, Diorre, Dyor, Deor, Dyorre, Deorre

Diron (American) Form of Darren, meaning "a great man / a gift from God"
Dirun, Diren, Diran, Dirin, Diryn, Dyron, Dyren

Dixon (English) The son of Dick
Dixen, Dixin, Dixyn, Dixan, Dixun

Doane (English) From the rolling hills
Doan

Dobber (American) An independent man
Dobbar, Dobbor, Dobbur, Dobbir, Dobbyr

Dobbs (English) A fiery man
Dobbes, Dobes, Dobs

Domevlo (African) One who doesn't judge others
Domivlo, Domyvlo

Domingo (Spanish) Born on a Sunday
Domyngo, Demingo, Demyngo

Dominic (Latin) A lord
Demenico, Dom, Domenic, Domenico, Domenique, Domini, Dominick, Dominico

Domnall (Gaelic) A world ruler
Domhnall, Domnull, Domhnull

Don (Scottish) Form of Donald, meaning "ruler of the world"
Donn, Donny, Donney, Donnie, Donni, Donnee, Donnea, Donne

Donald (Scottish) Ruler of the world
Don, Donold, Donuld, Doneld, Donild, Donyld

Donato (Italian) A gift from God

Donovan (Irish) A brown-haired chief
Donavan, Donavon, Donevon, Donovyn

Dor (Hebrew) Of this generation
Doram, Doriel, Dorli, Dorlie, Dorlee, Dorlea, Dorleigh, Dorly

Doran (Irish) A stranger; one who has been exiled
Doren, Dorin, Doryn

Dorsey (Gaelic) From the fortress near the sea
Dorsy, Dorsee, Dorsea, Dorsi, Dorsie

Dost (Arabic) A beloved friend
Doste, Daust, Dauste, Dawst, Dawste

Dotson (English) The son of Dot
Dotsen, Dotsan, Dotsin, Dotsyn, Dotsun, Dottson, Dottsun, Dottsin

Dove (American) A peaceful man
Dovi, Dovie, Dovy, Dovey, Dovee, Dovea

Drake (English) Resembling a dragon
Drayce, Drago, Drakie

Drew (Welsh) One who is wise
Drue, Dru

Driscoll (Celtic) A mediator; one who is sorrowful; a messenger
Dryscoll, Driscol, Dryscol, Driskoll, Dryskoll, Driskol, Dryskol, Driskell

Drummond (Scottish) One who lives on the ridge
Drummon, Drumond, Drumon, Drummund, Drumund, Drummun

Duane (Gaelic) A dark or swarthy man
Dewain, Dewayne, Duante, Duayne, Duwain, Duwaine, Duwayne, Dwain

Dublin (Irish) From the capital of Ireland
Dublyn, Dublen, Dublan, Dublon, Dublun

Duc (Vietnamese) One who has upstanding morals

Due (Vietnamese) A virtuous man

Duke (English) A title of nobility; a leader
Dooke, Dook, Duki, Dukie, Dukey, Duky, Dukee, Dukea

Dumi (African) One who inspires others
Dumie, Dumy, Dumey, Dumee, Dumea

Dumont (French) Man of the mountain
Dumonte, Dumount, Dumounte

Duncan (Scottish) A dark warrior
Dunkan, Dunckan, Dunc, Dunk, Dunck

Dundee (Scottish) From the town on the Firth of Tay
Dundea, Dundi, Dundie, Dundy, Dundey

Dunton (English) From the town on the hill
Duntun, Dunten, Duntan, Duntin, Duntyn

Durin (Norse) In mythology, one of the fathers of the dwarves
Duryn, Duren, Duran, Duron, Durun

Durjaya (Hindi) One who is difficult to defeat

Durrell (English) One who is strong and protective
Durrel, Durell, Durel

Dustin (English / German) From the dusty area / a courageous warrior
Dustyn, Dusten, Dustan, Duston, Dustun, Dusty, Dustey, Dusti

Duvall (French) From the valley
Duval, Duvale

Dwade (English) A dark traveler
Dwaid, Dwaide, Dwayd, Dwayde, Dwaed, Dwaede

Dwight (Flemish) A white- or blond-haired man
Dwite, Dwhite, Dwyght, Dwighte

Dyami (Native American) Resembling an eagle
Dyamie, Dyamy, Dyamey, Dyamee, Dyamea, Dyame

Dyer (English) A creative man
Dier, Dyar, Diar, Dy, Dye, Di, Die

Dylan (Welsh) Son of the sea
Dyllan, Dylon, Dyllon, Dylen, Dyllen, Dylun, Dyllun, Dylin

Dzigbode (African) One who is patient

E

Eagan (Irish) A fiery man
Eegan, Eagen, Eegen, Eagon, Eegon, Eagun, Eegun

Eagle (Native American) Resembling the bird
Eegle, Eagel, Eegel

Eamon (Irish) Form of Edmund, meaning "a wealthy protector"
Eaman, Eamen, Eamin, Eamyn, Eamun, Eamonn, Eames, Eemon

Ean (Gaelic) Form of John, meaning "God is gracious"
Eion, Eyan, Eyon, Eian

Earl (English) A nobleman
Earle, Erle, Erl, Eorl

Eastman (English) A man from the east
East, Easte, Eeste

Easton (English) Eastern place
Eastan, Easten, Eastyn

Eckhard (German) Of the brave sword point
Eckard, Eckardt, Eckhardt, Ekkehard, Ekkehardt, Ekhard, Ekhardt

Ed (English) Form of Edward, meaning "a wealthy protector"
Edd, Eddi, Eddie, Eddy, Eddey, Eddee, Eddea, Edi

Edan (Celtic) One who is full of fire
Edon, Edun

Edbert (English) One who is prosperous and bright
Edberte, Edburt, Edburte, Edbirt, Edbirte, Edbyrt, Edbyrte

Edenson (English) Son of Eden
Eadenson, Edensun, Eadensun, Edinson

Edgar (English) A powerful and wealthy spearman
Eadger, Edgardo, Edghur, Edger

Edison (English) Son of Edward
Eddison, Edisun, Eddisun, Edisen, Eddisen, Edisyn, Eddisyn, Edyson

Edlin (Anglo-Saxon) A wealthy friend
Edlinn, Edlinne, Edlyn, Edlynn, Edlynne, Eadlyn, Eadlin, Edlen

Edmund (English) A wealthy protector
Ed, Eddie, Edmond, Eamon

Edom (Hebrew) A red-haired man
Edum, Edam, Edem, Edim, Edym

Edred (Anglo-Saxon) A king
Edread, Edrid, Edryd

Edward (English) A wealthy protector
Ed, Eadward, Edik, Edouard, Eduard, Eduardo, Edvard, Edvardas, Edwardo

Edwardson (English) The son of Edward
Edwardsun, Eadwardsone, Eadwardsun

Edwin (English) A wealthy friend
Edwinn, Edwinne, Edwine, Edwyn, Edwynn, Edwynne, Edwen, Edwenn

Effiom (African) Resembling a crocodile
Efiom, Effyom, Efyom, Effeom, Efeom

Efrain (Spanish) Form of Ephraim, meaning "one who is fertile; productive"
Efraine, Efrayn, Efrayne, Efraen, Efraene, Efrane

Egesa (Anglo-Saxon) One who creates terror
Egessa, Egeslic, Egeslick, Egeslik

Eghert (German) An intelligent man
Egherte, Eghurt, Eghurte, Eghirt, Eghirte, Eghyrt

Eilert (Scandinavian) Of the hard point
Elert, Eilart, Elart, Eilort, Elort, Eilurt, Elurt, Eilirt

Eilon (Hebrew) From the oak tree
Eilan, Eilin, Eilyn, Eilen, Eilun

Einar (Scandinavian) A leading warrior
Einer, Ejnar, Einir, Einyr, Einor, Einur, Ejnir, Ejnyr

Einri (Teutonic) An intelligent man
Einrie, Einry, Einrey, Einree, Einrea

Eisig (Hebrew) One who laughs often
Eisyg

Eladio (Spanish) A man from Greece
Eladeo, Eladiyo, Eladeyo

Elbert (English / German) A well-born man / a bright man
Elberte, Elburt, Elburte, Elbirt, Elbirte, Ethelbert, Ethelburt, Ethelbirt

Eldan (English) From the valley of the elves

Eldon (English) From the sacred hill
Eldun

Eldorado (Spanish) The golden man

Eldred (English) An old, wise advisor
Eldrid, Eldryd, Eldrad, Eldrod, Edlrud, Ethelred

Eldrick (English) An old, wise ruler
Eldrik, Eldric, Eldryck, Eldryk, Eldryc, Eldrich

Eleazar (Hebrew) God will help
Elazar, Eleasar, Eliezer, Elazaro, Eleazaro, Elazer

Eli (Hebrew) One who has ascended; my God on High
Ely

Eliachim (Hebrew) God will establish
Eliakim, Elyachim, Elyakim, Eliakym

Elian (Spanish) A spirited man
Elyan, Elien, Elyen, Elion, Elyon, Eliun, Elyun

Elias (Hebrew) Form of Elijah, meaning "Jehovah is my god"
Eliyas

Elihu (Hebrew) My God is He
Elyhu, Elihue, Elyhue

Elijah (Hebrew) Jehovah is my God
Elija, Eliyahu, Eljah, Elja, Elyjah, Elyja, Elijuah, Elyjuah

Elimu (African) Having knowledge of science
Elymu, Elimue, Elymue, Elimoo, Elymoo

Elisha (Hebrew) God is my salvation
Elisee, Eliseo, Elisher, Eliso, Elisio, Elysha, Elysee, Elyseo

Elliott (English) Form of Elijah, meaning "Jehovah is my God"
Eliot, Eliott, Elliot, Elyot

Ellory (Cornish) Resembling a swan
Ellorey, Elloree, Ellorea, Ellori, Ellorie, Elory, Elorey

Ellsworth (English) From the nobleman's estate
Elsworth, Ellswerth, Elswerth, Ellswirth, Elswirth, Elzie

Elman (English) A nobleman
Elmann, Ellman, Ellmann

Elmo (English / Latin) A protector / an amiable man
Elmoe, Elmow, Elmowe

Elmot (American) A lovable man
Elmott, Ellmot, Ellmott

Elof (Swedish) The only heir
Eluf, Eloff, Eluff, Elov, Ellov, Eluv, Elluv

Elois (German) A famous warrior
Eloys, Eloyis, Elouis

Elpidio (Spanish) A fearless man; having heart
Elpydio, Elpideo, Elpydeo, Elpidios, Elpydios, Elpidius

Elroy (Irish / English) A red-haired young man / a king
Elroi, Elroye, Elric, Elryc, Elrik, Elryk, Elrick, Elryck

Elston (English) From the nobleman's town
Ellston, Elstun, Ellstun, Elson, Ellson, Elsun, Ellsun

Elton (English) From the old town
Ellton, Eltun, Elltun, Elten, Ellten, Eltin, Elltin, Eltyn

Eluwilussit (Native American) A holy man

Elvis (Scandinavian) One who is wise
Elviss, Elvys, Elvyss

Elzie (English) Form of Ellsworth, meaning "from the nobleman's estate"
Elzi, Elzy, Elzey, Elzee, Elzea, Ellzi, Ellzie, Ellzee

Emest (German) One who is serious
Emeste, Emesto, Emestio, Emestiyo, Emesteo, Emesteyo, Emo, Emst

Emil (Latin) One who is eager; an industrious man
Emelen, Emelio, Emile, Emilian, Emiliano, Emilianus, Emilio, Emilion

Emiliano (Spanish) Form of Emil, meaning "one who is eager"

Emmanuel (Hebrew) God is with us
Manuel, Manny, Em, Eman, Emmannuel

Emmett (German) A universal man
Emmet, Emmit, Emmitt, Emmot

Emrys (Welsh) An immortal man

Enapay (Native American) A brave man
Enapaye, Enapai, Enapae

Enar (Swedish) A great warrior
Ener, Enir, Enyr, Enor, Enur

Engelbert (German) As bright as an angel
Englebert, Englbert, Engelburt, Engleburt, Englburt, Englebirt, Engelbirt, Englbirt

Enoch (Hebrew) One who is dedicated to God
Enoc, Enok, Enock

Enrique (Spanish) The ruler of the estate
Enrico, Enriko, Enricko, Enriquez, Enrikay, Enreekay, Enrik, Enric

Enyeto (Native American) One who walks like a bear

Enzo (Italian) The ruler of the estate
Enzio, Enzeo, Enziyo, Enzeyo

Ephraim (Hebrew) One who is fertile; productive
Eff, Efraim, Efram, Efrem, Efrain

Eric (Scandinavian) Ever the ruler
Erek, Erich, Erick, Erik, Eriq, Erix, Errick, Eryk

Ernest (English) One who is sincere and determined; serious
Earnest, Ernesto, Ernestus, Ernst, Erno, Ernie, Erni, Erney

Eron (Spanish) Form of Aaron, meaning "one who is exalted"
Erun, Erin, Eran, Eren, Eryn

Erskine (Gaelic) From the high cliff
Erskin, Erskyne, Erskyn, Erskein, Erskeine, Erskien, Erskiene

Esam (Arabic) A safeguard
Essam

Esben (Scandinavian) Of God
Esbin, Esbyn, Esban, Esbon, Esbun

Esmé (French) One who is esteemed
Esmay, Esmaye, Esmai, Esmae, Esmeling, Esmelyng

Esmun (American) A kind man
Esmon, Esman, Esmen, Esmin, Esmyn

Esperanze (Spanish) Filled with hope
Esperance, Esperence, Esperenze, Esperanzo, Esperenzo

Estcott (English) From the eastern cottage
Estcot

Esteban (Spanish) One who is crowned in victory
Estebon, Estevan, Estevon, Estefan, Estefon, Estebe, Estyban, Estyvan

Ethan (Hebrew) One who is firm and steadfast
Ethen, Ethin, Ethyn, Ethon, Ethun, Eitan, Etan, Eithan

Ethanael (American) God has given me strength
Ethaniel, Ethaneal, Ethanail, Ethanale

Ethel (Hebrew) One who is noble
Ethal, Etheal

Etlelooaat (Native American) One who shouts

Eudocio (Greek) One who is respected
Eudoceo, Eudociyo, Eudoceyo, Eudoco

Eugene (Greek) A well-born man
Eugean, Eugenie, Ugene, Efigenio, Gene, Owen

Eulogio (Greek) A reasonable man
Eulogiyo, Eulogo, Eulogeo, Eulogeyo

Euodias (Greek) Having good fortune
Euodeas, Euodyas

Euphemios (Greek) One who is well-spoken
Eufemio, Eufemius, Euphemio, Eufemios, Euphemius, Eufemius

Euphrates (Turkish) From the great river
Eufrates, Euphraites, Eufraites, Euphraytes, Eufraytes

Eusebius (Greek) One who is devout
Esabio, Esavio, Esavius, Esebio, Eusabio, Eusaio, Eusebio, Eusebios

Eustace (Greek) Having an abundance of grapes
Eustache, Eustachios, Eustachius, Eustachy, Eustaquio, Eustashe, Eustasius, Eustatius

Evan (Welsh) Form of John, meaning "God is gracious"
Evann, Evans, Even, Evin, Evon, Evyn, Evian, Evien

Evander (Greek) A benevolent man
Evandor, Evandar, Evandir, Evandur, Evandyr

Everett (English) Form of Everhard, meaning "as strong as a bear"

Evett (American) A bright man
Evet, Evatt, Evat, Evitt, Evit, Evytt, Evyt

Eyal (Hebrew) Having great strength

Eze (African) A king

Ezeji (African) The king of yams
Ezejie, Ezejy, Ezejey, Ezejee, Ezejea

Ezekiel (Hebrew) Strengthened by God
Esequiel, Ezechiel, Eziechiele, Eziequel, Ezequiel, Ezekial, Ezekyel, Esquevelle, Zeke

Fairbairn (Scottish) A fair-haired boy
Fayrbairn, Faerbairn, Fairbaern, Fayrbaern, Faerbaern, Fairbayrn, Fayrbayrn, Faerbayrn

Fairbanks (English) From the bank along the path
Fayrbanks, Faerbanks, Farebanks

Faisal (Arabic) One who is decisive; resolute
Faysal, Faesal, Fasal, Feisal, Faizal, Fasel, Fayzal, Faezal

Fakhir (Arabic) A proud man
Fakheer, Fakhear, Fakheir, Fakhier, Fakhyr, Faakhir, Faakhyr, Fakhr

Fakih (Arabic) A legal expert
Fakeeh, Fakeah, Fakieh, Fakeih, Fakyh

Falco (Latin) Resembling a falcon; one who works with falcons
Falcon, Falconer, Falconner, Falk, Falke, Falken, Falkner, Faulconer

Fang (Scottish) From the sheep pen
Faing, Fayng, Faeng

Faraji (African) One who provides consolation
Farajie, Farajy, Farajey, Farajee, Farajea

Fardoragh (Irish) Having dark features

Farha (Arabic) Filled with happiness
Farhah, Farhad, Farhan, Farhat, Farhani, Farhanie, Farhany, Farhaney

Fariq (Arabic) One who holds rank as lieutenant general
Fareeq, Fareaq, Fareiq, Farieq, Faryq, Farik, Fareek, Fareak

Farnell (English) From the fern hill
Farnel, Farnall, Farnal, Fernauld, Farnauld, Fernald, Farnald

Farold (English) A mighty traveler
Farould, Farald, Farauld, Fareld

Farran (Irish / Arabic / English) Of the land / a baker / one who is adventurous
Fairran, Fayrran, Faerran, Farren, Farrin, Farron, Ferrin, Ferron

Farrar (English) A blacksmith
Farar, Farrer, Farrier, Ferrar, Ferrars, Ferrer, Ferrier, Farer

Farro (Italian) Of the grain
Farroe, Faro, Faroe, Farrow, Farow

Fatik (Indian) Resembling a crystal
Fateek, Fateak, Fatyk, Fatiek, Fateik

Faust (Latin) Having good luck
Fauste, Faustino, Fausto, Faustos, Faustus, Fauston, Faustin, Fausten

Fawcett (American) An audacious man
Fawcet, Fawcette, Fawcete, Fawce, Fawci, Fawcie, Fawcy, Fawcey

Fawwaz (Arabic) A successful man
Fawaz, Fawwad, Fawad

Fay (Irish) Resembling a raven
Faye, Fai, Fae, Feich

Februus (Latin) A pagan god

Fedor (Russian) A gift from God
Faydor, Feodor, Fyodor, Fedyenka, Fyodr, Fydor, Fjodor

Feivel (Hebrew) The brilliant one
Feival, Feivol, Feivil, Feivyl, Feivul, Feiwel, Feiwal, Feiwol

Felim (Gaelic) One who is always good
Felym, Feidhlim, Felimy, Felimey, Felimee, Felimea, Felimi, Felimie

Felipe (Spanish) Form of Phillip, meaning "one who loves horses"
Felippe, Filip, Filippo, Fillip, Flip, Fulop, Fullop, Fulip

Felix (Latin) One who is happy and prosperous

Felton (English) From the town near the field
Feltun, Felten, Feltan, Feltyn, Feltin

Fenn (English) From the marsh
Fen

Ferdinand (German) A courageous voyager
Ferdie, Ferdinando, Fernando

Fergus (Gaelic) The first and supreme choice
Fearghas, Fearghus, Feargus, Fergie, Ferguson, Fergusson, Furgus, Fergy

Ferrell (Irish) A brave man; a hero
Ferell, Ferel, Ferrel

Fiacre (Celtic) Resembling a raven
Fyacre, Fiacra, Fyacra, Fiachra, Fyachra, Fiachre, Fyachre

Fielding (English) From the field
Fieldyng, Fielder, Field, Fielde, Felding, Feldyng, Fields

Fiero (Spanish) A fiery man
Fyero

Finbar (Irish) A fair-haired man
Finnbar, Finnbarr, Fionn, Fionnbharr, Fionnbar, Fionnbarr, Fynbar, Fynnbar

Finch (English) Resembling the small bird
Fynch, Finche, Fynche, Finchi, Finchie, Finchy, Finchey, Finchee

Fineas (Egyptian) A dark-skinned man
Fyneas, Finius, Fynius

Finian (Irish) A handsome man; fair
Finan, Finnian, Fionan, Finien, Finnien, Finghin, Finneen, Fineen

Finn (Gaelic) A fair-haired
man
Fin, Fynn, Fyn, Fingal, Fingall

Finnegan (Irish) A fair-haired
man
*Finegan, Finnegen, Finegen,
Finnigan, Finigan*

Finnley (Gaelic) A fair-haired
hero
*Findlay, Findley, Finly, Finlay,
Finlee, Finnly, Finnley*

Fiorello (Italian) Resembling a
little flower
*Fiorelo, Fiorelio, Fioreleo,
Fiorellio, Fiorelleo*

Fisher (English) A fisherman
Fischer, Fysher

Fitch (English) Resembling an
ermine
Fytch, Fich, Fych, Fitche, Fytche

Fitzgerald (English) The son of
Gerald
Fytzgerald

Flann (Irish) One who has a
ruddy complexion
*Flan, Flainn, Flannan,
Flannery, Flanneri, Flannerie,
Flannerey*

Fletcher (English) One who
makes arrows
Fletch, Fletche, Flecher

Flynn (Irish) One who has a
ruddy complexion
*Flyn, Flinn, Flin, Flen, Flenn,
Floinn*

Fogarty (Irish) One who has
been exiled
*Fogartey, Fogartee, Fogartea,
Fogarti, Fogartie, Fogerty,
Fogertey, Fogerti*

Foley (English) A creative man
Foly, Folee, Foli, Folie

Folker (German) A guardian of
the people
*Folkar, Folkor, Folkur, Folkir,
Folkyr, Folke, Folko, Folkus*

Fonso (German) Form of
Alfonso, meaning "prepared
for battle; eager and ready"
*Fonzo, Fonsie, Fonzell, Fonzie,
Fonsi, Fonsy, Fonsey, Fonsee*

Fontaine (French) From the
water source
*Fontayne, Fontaene, Fontane,
Fonteyne, Fontana, Fountain*

Ford (English) From the river
crossing
*Forde, Forden, Fordan, Fordon,
Fordun, Fordin, Fordyn, Forday*

Fouad (Arabic) One who
has heart
Fuad

Francisco (Spanish) A man from France
Francesco, Franchesco, Fransisco

Frank (Latin) Form of Francis, meaning "a man from France; one who is free"
Franco, Frankie

Fred (German) Form of Frederick, meaning "a peaceful ruler"
Freddi, Freddie, Freddy, Freddey, Freddee, Freddea, Freddis, Fredis

Frederick (German) A peaceful ruler
Fred, Fredrick, Federico, Federigo, Fredek, Frederic, Frederich, Frederico, Frederik, Fredric

Fremont (French) The protector of freedom
Freemont, Fremonte

Frigyes (Hungarian) A mighty and peaceful ruler

Frode (Norse) A wise man
Froad, Froade

Froyim (Hebrew) A kind man
Froiim

Fu (Chinese) A wealthy man

Fudail (Arabic) Of high moral character
Fudaile, Fudayl, Fudayle, Fudale, Fudael, Fudaele

Fulbright (English) A brilliant man
Fullbright, Fulbrite, Fullbrite, Fulbryte, Fullbryte, Fulbert, Fullbert

Fulki (Indian) A spark
Fulkie, Fulkey, Fulky, Fulkee, Fulkea

Fullerton (English) From Fuller's town
Fullertun, Fullertin, Fullertyn, Fullertan, Fullerten

Fursey (Gaelic) The name of a missionary saint
Fursy, Fursi, Fursie, Fursee, Fursea

Fyfe (Scottish) A man from Fifeshire
Fife, Fyffe, Fiffe, Fibh

Fyren (Anglo-Saxon) A wicked man
Fyrin, Fyryn, Fyran, Fyron, Fyrun

G

Gabai (Hebrew) A delightful man

Gabbana (Italian) A creative man
Gabbanah, Gabana, Gabanah, Gabbanna, Gabanna

Gabor (Hebrew) God is my strength
Gabur, Gabar, Gaber, Gabir, Gabyr

Gabra (African) An offering
Gabre

Gabriel (Hebrew) A hero of God
Gabrian, Gabriele, Gabrielli, Gabriello, Gaby, Gab, Gabbi, Gabbie

Gad (Hebrew / Native American) Having good fortune / from the juniper tree
Gadi, Gadie, Gady, Gadey, Gadee, Gadea

Gadiel (Arabic) God is my fortune
Gadiell, Gadiele, Gadielle, Gaddiel, Gaddiell, Gadil, Gadeel, Gadeal

Gaffney (Irish) Resembling a calf
Gaffny, Gaffni, Gaffnie, Gaffnee, Gaffnea

Gage (French) Of the pledge
Gaige, Gaege, Gauge

Gahuj (African) A hunter

Gair (Gaelic) A man of short stature
Gayr, Gaer, Gaire, Gayre, Gaere, Gare

Gaius (Latin) One who rejoices
Gaeus

Galal (Arabic) A majestic man
Galall, Gallal, Gallall

Galbraith (Irish) A foreigner; a Scot
Galbrait, Galbreath, Gallbraith, Gallbreath, Galbraithe, Gallbraithe, Galbreathe, Gallbreathe

Gale (Irish / English) A foreigner / one who is cheerful
Gail, Gaill, Gaille, Gaile, Gayl, Gayle, Gaylle, Gayll

Galen (Greek) A healer; one who is calm
Gaelan, Gaillen, Galan, Galin, Galyn, Gaylen, Gaylin, Gaylinn

Gali (Hebrew) From the fountain
Galie, Galy, Galey, Galee, Galea, Galeigh

Galip (Turkish) A victorious man
Galyp, Galup, Galep, Galap, Galop

Gallagher (Gaelic) An eager helper
Gallaghor, Gallaghar, Gallaghur, Gallaghir, Gallaghyr, Gallager, Gallagar, Gallagor

Galt (English) From the high, wooded land
Galte, Gallt, Gallte

Galtero (Spanish) Form of Walter, meaning "the commander of the army"
Galterio, Galteriyo, Galtereo, Galtereyo, Galter, Galteros, Galterus, Gualterio

Gamaliel (Hebrew) God's reward
Gamliel, Gamalyel, Gamlyel, Gamli, Gamlie, Gamly, Gamley, Gamlee

Gameel (Arabic) A handsome man
Gameal, Gamil, Gamiel, Gameil, Gamyl

Gamon (American) One who enjoys playing games
Gamun, Gamen, Gaman, Gamin, Gamyn, Gammon, Gammun, Gamman

Gan (Chinese) A wanderer

Gann (English) One who defends with a spear
Gan

Gannon (Gaelic) A fair-skinned man
Gannun, Gannen, Gannan, Gannin, Gannyn, Ganon, Ganun, Ganin

Garcia (Spanish) One who is brave in battle
Garce, Garcy, Garcey, Garci, Garcie, Garcee, Garcea

Gared (English) Form of Gerard, meaning "one who is mighty with a spear"
Garad, Garid, Garyd, Garod, Garud

Garrett (English) Form of Gerard, meaning "one who is mighty with a spear"
Garett, Garret, Garretson, Garritt, Garrot, Garrott, Gerrit, Gerritt

Garrison (French) Prepared
Garris, Garrish, Garry, Gary

Garson (English) The son of Gar (Garrett, Garrison, etc.)
Garrson, Garsen, Garrsen, Garsun, Garrsun, Garsone, Garrsone

Garth (Scandinavian) The keeper of the garden
Garthe, Gart, Garte

Garvey (Gaelic) A rough but peaceful man
Garvy, Garvee, Garvea, Garvi, Garvie, Garrvey, Garrvy, Garrvee

Garvin (English) A friend with a spear
Garvyn, Garven, Garvan, Garvon, Garvun

Gary (English) One who wields a spear
Garey, Gari, Garie, Garea, Garee, Garry, Garrey, Garree

Gassur (Arabic) A courageous man
Gassor, Gassir, Gassyr, Gassar, Gasser

Gaston (French) A man from Gascony
Gastun, Gastan, Gasten, Gascon, Gascone, Gasconey, Gasconi, Gasconie

Gate (American) One who is close-minded
Gates, Gait, Gaite, Gaits

Gavin (Welsh) A little white falcon
Gavan, Gaven, Gavino, Gavyn, Gavynn, Gavon, Gavun, Gavyno

Gazali (African) A mystic
Gazalie, Gazaly, Gazaley, Gazalee, Gazalea, Gazaleigh

Geirleif (Norse) A descendant of the spear
Geirleaf, Geerleif, Geerleaf

Geirstein (Norse) One who wields a rock-hard spear
Geerstein, Gerstein

Gellert (Hungarian) A mighty soldier
Gellart, Gellirt, Gellyrt, Gellort, Gellurt

Genaro (Latin) A dedicated man
Genaroh, Genaroe, Genarow, Genarowe

Gene (English) Form of Eugene, meaning "a well-born man"
Genio, Geno, Geneo, Gino, Ginio, Gineo

Genet (African) From Eden
Genat, Genit, Genyt, Genot, Genut

Genoah (Italian) From the city of Genoa
Genoa, Genovise, Genovize

Geoffrey (English) Form of Jeffrey, meaning "a man of peace"
Geffrey, Geoff, Geoffery, Geoffroy, Geoffry, Geofrey, Geofferi, Geofferie

George (Greek) One who works the earth; a farmer
Georas, Geordi, Geordie, Georg, Georges, Georgi, Georgie, Georgio, Yegor, Jurgen, Joren

Gerald (German) One who rules with the spear
Jerald, Garald, Garold, Gearalt, Geralde, Geraldo, Geraud, Gere, Gerek

Gerard (French) One who is mighty with a spear
Gerord, Gerrard, Gared, Garrett

Germain (French / Latin) A man from Germany / one who is brotherly
Germaine, German, Germane, Germanicus, Germano, Germanus, Germayn, Germayne

Gerry (German) Short form of names beginning with Ger-, such as Gerald or Gerard
Gerrey, Gerri, Gerrie, Gerrea, Gerree

Gershom (Hebrew) One who has been exiled
Gersham, Gershon, Gershoom, Gershem, Gershim, Gershym, Gershum, Gersh

Getachew (African) Their master

Ghazi (Arabic) An invader; a conqueror
Ghazie, Ghazy, Ghazey, Ghazee, Ghazea

Ghoukas (Armenian) Form of Lucas, meaning "a man from Lucania"
Ghukas

Giancarlo (Italian) One who is gracious and mighty
Gyancarlo

Gideon (Hebrew) A mighty warrior; one who fells trees
Gideone, Gidi, Gidon, Gidion, Gid, Gidie, Gidy, Gidey

Gilam (Hebrew) The joy of the people
Gylam, Gilem, Gylem, Gilim, Gylim, Gilym, Gylym, Gilom

Gilbert (French / English) Of the bright promise / one who is trustworthy
Gib, Gibb, Gil, Gilberto, Gilburt, Giselbert, Giselberto, Giselbertus

Gildas (Irish / English) One who serves God / the golden one
Gyldas, Gilda, Gylda, Gilde, Gylde, Gildea, Gyldea, Gildes

Giles (Greek) Resembling a young goat
Gyles, Gile, Gil, Gilles, Gillis, Gilliss, Gyle, Gyl

Gill (Gaelic) A servant
Gyll, Gilly, Gilley, Gillee, Gillea, Gilli, Gillie, Ghill

Gillivray (Scottish) A servant
of God
Gillivraye, Gillivrae, Gillivrai

Gilmat (Scottish) One who
wields a sword
Gylmat, Gilmet, Gylmet

Gilmer (English) A famous
hostage
*Gilmar, Gilmor, Gilmur,
Gilmir, Gilmyr, Gillmer,
Gillmar, Gillmor*

Gilon (Hebrew) Filled with joy
*Gilun, Gilen, Gilan, Gilin,
Gilyn, Gilo*

Ginton (Arabic) From the gar-
den
*Gintun, Gintan, Ginten,
Gintin, Gintyn*

Giovanni (Italian) Form of
John, meaning "God is gra-
cious"
*Geovani, Geovanney, Geovanni,
Geovanny, Geovany, Giannino,
Giovan, Giovani, Yovanny*

Giri (Indian) From the mountain
Girie, Giry, Girey, Giree, Girea

Girvan (Gaelic) The small
rough one
*Gyrvan, Girven, Gyrven,
Girvin, Gyrvin, Girvyn, Gyrvyn,
Girvon*

Giulio (Italian) One who is
youthful
Giuliano, Giuleo

Giuseppe (Italian) Form of
Joseph, meaning "God will
add"
*Giuseppi, Giuseppie, Giuseppy,
Giuseppee, Giuseppea,
Giuseppey, Guiseppe, Guiseppi*

Glade (English) From the
clearing in the woods
*Glayd, Glayde, Glaid, Glaide,
Glaed, Glaede*

Glaisne (Irish) One who is
calm; serene
*Glaisny, Glaisney, Glaisni,
Glaisnie, Glaisnee, Glasny,
Glasney, Glasni*

Glasgow (Scottish) From the
city in Scotland
Glasgo

Glen (Gaelic) From the secluded
narrow valley
*Glenn, Glennard, Glennie,
Glennon, Glenny, Glin, Glinn,
Glyn*

Glover (English) One who
makes gloves
*Glovar, Glovir, Glovyr, Glovur,
Glovor*

Gobind (Sanskrit) The cow finder
Gobinde, Gobinda, Govind, Govinda, Govinde

Goby (American) An audacious man
Gobi, Gobie, Gobey, Gobee, Gobea

Godfrey (German) God is peace
Giotto, Godefroi, Godfry, Godofredo, Goffredo, Gottfrid, Gottfried, Godfried

Godfried (German) God is peace
Godfreed, Gjord

Gogo (African) A grandfatherly man

Goldwin (English) A golden friend
Goldwine, Goldwinn, Goldwinne, Goldwen, Goldwenn, Goldwenne, Goldwyn, Goldwynn

Goode (English) An upstanding man
Good, Goodi, Goodie, Goody, Goodey, Goodee, Goodea

Gordon (Gaelic) From the great hill; a hero
Gorden, Gordin, Gordyn, Gordun, Gordan, Gordi, Gordie, Gordee

Gormley (Irish) The blue spearman
Gormly, Gormlee, Gormlea, Gormleah, Gormleigh, Gormli, Gormlie, Gormaly

Goro (Japanese) The fifth-born child

Gotzon (Basque) A heavenly messenger; an angel

Gower (Welsh) One who is pure; chaste
Gwyr, Gowyr, Gowir, Gowar, Gowor, Gowur

Gozal (Hebrew) Resembling a baby bird
Gozall, Gozel, Gozell, Gozale, Gozele

Grady (Gaelic) One who is famous; noble
Gradey, Gradee, Gradea, Gradi, Gradie, Graidy, Graidey, Graidee

Graham (English) From the graveled area; from the gray home
Graem

Grand (English) A superior man
Grande, Grandy, Grandey, Grandi, Grandie, Grandee, Grandea, Grander

Granger (English) A farmer
Grainger, Graynger, Graenger, Grange, Graynge, Graenge, Grainge, Grangere

Grant (English) A tall man;
a great man
Grante, Graent

Gray (English) A gray-haired
man
Graye, Grai, Grae, Greye, Grey, Graylon, Graylen, Graylin

Grayson (English) The son of
a gray-haired man
Graysen, Graysun, Graysin, Greyson, Graysan, Graison, Graisun, Graisen

Greenwood (English) From
the green forest
Greenwode

Gregory (Greek) One who is
vigilant; watchful
Greg, Greggory, Greggy, Gregori, Gregorie, Gregry, Grigori

Gremian (Anglo-Saxon) One
who enrages others
Gremien, Gremean, Gremyan

Gridley (English) From the flat
meadow
Gridly, Gridlee, Gridlea, Gridleah, Gridleigh, Gridli, Gridlie

Griffin (Latin) Having a
hooked nose
Griff, Griffen, Griffon, Gryffen, Gryffin, Gryphen

Griffith (Welsh) A mighty chief
Griffyth, Gryffith, Gryffyth

Grimsley (English) From the
dark meadow
Grimsly, Grimslee, Grimslea, Grimsleah, Grimsleigh, Grimsli, Grimslie

Griswold (German) From the
gray forest
Griswald, Gryswold, Gryswald, Greswold, Greswald

Guban (African) One who has
been burnt
Guben, Gubin, Gubyn, Gubon, Gubun

Guerdon (English) A warring
man
Guerdun, Guerdan, Guerden, Guerdin, Guerdyn

Guido (Italian) One who acts
as a guide
Guidoh, Gwedo, Gwido, Gwydo, Gweedo

Guillaume (French) Form of
William, meaning "the deter-
mined protector"
Gillermo, Guglielmo, Guilherme, Guillermo, Gwillyn, Gwilym, Guglilmo

Gulshan (Hindi) From the gardens

Gunner (Scandinavian) A bold warrior
Gunnar, Gunnor, Gunnur, Gunnir, Gunnyr

Gunnolf (Norse) A warrior wolf
Gunolf, Gunnulf, Gunulf

Gur (Hebrew) Resembling a lion cub
Guryon, Gurion, Guriel, Guriell, Guryel, Guryell, Guri, Gurie

Gurpreet (Indian) A devoted follower
Gurpreat, Gurpriet, Gurpreit, Gurprit, Gurpryt

Gurutz (Basque) Of the holy cross
Guruts

Gus (German) A respected man; one who is exalted
Guss

Gustav (Scandinavian) Of the staff of the gods
Gus, Gustave, Gussie, Gustaf, Gustof, Tavin

Guwayne (American) Form of Wayne, meaning "one who builds wagons"
Guwayn, Guwain, Guwaine, Guwaen, Guwaene, Guwane

Gwalchmai (Welsh) A battle hawk

Gwandoya (African) Suffering a miserable fate

Gwydion (Welsh) In mythology, a magician
Gwydeon, Gwydionne, Gwydeonne

Gylfi (Scandinavian) A king
Gylfie, Gylfee, Gylfea, Gylfi, Gylfie, Gylphi, Gylphie, Gylphey

Gypsy (English) A wanderer; a nomad
Gipsee, Gipsey, Gipsy, Gypsi, Gypsie, Gypsey, Gypsee, Gipsi

H

Hadden (English) From the heather-covered hill
Haddan, Haddon, Haddin, Haddyn, Haddun

Hadriel (Hebrew) The splendor of God
Hadryel, Hadriell, Hadryell

Hadwin (English) A friend in war
Hadwinn, Hadwinne, Hadwen, Hadwenn, Hadwenne, Hadwyn, Hadwynn, Hadwynne

Hafiz (Arabic) A protector
Haafiz, Hafeez, Hafeaz, Hafiez, Hafeiz, Hafyz, Haphiz, Haaphiz

Hagar (Hebrew) A wanderer

Hagen (Gaelic) One who is youthful
Haggen, Hagan, Haggan, Hagin, Haggin, Hagyn, Haggyn, Hagon

Hagop (Armenian) Form of James, meaning "he who supplants"
Hagup, Hagap, Hagep, Hagip, Hagyp

Hagos (African) Filled with happiness

Hahnee (Native American) A beggar
Hahnea, Hahni, Hahnie, Hahny, Hahney

Haim (Hebrew) A giver of life
Hayim, Hayyim

Haines (English) From the vined cottage; from the hedged enclosure
Haynes, Haenes, Hanes, Haine, Hayne, Haene, Hane

Hajari (African) One who takes flight
Hajarie, Hajary, Hajarey, Hajaree, Hajarea

Haji (African) Born during the hajj
Hajie, Hajy, Hajey, Hajee, Hajea

Hakan (Norse / Native American) One who is noble / a fiery man

Hakim (Arabic) One who is wise; intelligent
Hakeem, Hakeam, Hakeim, Hakiem, Hakym

Hal (English) A form of Henry, meaning "the ruler of the house"; a form of Harold, meaning "the ruler of an army"

Halford (English) From the hall by the ford
Hallford, Halfurd, Hallfurd, Halferd, Hallferd

Halil (Turkish) A beloved friend
Haleel, Haleal, Haleil, Haliel, Halyl

Halla (African) An unexpected gift
Hallah, Hala, Halah

Hallberg (Norse) From the rocky mountain
Halberg, Hallburg, Halburg

Halle (Norse) As solid as a rock

Halley (English) From the hall near the meadow
Hally, Halli, Hallie, Halleigh, Hallee, Halleah, Hallea

Halliwell (English) From the holy spring
Haligwell

Hallward (English) The guardian of the hall
Halward, Hallwerd, Halwerd, Hallwarden, Halwarden, Hawarden, Haward, Hawerd

Hamid (Arabic / Indian) A praiseworthy man / a beloved friend
Hameed, Hamead, Hameid, Hamied, Hamyd, Haamid

Hamidi (Swahili) One who is commendable
Hamidie, Hamidy, Hamidey, Hamidee, Hamidea, Hamydi, Hamydie, Hamydee

Hamilton (English) From the flat-topped hill
Hamylton, Hamiltun, Hamyltun, Hamilten, Hamylten, Hamelton, Hameltun, Hamelten

Hamlet (German) From the little home
Hamlett, Hammet, Hammett, Hamnet, Hamnett, Hamlit, Hamlitt, Hamoelet

Hammer (German) One who makes hammers; a carpenter
Hammar, Hammor, Hammur, Hammir, Hammyr

Hancock (English) One who owns a farm
Hancok, Hancoc

Hanford (English) From the high ford
Hanferd, Hanfurd, Hanforde, Hanferde, Hanfurde

Hanisi (Swahili) Born on a Thursday
Hanisie, Hanisy, Hanisey, Hanisee, Hanisea, Hanysi, Hanysie, Hanysy

Hank (English) Form of Henry, meaning "the ruler of the house"
Hanke, Hanks, Hanki, Hankie, Hankee, Hankea, Hanky, Hankey

Hanley (English) From the high meadow
Hanly, Hanleigh, Hanleah, Hanlea, Hanlie, Hanli

Hanoch (Hebrew) One who is
dedicated
Hanock, Hanok, Hanoc

Hanraoi (Irish) Form of
Henry, meaning "the ruler of
the house"

Hansraj (Hindi) The swan
king

Hardik (Indian) One who has
heart
*Hardyk, Hardick, Hardyck,
Hardic, Hardyc*

Hare (English) Resembling a
rabbit

Hari (Indian) Resembling a
lion
*Harie, Hary, Harey, Haree,
Harea*

Harim (Arabic) A superior
man
*Hareem, Haream, Hariem,
Hareim, Harym*

Harkin (Irish) Having dark red
hair
*Harkyn, Harken, Harkan,
Harkon, Harkun*

Harlemm (American) A
soulful man
*Harlam, Harlom, Harlim,
Harlym, Harlem*

Harlow (English) From the
army on the hill
Harlowe, Harlo, Harloe

Harold (Scandinavian) The
ruler of an army
*Hal, Harald, Hareld, Harry,
Darold*

Harper (English) One who
plays or makes harps
*Harpur, Harpar, Harpir,
Harpyr, Harpor, Hearpere*

Harrington (English) From
Harry's town; from the
herring town
*Harringtun, Harryngton,
Harryngtun, Harington,
Haringtun, Haryngton,
Haryntun*

Harrison (English) The son of
Harry
*Harrisson, Harris, Harriss,
Harryson*

Harshad (Indian) A bringer
of joy
*Harsh, Harshe, Harsho,
Harshil, Harshyl, Harshit,
Harshyt*

Hartford (English) From the
stag's ford
*Harteford, Hartferd, Harteferd,
Hartfurd, Hartefurd, Hartforde,
Harteforde, Hartferde*

Haru (Japanese) Born during the spring

Harvey (English / French) One who is ready for battle / a strong man
Harvy, Harvi, Harvie, Harvee, Harvea, Harv, Harve, Hervey

Hasim (Arabic) One who is decisive
Haseem, Haseam, Hasiem, Haseim, Hasym

Haskel (Hebrew) An intelligent man
Haskle, Haskell, Haskil, Haskill, Haske, Hask

Hasso (German) Of the sun
Hassoe, Hassow, Hassowe

Hassun (Native American) As solid as a stone

Hastiin (Native American) A man

Hawes (English) From the hedged place
Haws, Hayes, Hays, Hazin, Hazen, Hazyn, Hazon, Hazan

Hawiovi (Native American) One who descends on a ladder
Hawiovie, Hawiovy, Hawiovey, Hawiovee, Hawiovea

Hawkins (English) Resembling a small hawk
Haukins, Hawkyns, Haukyn

Hawthorne (English) From the hawthorn tree
Hawthorn

Hayden (English) From the hedged valley
Haydan, Haydon, Haydun, Haydin, Haydyn, Haden, Hadan, Hadon

Haye (Scottish) From the stockade
Hay, Hae, Hai

Hazaiah (Hebrew) God will decide
Hazaia, Haziah, Hazia

Hazleton (English) From the hazel-tree town
Hazelton, Hazletun, Hazelton, Hazleten, Hazelten

Heath (English) From the untended land of flowering shrubs
Heathe, Heeth, Heethe

Heaton (English) From the town on high ground
Heatun, Heeton, Heetun, Heaten, Heeten

Heber (Hebrew) A partner or companion
Heeber, Hebar, Heebar, Hebor, Heebor, Hebur, Heebur, Hebir

Hector (Greek) One who is steadfast; in mythology, the prince of Troy
Hecter, Hekter, Heckter

Helio (Greek) Son of the sun
Heleo, Helios, Heleos

Hem (Indian) The golden son

Hemendu (Indian) Born beneath the golden moon
Hemendue, Hemendoo

Hemi (Maori) Form of James, meaning "he who supplants"
Hemie, Hemy, Hemee, Hemea, Hemey

Henderson (Scottish) The son of Henry
Hendrie, Hendries, Hendron, Hendri, Hendry, Hendrey, Hendree, Hendrea

Hendrick (English) Form of Henry, meaning "the ruler of the house"
Hendryck, Hendrik, Hendryk, Hendric, Hendryc, Hendrix

Henley (English) From the high meadow
Henly, Henleigh, Henlea, Henleah, Henlee, Henli, Henlie

Henry (German) The ruler of the house
Hal, Hank, Harry, Henny, Henree, Henri, Hanraoi, Hendrick, Henrik

Heraldo (Spanish) Of the divine

Hercules (Greek) In mythology, a son of Zeus who possessed superhuman strength
Herakles, Hercule, Herculi, Herculie, Herculy, Herculey, Herculee

Herman (German) A soldier
Hermon, Hermen, Hermun, Hermin, Hermyn, Hermann, Hermie

Herne (English) Resembling a heron
Hern, Hearn, Hearne

Hero (Greek) The brave defender
Heroe, Herow, Herowe

Hershel (Hebrew) Resembling a deer
Hersch, Herschel, Herschell, Hersh, Hertzel, Herzel, Herzl, Heschel

Herwin (Teutonic) A friend of war
Herwinn, Herwinne, Herwen, Herwenn, Herwenne, Herwyn, Herwynn, Herwynne

Hesed (Hebrew) A kind man

Hesutu (Native American) A rising yellow-jacket nest
Hesutou, Hesoutou

Hewson (English) The son of Hugh
Hewsun

Hiawatha (Native American) He who makes rivers
Hiawathah, Hyawatha, Hiwatha, Hywatha

Hickok (American) A famous frontier marshal
Hickock, Hickoc, Hikock, Hikoc, Hikok, Hyckok, Hyckock, Hyckoc

Hidalgo (Spanish) The noble one
Hydalgo

Hideaki (Japanese) A clever man; having wisdom
Hideakie, Hideaky, Hideakey, Hideakee, Hideakea

Hietamaki (Finnish) From the sand hill
Hietamakie, Hietamaky, Hietamakey, Hietamakee, Hietamakea

Hieu (Vietnamese) A pious man

Hikmat (Islamic) Filled with wisdom
Hykmat

Hildefuns (German) One who is ready for battle
Hildfuns, Hyldefuns, Hyldfuns

Hillel (Hebrew) One who is praised
Hyllel, Hillell, Hyllell, Hilel, Hylel, Hilell, Hylell

Hiranmay (Indian) The golden one
Hiranmaye, Hiranmai, Hiranmae, Hyranmay, Hyranmaye, Hyranmai, Hyranmae

Hiroshi (Japanese) A generous man
Hiroshie, Hiroshy, Hiroshey, Hiroshee, Hiroshea, Hyroshi, Hyroshie, Hyroshey

Hirsi (African) An amulet
Hirsie, Hirsy, Hirsey, Hirsee, Hirsea

Hisoka (Japanese) One who is secretive
Hysoka, Hisokie, Hysokie, Hisoki, Hysoki, Hisokey, Hysokey, Hisoky

Hitakar (Indian) One who wishes others well
Hitakarin, Hitakrit

Hobart (American) Form of Hubert, meaning "having a shining intellect"
Hobarte, Hoebart, Hoebarte, Hobert, Hoberte, Hoburt, Hoburte, Hobirt

Hohberht (German) One who is high and bright
Hohbert, Hohburt, Hohbirt, Hohbyrt, Hoh

Holcomb (English) From the deep valley
Holcom, Holcombe

Holden (English) From a hollow in the valley
Holdan, Holdyn, Holdon

Holland (American) From the Netherlands
Hollend, Hollind, Hollynd, Hollande, Hollende, Hollinde, Hollynde

Hollis (English) From the holly tree
Hollys, Holliss, Hollyss, Hollace, Hollice, Holli, Hollie, Holly

Holman (English) A man from the valley
Holmann, Holmen, Holmin, Holmyn, Holmon, Holmun

Holt (English) From the forest
Holte, Holyt, Holyte, Holter, Holtar, Holtor, Holtur, Holtir

Honaw (Native American) Resembling a bear
Honawe, Honau

Hondo (African) A warring man
Hondoh, Honda, Hondah

Honesto (Spanish) One who is honest
Honestio, Honestiyo, Honesteo, Honesteyo, Honestoh

Honon (Native American) Resembling a bear
Honun, Honen, Honan, Honin, Honyn

Honovi (Native American) Having great strength
Honovie, Honovy, Honovey, Honovee, Honovea

Honza (Czech) A gift from God

Horst (German) From the thicket
Horste, Horsten, Horstan, Horstin, Horstyn, Horston, Horstun, Horstman

Hoshi (Japanese) Resembling a star
Hoshiko, Hoshyko, Hoshie, Hoshee, Hoshea, Hoshy, Hoshey

Hototo (Native American) One who whistles; a warrior spirit that sings

Houston (Gaelic / English) From Hugh's town / from the town on the hill
Huston, Houstyn, Hustin, Husten, Hustin, Houstun

Howard (English) The guardian of the home
Howerd, Howord, Howurd, Howird, Howyrd, Howi, Howie, Howy

Howi (Native American) Resembling a turtle dove

Hrothgar (Anglo-Saxon) A king
Hrothgarr, Hrothegar, Hrothegarr, Hrothgare, Hrothegare

Hubert (German) Having a shining intellect
Hobart, Huberte, Huburt, Huburte, Hubirt, Hubirte, Hubyrt, Hubyrte, Hubie, Uberto

Hudson (English) The son of Hugh; from the river
Hudsun, Hudsen, Hudsan, Hudsin, Hudsyn

Humam (Arabic) A generous and brave man

Hungan (Haitian) A spirit master or priest
Hungen, Hungon, Hungun, Hungin, Hungyn

Hungas (Irish) A vigorous man

Hunter (English) A great huntsman and provider
Huntar, Huntor, Huntur, Huntir, Huntyr, Hunte, Hunt, Hunting

Huslu (Native American) Resembling a hairy bear
Huslue, Huslou

Husto (Spanish) A righteous man
Hustio, Husteo, Hustiyo, Husteyo

Huynh (Vietnamese) An older brother

I

Iakovos (Hebrew) Form of Jacob, meaning "he who supplants"
Iakovus, Iakoves, Iakovas, Iakovis, Iakovys

Ian (Gaelic) Form of John, meaning "God is gracious"
Iain, Iaine, Iayn, Iayne, Iaen, Iaene, Iahn

Iavor (Bulgarian) From the sycamore tree
Iaver, Iavur, Iavar, Iavir, Iavyr

Ibrahim (Arabic) Form of Abraham, meaning "father of a multitude; father of nations"
Ibraheem, Ibraheim, Ibrahiem, Ibraheam, Ibrahym

Ichabod (Hebrew) The glory has gone
Ikabod, Ickabod, Icabod, Ichavod, Ikavod, Icavod, Ickavod, Icha

Ichtaca (Nahuatl) A secretive man
Ichtaka, Ichtacka

Ida (Anglo-Saxon) A king
Idah

Idi (African) Born during the holiday of Idd
Idie, Idy, Idey, Idee, Idea

Ido (Arabic / Hebrew) A mighty man / to evaporate
Iddo, Idoh, Iddoh

Idris (Welsh) An eager lord
Idrys, Idriss, Idrisse, Idryss, Idrysse

Iefan (Welsh) Form of John, meaning "God is gracious"
Iefon, Iefen, Iefin, Iefyn, Iefun, Ifan, Ifon, Ifen

Ifor (Welsh) An archer
Ifore, Ifour, Ifoure

Igasho (Native American) A wanderer
Igashoe, Igashow, Igashowe

Ignatius (Latin) A fiery man; one who is ardent
Ignac, Ignace, Ignacio, Ignacius, Ignatious, Ignatz, Ignaz, Ignazio

Igor (Scandinavian / Russian) A hero / Ing's soldier
Igoryok

Ihit (Indian) One who is honored
Ihyt, Ihitt, Ihytt

Ihsan (Arabic) A charitable man
Ihsann, Ihsen, Ihsin, Ihsyn, Ihson, Ihsun

Ike (Hebrew) Form of Isaac, meaning "full of laughter"
Iki, Ikie, Iky, Ikey, Ikee, Ikea

Iker (Basque) A visitor
Ikar, Ikir, Ikyr, Ikor, Ikur

Ilario (Italian) A cheerful man
Ilareo, Ilariyo, Ilareyo, Ilar, Ilarr, Ilari, Ilarie, Ilary

Iluminado (Spanish) One who shines brightly
Illuminado, Iluminato, Illuminato, Iluminados, Iluminatos, Illuminados, Illuminatos

Imaran (Indian) Having great strength
Imaren, Imaron, Imarun, Imarin, Imaryn

Inaki (Basque) An ardent man
Inakie, Inaky, Inakey, Inakee, Inakea, Inacki, Inackie, Inackee

Ince (Hungarian) One who is innocent
Inse

Ingemar (Scandinavian) The son of Ing
Ingamar, Ingemur, Ingmar, Ingmur, Ingar, Ingemer, Ingmer

Inger (Scandinavian) One who is fertile
Inghar, Ingher

Ingo (Scandinavian / Danish) A lord / from the meadow
Ingoe, Ingow, Ingowe

Ingram (Scandinavian) A raven of peace
Ingra, Ingrem, Ingrim, Ingrym, Ingrum, Ingrom, Ingraham, Ingrahame, Ingrams

Iniko (African) Born during troubled times
Inicko, Inico, Inyko, Inycko, Inyco

Iranga (Sri Lankan) One who is special

Irenbend (Anglo-Saxon) From the iron bend
Ironbend

Irwin (English) A friend of the wild boar
Irwinn, Irwinne, Irwyn, Irwynne, Irwine, Irwen, Irwenn, Irwenne

Isaac (Hebrew) Full of laughter
Ike, Isaack, Isaak, Isac, Isacco, Isak, Issac, Itzak

Isaiah (Hebrew) God is my salvation
Isa, Isaia, Isais, Isia, Isiah, Issiah, Izaiah, Iziah

Iseabail (Hebrew) One who is devoted to God
Iseabaile, Iseabayl, Iseabyle, Iseabael, Iseabaele

Isham (English) From the iron one's estate
Ishem, Ishom, Ishum, Ishim, Ishym, Isenham

Isidore (Greek) A gift of Isis
Isador, Isadore, Isidor, Isidoro, Isidorus, Isidro

Iskander (Arabic) Form of
Alexander, meaning "a helper
and defender of mankind"
*Iskinder, Iskandar, Iskindar,
Iskynder, Iskyndar, Iskender,
Iskendar*

Israel (Hebrew) God perse-
veres
Israeli, Israelie, Isreal, Izrael

Istvan (Hungarian) One who
is crowned
*Istven, Istvin, Istvyn, Istvon,
Istvun*

Iulian (Romanian) A youthful
man
Iulien, Iulio, Iuleo

Ivan (Slavic) Form of John,
meaning "God is gracious"
*Ivann, Ivanhoe, Ivano, Iwan,
Iban, Ibano, Ivanti, Ivantie*

Ives (Scandinavian) The
archer's bow; of the yew wood
*Ivair, Ivar, Iven, Iver, Ivo, Ivon,
Ivor, Ivaire*

Ivy (English) Resembling the
evergreen vining plant
Ivee, Ivey, Ivie, Ivi, Ivea

Iyar (Hebrew) Surrounded by
light
Iyyar, Iyer, Iyyer

J

Ja (Korean / African) A handsome man / one who is
magnetic

Jabari (African) A valiant man
*Jabarie, Jabary, Jabarey,
Jabaree, Jabarea*

Jabbar (Indian) One who
consoles others
Jabar

Jabin (Hebrew) God has built;
one who is perceptive

Jabon (American) A fiesty man
*Jabun, Jabin, Jabyn, Jaben,
Jaban*

Jace (Hebrew) God is my
salvation
*Jacen, Jacey, Jacian, Jacy, Jaice,
Jayce, Jaece, Jase*

Jacinto (Spanish) Resembling
a hyacinth
*Jacynto, Jacindo, Jacyndo,
Jacento, Jacendo, Jacenty,
Jacentey, Jacentee*

Jack (English) Form of John,
meaning "God is gracious"
*Jackie, Jackman, Jacko, Jacky,
Jacq, Jacqin, Jak, Jaq*

Jackson (English) The son of Jack or John
Jacksen, Jacksun, Jacson, Jakson, Jaxen, Jaxon, Jaxun, Jaxson

Jacob (Hebrew) He who supplants
Jake, James, Kuba, Iakovos, Yakiv, Yankel, Yaqub, Jaco, Jacobo, Jacobi, Jacoby, Jacobie, Jacobey, Jacobo

Jacoby (Hebrew) Form of Jacob, meaning "he who supplants"

Jadal (American) One who is punctual
Jadall, Jadel, Jadell

Jade (Spanish) Resembling the green gemstone
Jadee, Jadie, Jayde, Jaden

Jaden (Hebrew / English) One who is thankful to God; God has heard / form of Jade, meaning "resembling the green gemstone"
Jaiden, Jadyn, Jaeden, Jaidyn, Jayden, Jaydon

Jagan (English) One who is self-confident
Jagen, Jagin, Jagyn, Jagon, Jagun, Jago

Jahan (Indian) Man of the world
Jehan, Jihan, Jag, Jagat, Jagath

Jaidayal (Indian) The victory of kindness
Jadayal, Jaydayal, Jaedayal

Jaime (Spanish) Form of James, meaning "he who supplants"
Jamie, Jaimee, Jaimey, Jaimi, Jaimie, Jaimy, Jamee

Jaimin (French) One who is loved
Jaimyn, Jamin, Jamyn, Jaymin, Jaymyn, Jaemin, Jaemyn

Jairdan (American) One who enlightens others
Jardan, Jayrdan, Jaerdan, Jairden, Jarden, Jayrden, Jaerden

Jaja (African) A gift from God

Jajuan (American) One who loves God

Jake (English) Form of Jacob, meaning "he who supplants"
Jaik, Jaike, Jayk, Jayke, Jakey, Jaky

Jakome (Basque) Form of James, meaning "he who supplants"
Jackome, Jakom, Jackom, Jacome

Jalen (American) One who heals others; one who is tranquil
Jaylon, Jaelan, Jalon, Jaylan, Jaylen, Jalan, Jaylin

Jamal (Arabic) A handsome man
Jamail, Jahmil, Jam, Jamaal, Jamy, Jamar

Jamar (American) Form of Jamal, meaning "a handsome man"
Jamarr, Jemar, Jemarr, Jimar, Jimarr, Jamaar, Jamari, Jamarie

James (Hebrew) Form of Jacob, meaning "he who supplants"
Jaimes, Jaymes, Jame, Jaym, Jaim, Jaem, Jaemes, Jamese, Jim, Jaime, Diego, Hagop, Hemi, Jakome

Jameson (English) The son of James
Jaimison, Jamieson, Jaymeson, Jamison, Jaimeson, Jaymison, Jaemeson, Jaemison

Jamin (Hebrew) The right hand of favor
Jamian, Jamiel, Jamon, Jaymin, Jaemin, Jaymon

Janesh (Hindi) A leader of the people
Janeshe

Japheth (Hebrew) May he expand; in the Bible, one of Noah's sons
Jaypheth, Jaepheth, Jaipheth, Jafeth, Jayfeth

Jarah (Hebrew) One who is as sweet as honey
Jarrah, Jara, Jarra

Jared (Hebrew) Of the descent; descending
Jarad, Jarod, Jarrad, Jarryd, Jarred, Jarrod, Jaryd, Jerod, Jerrad, Jered

Jarman (German) A man from Germany
Jarmann, Jerman, Jermann

Jaron (Israeli) A song of rejoicing
Jaran, Jaren, Jarin, Jarran, Jarren, Jarrin, Jarron, Jaryn

Jaroslav (Slavic) Born with the beauty of spring
Jaroslaw

Jarrett (English) One who is strong with the spear
Jaret, Jarret, Jarrott, Jerett, Jarritt, Jaret

Jason (Hebrew / Greek) God is my salvation / a healer; in mythology, the leader of the Argonauts
Jacen, Jaisen, Jaison, Jasen, Jasin, Jasun, Jayson, Jaysen

Jaspar (Persian) One who holds the treasure
Jasper, Jaspir, Jaspyr, Jesper, Jespar, Jespir, Jespyr

Jatan (Indian) One who is nurturing

Javan (Hebrew) Man from Greece; in the Bible, Noah's grandson
Jayvan, Jayven, Jayvon, Javon, Javern, Javen

Javier (Spanish) The owner of a new house
Javiero

Jax (American) Form of Jackson, meaning "son of Jack or John"

Jay (Latin / Sanskrit) Resembling a jaybird / one who is victorious
Jae, Jai, Jaye, Jayron, Jayronn, Jey

Jayce (American) Form of Jason, meaning "God is my salvation"
Jayse, Jace, Jase

Jean (French) Form of John, meaning "God is gracious"
Jeanne, Jeane, Jene, Jeannot, Jeanot

Jedidiah (Hebrew) One who is loved by God
Jedadiah, Jedediah, Jed, Jedd, Jedidiya, Jedidiyah, Jedadia, Jedadiya

Jeffrey (English) A man of peace
Jeff, Geoffrey, Jeffery, Jeffree

Jelani (African) One who is mighty; strong
Jelanie, Jelany, Jelaney, Jelanee, Jelanea

Jennett (Hindi) One who is heaven-sent
Jenett, Jennet, Jenet, Jennitt, Jenitt, Jennit, Jenit

Jerald (English) Form of Gerald, meaning "one who rules with the spear"
Jeraldo, Jerold, Jerrald, Jerrold

Jeremiah (Hebrew) One who is exalted by the Lord
Jeremia, Jeremias, Jeremija, Jeremiya, Jeremyah, Jeramiah, Jeramia, Jerram, Geremia

Jeremy (Hebrew) Form of Jeremiah, meaning "one who is exalted by the Lord"
Jeramey, Jeramie, Jeramy, Jerami, Jereme, Jeromy

Jermaine (French / Latin) A man from Germany / one who is brotherly
Jermain, Jermane, Jermayne, Jermin, Jermyn, Jermayn, Jermaen, Jermaene

Jerome (Greek) Of the sacred name
Jairome, Jeroen, Jeromo, Jeronimo, Jerrome, Jerom, Jerolyn, Jerolin, Hieronim

Jerram (Hebrew) Form of Jeremiah, meaning "one who is exalted by the Lord"
Jeram, Jerrem, Jerem, Jerrym, Jerym

Jesimiel (Hebrew) The Lord establishes
Jessimiel

Jesse (Hebrew) God exists; a gift from God; God sees all
Jess, Jessey, Jesiah, Jessie, Jessy, Jese, Jessi, Jessee

Jesus (Hebrew) God is my salvation
Jesous, Jesues, Jesús, Xesus

Jett (English) Resembling the jet-black lustrous gemstone
Jet, Jette

Jibril (Arabic) Refers to the archangel Gabriel
Jibryl, Jibri, Jibrie, Jibry, Jibrey, Jibree

Jim (English) Form of James, meaning "he who supplants"
Jimi, Jimmee, Jimmey, Jimmie, Jimmy, Jimmi, Jimbo

Jivan (Hindi) A giver of life
Jivin, Jiven, Jivyn, Jivon

Joab (Hebrew) The Lord is my father
Joabb, Yoav

Joachim (Hebrew) One who is established by God; God will judge
Jachim, Jakim, Joacheim, Joaquim, Joaquin, Josquin, Joakim, Joakeen

Joe (English) Form of Joseph, meaning "God will add"
Jo, Joemar, Jomar, Joey, Joie, Joee, Joeye

Joel (Hebrew) Jehovah is God; God is willing

Johan (German) Form of John, meaning "God is gracious"

John (Hebrew) God is gracious; in the Bible, one of the Apostles
Sean, Jack, Juan, Ian, Ean, Evan, Giovanni, Hanna, Hovannes, Iefan, Ivan, Jean, Xoan, Yochanan, Yohan, Johnn, Johnny, Jhonny

Jonah (Hebrew) Resembling a dove; in the Bible, the man swallowed by a whale

Jonas (Greek) Form of Jonah, meaning "resembling a dove"

Jonathan (Hebrew) A gift of God
Johnathan, Johnathon, Jonathon, Jonatan, Jonaton, Jonathen, Johnathen, Jonaten, Yonatan

Jordan (Hebrew) Of the down-flowing river; in the Bible, the river where Jesus was baptized
Johrdan, Jordain, Jordaine, Jordane, Jordanke, Jordann, Jorden, Jordaen

Jorge (Spanish) Form of George, meaning "one who works the earth; a farmer"

Jose (Spanish) Form of Joseph, meaning "God will add"
José, Joseito, Joselito

Joseph (Hebrew) God will add
Joe, Guiseppe, Yosyp, Jessop, Jessup, Joop, Joos, José, Jose, Josef, Joseito

Joshua (Hebrew) God is salvation
Josh, Joshuah, Josua, Josue, Joushua, Jozua, Joshwa, Joshuwa

Josiah (Hebrew) God will help
Josia, Josias, Joziah, Jozia, Jozias

Journey (American) One who likes to travel
Journy, Journi, Journie, Journee, Journye, Journea

Juan (Spanish) Form of John, meaning "God is gracious"
Juanito, Juwan, Jwan

Judah (Hebrew) One who praises God
Juda, Jude, Judas, Judsen, Judson, Judd, Jud

Jude (Latin) Form of Judah, meaning "one who praises God"

Julian (Greek) The child of Jove; one who is youthful
Juliano, Julianus, Julien, Julyan, Julio, Jolyon, Jullien, Julen

Julius (Greek) One who is youthful
Juleus, Yuliy

Juma (African) Born on a Friday
Jumah

Jumbe (African) Having great strength
Jumbi, Jumbie, Jumby, Jumbey, Jumbee

Jumoke (African) One who is dearly loved
Jumok, Jumoak

Jun (Japanese) One who is obedient

Junaid (Arabic) A warrior
Junaide, Junayd, Junayde

Jung (Korean) A righteous man

Justice (English) One who upholds moral rightness and fairness
Justyce, Justiss, Justyss, Justis, Justus, Justise

Justin (Latin) One who is just and upright
Joost, Justain, Justan, Just, Juste, Justen, Justino, Justo

Kabir (Indian) A spiritual leader
Kabeer, Kabear, Kabier, Kabeir, Kabyr, Kabar

Kabonesa (African) One who is born during difficult times

Kacey (Irish) A vigilant man; one who is alert
Kacy, Kacee, Kacea, Kaci, Kacie, Kasey, Kasy, Kasi

Kaden (Arabic) A beloved companion
Kadan, Kadin, Kadon, Kaidan, Kaiden, Kaidon, Kaydan, Kayden

Kadmiel (Hebrew) One who stands before God
Kamiell

Kaemon (Japanese) Full of joy; one who is right-handed
Kamon, Kaymon, Kaimon

Kagen (Irish) A fiery man; a thinker
Kaigen, Kagan, Kaigan, Kaygen, Kaygan, Kaegen, Kaegan

Kahoku (Hawaiian) Resembling a star
Kahokue, Kahokoo, Kahokou

Kai (Hawaiian / Welsh / Greek) Of the sea / the keeper of the keys / of the earth
Kye

Kaimi (Hawaiian) The seeker
Kaimie, Kaimy, Kaimey, Kaimee, Kaimea

Kalama (Hawaiian) A source of light
Kalam, Kalame

Kale (English) Form of Charles, meaning "one who is manly and strong / a free man"

Kaleb (Hebrew) Resembling an aggressive dog
Kaileb, Kaeleb, Kayleb, Kalob, Kailob, Kaelob

Kalidas (Hindi) A poet or musician; a servant of Kali
Kalydas

Kalki (Indian) Resembling a white horse
Kalkie, Kalky, Kalkey, Kalkee, Kalkea

Kalkin (Hindi) The tenth-born child
Kalkyn, Kalken, Kalkan, Kalkon, Kalkun

Kamden (English) From the winding valley
Kamdun, Kamdon, Kamdan, Kamdin, Kamdyn

Kane (Gaelic) The little warrior
Kayn, Kayne, Kaen, Kaene, Kahan, Kahane

Kang (Korean) A healthy man

Kano (Japanese) A powerful man
Kanoe, Kanoh

Kantrava (Indian) Resembling a roaring animal

Kaper (American) One who is capricious
Kahper, Kapar, Kahpar

Kapono (Hawaiian) A righteous man

Karcsi (French) A strong, manly man
Karcsie, Karcsy, Karcsey, Karcsee, Karcsea

Karl (German) A free man
Carl, Karel, Karlan, Karle, Karlens, Karli, Karlin, Karlo, Karlos

Karman (Gaelic) The lord of the manor
Karmen, Karmin, Karmyn, Karmon, Karmun

Karson (Scottish) Form of Carson, meaning son of a marsh dweller
Karsen

Karter (English) Form of Carter, meaning one who drives a cart

Kashvi (Indian) A shining man
Kashvie, Kashvy, Kashvey, Kashvee, Kashvea

Kasib (Arabic) One who is fertile
Kaseeb, Kaseab, Kasieb, Kaseib, Kasyb

Kasim (Arabic) One who is divided
Kassim, Kaseem, Kasseem, Kaseam, Kasseam, Kasym, Kassym

Kasimir (Slavic) One who demands peace
Kasimeer, Kasimear, Kasimier, Kasimeir, Kasimyr, Kaz, Kazimierz

Kason (Basque) Protected by a helmet
Kasin, Kasyn, Kasen, Kasun, Kasan

Katzir (Hebrew) The harvester
Katzyr, Katzeer, Katzear, Katzier, Katzeir

Kaushal (Indian) One who is skilled
Kaushall, Koshal, Koshall

Kazim (Arabic) An even-tempered man
Kazeem, Kazeam, Kaziem, Kazeim, Kazym

Keahi (Hawaiian) Of the flames
Keahie, Keahy, Keahey, Keahee, Keahea

Kealoha (Hawaiian) From the bright path
Keeloha, Kieloha

Kean (Gaelic / English) A warrior / one who is sharp
Keane, Keen, Keene, Kein, Keine, Keyn, Keyne, Kien

Keandre (American) One who is thankful
Kiandre, Keandray, Kiandray, Keandrae, Kiandrae, Keandrai, Kiandrai

Keanu (Hawaiian) Of the mountain breeze
Keanue, Kianu, Kianue, Keanoo, Kianoo, Keanou

Keaton (English) From the town of hawks
Keatun, Keeton, Keetun, Keyton, Keytun

Kedar (Arabic) A powerful man
Keder, Kedir, Kedyr, Kadar, Kader, Kadir, Kadyr

Kefir (Hebrew) Resembling a young lion
Kefyr, Kefeer, Kefear, Kefier, Kefeir

Keegan (Gaelic) A small and fiery man
Kegan, Keigan, Keagan, Keagen, Keegen

Keith (Scottish) Man from the forest
Keithe, Keath, Keathe, Kieth, Kiethe, Keyth, Keythe, Keithen

Kellach (Irish) One who suffers strife during battle
Kelach, Kellagh, Kelagh, Keallach

Kellen (Gaelic / German) One who is slender / from the swamp
Kellan, Kellon, Kellun, Kellin

Kelley (Celtic / Gaelic) A warrior / one who defends
Kelly, Kelleigh, Kellee, Kellea, Kelleah, Kelli, Kellie

Kendi (African) One who is much loved
Kendie, Kendy, Kendey, Kendee, Kendea

Kendrick (English / Gaelic) A royal ruler / the champion
Kendric, Kendricks, Kendrik, Kendrix, Kendryck, Kenrick, Kenrik, Kenricks

Kenley (English) From the king's meadow
Kenly, Kenlee, Kenleigh, Kenlea, Kenleah, Kenli, Kenlie

Kenn (Welsh) Of the bright waters

Kennedy (Gaelic) A helmeted chief
Kennedi, Kennedie, Kennedey, Kennedee, Kennedea, Kenadie, Kenadi, Kenady

Kenneth (Irish) Born of the fire; an attractive man
Kennet, Kennett, Kennith, Kennit, Kennitt

Kent (English) From the edge or border
Kentt, Kennt, Kentrell

Kenton (English) From the king's town
Kentun, Kentan, Kentin, Kenten, Kentyn

Kenyon (Gaelic) A blond-haired man
Kenyun, Kenyan, Kenyen, Kenyin

Kepler (German) One who makes hats
Keppler, Kappler, Keppel, Keppeler

Kershet (Hebrew) Of the rainbow

Kesler (American) An energetic man; one who is independent
Keslar, Keslir, Keslyr, Keslor, Keslur

Keung (Chinese) A universal spirit

Kevin (Gaelic) A beloved and handsome man
Kevyn, Kevan, Keven, Keveon, Kevinn, Kevion, Kevis, Kevon

Khairi (Swahili) A kingly man
*Khairie, Khairy, Khairey,
Khairee, Khairea*

Khalon (American) A strong
warrior
*Khalun, Khalen, Khalan,
Khalin, Khalyn*

Khayri (Arabic) One who is
charitable
*Khayrie, Khayry, Khayrey,
Khayree, Khayrea*

Khushi (Indian) Filled with
happiness
*Khushie, Khushey, Khushy,
Khushee*

Kibbe (Native American) A
nocturnal bird
Kybbe

Kibo (African) From the highest mountain peak
Keybo, Keebo, Keabo, Keibo, Kiebo

Kiefer (German) One who
makes barrels
*Keefer, Keifer, Kieffer, Kiefner,
Kieffner, Kiefert, Kuefer, Kueffner*

Kieran (Gaelic) Having dark
features; the little dark one
*Keiran, Keiron, Kernan, Kieren,
Kiernan, Kieron, Kierren, Kierrien,
Kierron, Keeran, Keeron, Keernan,
Keeren, Kearan, Kearen,
Kearon, Kearnan*

Kim (Vietnamese) As precious
as gold
Kym

Kimoni (African) A great man
*Kimonie, Kimony, Kimoney,
Kimonee, Kymoni, Kymonie,
Kymony, Kymoney*

Kincaid (Celtic) The leader
during battle
*Kincade, Kincayd, Kincayde,
Kincaide, Kincaed, Kincaede,
Kinkaid, Kinkaide*

Kindin (Basque) The fifth-born
child
*Kinden, Kindan, Kindyn,
Kindon, Kindun*

Kindle (American) To set
aflame
Kindel, Kyndle, Kyndel

King (English) The royal ruler
Kyng, Kingsley

Kingston (English) From the
king's town
Kingstun, Kinston, Kindon

Kinnard (Irish) From the tall
hill
*Kinard, Kinnaird, Kinaird,
Kynnard, Kynard, Kynnaird,
Kynaird*

Kinsey (English) The victori-
ous prince
*Kynsey, Kinsi, Kynsi, Kinsie,
Kynsie, Kinsee, Kynsee, Kinsea*

Kione (African) One who has come from nowhere

Kioshi (Japanese) One who is quiet
Kioshe, Kioshie, Kioshy, Kioshey, Kioshee, Kyoshi, Kyoshe, Kyoshie

Kipp (English) From the small pointed hill
Kip, Kipling, Kippling, Kypp, Kyp, Kiplyng, Kipplyng, Kippi

Kiri (Vietnamese) Resembling the mountains
Kirie, Kiry, Kirey, Kiree, Kirea

Kirk (Norse) A man of the church
Kyrk, Kerk, Kirklin, Kirklyn

Kirkland (English) From the church's land
Kirklan, Kirklande, Kyrkland, Kyrklan, Kyrklande

Kirkley (English) From the church's meadow
Kirkly, Kirkleigh, Kirklea, Kirkleah, Kirklee, Kirkli, Kirklie

Kit (English) Form of Christopher, meaning "one who bears Christ inside"
Kitt, Kyt, Kytt

Kitchi (Native American) A brave young man
Kitchie, Kitchy, Kitchey, Kitchee, Kitchea

Kitoko (African) A handsome man
Kytoko

Kivi (Finnish) As solid as stone
Kivie, Kivy, Kivey, Kivee, Kivea

Knight (English) A noble solidier
Knights

Knox (English) From the rounded hill

Kobe (African / Hungarian) Tortoise / Form of Jacob, meaning "he who supplants"
Kobi, Koby

Kody (English) One who is helpful
Kodey, Kodee, Kodea, Kodi, Kodie

Koen (German) An honest advisor
Koenz, Kunz, Kuno

Kohana (Native American / Hawaiian) One who is swift / the best

Kohler (German) One who mines coal
Koler

Kojo (African) Born on a Monday
Kojoe, Koejo, Koejoe

Koka (Hawaiian) A man from Scotland

Kolton (American) Form of Colton, meaning from the coal town
Kolten, Koltan

Konane (Hawaiian) Born beneath the bright moon
Konain, Konaine, Konayn, Konayne, Konaen, Konaene

Konnor (English) A wolf lover; one who is strong-willed
Konnur, Konner, Konnar, Konnir, Konnyr

Kordell (English) One who makes cord
Kordel, Kord, Kordale

Koresh (Hebrew) One who digs in the earth; a farmer
Koreshe

Kory (Irish) From the hollow; of the churning waters
Korey, Kori, Korie, Koree, Korea, Korry, Korrey, Korree

Kozma (Greek) One who is decorated
Kozmah

Kozue (Japanese) Of the tree branches
Kozu, Kozoo, Kozou

Kraig (Gaelic) From the rocky place; as solid as a rock
Kraige, Krayg, Krayge, Kraeg, Kraege, Krage

Kramer (German) A shop-keeper
Kramar, Kramor, Kramir, Kramur, Kramyr, Kraymer, Kraimer, Kraemer

Krany (Czech) A man of short stature
Kraney, Kranee, Kranea, Krani, Kranie

Krikor (Armenian) A vigilant watchman
Krykor, Krikur, Krykur

Kristian (Scandinavian) An annointed Christian
Kristan, Kristien, Krist, Kriste, Krister, Kristar, Khristian, Khrist

Kristopher (Scandinavian) A follower of Christ
Khristopher, Kristof, Kristofer, Kristoff, Kristoffer, Kristofor, Kristophor, Krystof

Kuba (Polish) Form of Jacob, meaning "he who supplants"
Kubas

Kuleen (Indian) A high-born man
Kulin, Kulein, Kulien, Kulean, Kulyn

Kumar (Indian) A prince;
a male child

Kuri (Japanese) Resembling
a chestnut
*Kurie, Kury, Kurey, Kuree,
Kurea*

Kuron (African) One who gives
thanks
*Kurun, Kuren, Kuran, Kurin,
Kuryn*

Kurt (German) A brave
counselor
Kurte

Kushal (Indian) A talented
man; adroit
Kushall

Kwaku (African) Born on a
Wednesday
*Kwakue, Kwakou, Kwako,
Kwakoe*

Kwan (Korean) Of a bold
character
Kwon

Kwintyn (Polish) The fifth-
born child
*Kwentyn, Kwinton, Kwenton,
Kwintun, Kwentun, Kwintan,
Kwentan, Kwinten*

Kyle (Gaelic) From the narrow
channel
*Kile, Kiley, Kye, Kylan, Kyrell,
Kylen, Kily, Kili*

Kylemore (Gaelic) From the
great wood
Kylmore, Kylemor, Kylmor

Kyrone (English) Form of
Tyrone, meaning "from
Owen's land"
*Kyron, Keirohn, Keiron,
Keirone, Keirown, Kirone*

L

Lacey (French) Man from
Normandy; as delicate as lace
Lacy, Laci, Lacie, Lacee, Lacea

Lachlan (Gaelic) From the land
of lakes
*Lachlen, Lachlin, Lachlyn,
Locklan, Locklen, Locklin,
Locklyn, Loklan*

Lachman (Gaelic) A man from
the lake
*Lachmann, Lockman,
Lockmann, Lokman, Lokmann,
Lakman, Lakmann*

Ladan (Hebrew) One who is
alert and aware
*Laden, Ladin, Ladyn, Ladon,
Ladun*

Ladislas (Slavic) A glorious
ruler
*Lacko, Ladislaus, Laslo, Laszlo,
Lazlo, Ladislav, Ladislauv,
Ladislao*

Lagrand (American) A
majestic man
Lagrande

Laibrook (English) One who
lives on the road near the
brook
*Laebrook, Laybrook, Laibroc,
Laebroc, Laybroc, Laibrok,
Laebrok, Laybrok*

Laird (Scottish) The lord of the
manor
*Layrd, Laerd, Lairde, Layrde,
Laerde*

Laken (American) Man from
the lake
*Laike, Laiken, Laikin, Lakin,
Lakyn, Lakan, Laikyn, Laeken*

Lalam (Indian) The best
Lallam, Lalaam, Lallaam

Lam (Vietnamese) Having a
full understanding

Laman (Arabic) A bright and
happy man
Lamaan, Lamann, Lamaann

Lamar (German / French)
From the renowned land / of
the sea
*Lamarr, Lamarre, Lemar,
Lemarr*

Lambert (Scandinavian) The
light of the land
*Lambart, Lamberto, Lambirt,
Landbert, Lambirto, Lambrecht,
Lambret, Lambrett*

Lambi (Norse) In mythology,
the son of Thorbjorn
*Lambie, Lamby, Lambey,
Lambe, Lambee*

Lameh (Arabic) A shining man

Lamorak (English) In
Arthurian legend, the brother
of Percival
*Lamerak, Lamurak, Lamorac,
Lamerac, Lamurac, Lamorack,
Lamerack, Lamurack*

Lance (English) Form of
Lancelot, meaning an
attendant, a knight of the
Round Table

Lander (English) One who
owns land
*Land, Landers, Landis, Landiss,
Landor, Lande, Landry, Landri*

Landon (English) From the
long hill
*Landyn, Landan, Landen,
Landin, Lando, Langdon,
Langden, Langdan*

Lane (English) One who takes the narrow path
Laine, Lain, Laen, Laene, Layne, Layn

Langhorn (English) Of the long horn
Langhorne, Lanhorn, Lanhorne

Langston (English) From the tall man's town
Langsten, Langstun, Langstown, Langstin, Langstyn, Langstan, Langton, Langtun

Langundo (Native American / Polynesian) A peaceful man / one who is graceful

Langworth (English) One who lives near the long paddock
Langworthe, Lanworth, Lanworthe

Lanier (French) One who works with wool

Lantos (Hungarian) One who plays the lute
Lantus

Lapidos (Hebrew) One who carries a torch
Lapydos, Lapidot, Lapydot, Lapidoth, Lapydoth, Lapidus, Lapydus

Lar (Anglo-Saxon) One who teaches others

Larson (Scandinavian) The son of Lawrence
Larsan, Larsen, Larsun, Larsin, Larsyn

Lasalle (French) From the hall
Lasall, Lasal, Lasale

Lashaun (American) An enthusiastic man
Lashawn, Lasean, Lashon, Lashond

Lassit (American) One who is open-minded
Lassyt, Lasset

Lathan (American) Form of Nathan, meaning "a gift from God"
Lathen, Lathun, Lathon, Lathin, Lathyn, Latan, Laten, Latun

Latimer (English) One who serves as an interpreter
Latymer, Latimor, Latymor, Latimore, Latymore, Lattemore, Lattimore

Laurian (English) One who lives near the laurel trees
Laurien, Lauriano, Laurieno, Lawrian, Lawrien, Lawriano, Lawrieno

Lave (Italian) Of the burning rock
Lava

Lawler (Gaelic) A soft-spoken man; one who mutters
Lauler, Lawlor, Loller, Lawlar, Lollar, Loller, Laular, Laulor

Lawley (English) From the meadow near the hill
Lawly, Lawli, Lawlie, Lawleigh, Lawlee, Lawlea, Lawleah

Lawrence (Latin) Man from Laurentum; crowned with laurel
Larance, Laranz, Larenz, Larrance, Larrence, Larrens, Larrey, Larry

Laziz (Arabic) One who is pleasant
Lazeez, Lazeaz, Laziez, Lazeiz, Lazyz

Leaman (American) A powerful man
Leeman, Leamon, Leemon, Leamond, Leamand

Lear (Greek) Of the royalty
Leare, Leer, Leere

Leather (American) As tough as hide
Lether

Leavitt (English) A baker
Leavit, Leavytt, Leavyt, Leavett, Leavet

Leben (English) Filled with hope

Lech (Slavic) In mythology, the founder of the Polish people
Leche

Lee (English) From the meadow
Leigh, Lea, Leah, Ley

Leeto (African) One who embarks on a journey
Leato, Leito, Lieto

Legend (American) One who is memorable
Legende, Legund, Legunde

Leighton (English) From the town near the meadow
Leightun, Layton, Laytun, Leyton, Leytun

Lekhak (Hindi) An author
Lekhan

Leland (English) From the meadow land

Lema (African) One who is cultivated
Lemah, Lemma, Lemmah

Len (Native American) One who plays the flute

Lencho (African) Resembling a lion
Lenchos, Lenchio, Lenchiyo, Lencheo, Lencheyo

Lennon (English) Son of love
Lennan

Lennor (English) A courageous man

Lennox (Scottish) One who owns many elm trees
Lenox, Lenoxe, Lennix, Lenix, Lenixe

Lensar (English) One who stays with his parents
Lenser, Lensor, Lensur

Lenton (American) A pious man
Lentin, Lentyn, Lentun, Lentan, Lenten, Lent, Lente

Leo (Latin) Having the strength of a lion
Lio, Lyo, Leon

Leon (Greek) Form of Leo, meaning "resembling a lion"

Leonard (German) Having the strength of a lion
Len, Lenard, Lenn, Lennard, Lennart, Lennerd, Leonardo

Leor (Latin) One who listens well
Leore

Lerato (Latin) The song of my soul
Leratio, Lerateo

Leron (French / Arabic) The circle / my song
Lerun, Leran, Leren, Lerin, Leryn

Leroy (French) The king
Leroi, Leeroy, Leeroi, Learoy, Learoi

Levi (Hebrew) We are united as one; in the Bible, one of Jacob's sons
Levie, Levin, Levyn, Levy, Levey, Levee

Li (Chinese) Having great strength

Liam (Gaelic) Form of William, meaning "the determined protector"

Lian (Chinese) Of the willow

Liang (Chinese) A good man
Lyang

Lidmann (Anglo-Saxon) A man of the sea; a sailor
Lidman, Lydmann, Lydman

Lif (Scandinavian) An energetic man; lively

Lihau (Hawaiian) A spirited man

Like (Asian) A soft-spoken man
Lyke

Lilo (Hawaiian) One who is generous
Lylo, Leelo, Lealo, Leylo, Lielo, Leilo

Lincoln (English) From the village near the lake
Lincon, Lyncon, Linc, Lynk, Lync

Lindford (English) From the linden-tree ford
Linford, Lindforde, Linforde, Lyndford, Lynford, Lyndforde, Lynforde

Lindhurst (English) From the village by the linden trees
Lyndhurst, Lindenhurst, Lyndenhurst, Lindhirst, Lindherst, Lyndhirst, Lyndherst, Lindenhirst

Lindley (English) From the meadow of linden trees
Lindly, Lindleigh, Lindlea, Lindleah, Lindlee, Lindli

Lindman (English) One who lives near the linden trees
Lindmann, Lindmon

Line (English) From the bank

Lipût (Hungarian) A brave young man

Lisimba (African) One who has been attacked by a lion
Lisymba, Lysimba, Lysymba

Liu (Asian) One who is quiet; peaceful

Llewellyn (Welsh) Resembling a lion
Lewellen, Lewellyn, Llewellen, Llewelyn, Llwewellin, Llew, Llewe, Llyweilun

Lochan (Hindi / Irish) The eyes / one who is lively

Logan (Gaelic) From the little hollow
Logann, Logen, Login, Logyn, Logenn, Loginn, Logynn

Loman (Gaelic) One who is small and bare
Lomann, Loeman, Loemann

Lombard (Latin) One who has a long beard
Lombardi, Lombardo, Lombardie, Lombardy, Lombardey, Lombardee

London (English) From the capital of England
Lundon, Londen, Lunden

Lonzo (Spanish) One who is ready for battle
Lonzio, Lonzeo

Lootah (Native American) Refers to the color red
Loota, Loutah, Louta, Lutah, Luta

Lorcan (Irish) The small fierce one
Lorcen, Lorcin, Lorcyn, Lorcon, Lorcun, Lorkan, Lorken, Lorkin

Lord (English) One who has authority and power
Lorde, Lordly, Lordley, Lordlee, Lordlea, Lordleigh, Lordli, Lordlie

Lore (Basque / English) Resembling a flower / form of Lawrence, meaning "man from Laurentum; crowned with laurel"
Lorea

Lorimer (Latin) One who makes harnesses
Lorrimer, Lorimar, Lorrimar, Lorymar, Lorrymar, Lorymer, Lorrymer

Louis (German) A famous warrior
Lew, Lewes, Lewis, Lodewick, Lodovico, Lou, Louie, Lucho, Luis

Lucas (English) A man from Lucania
Lukas, Loucas, Loukas, Luckas, Louckas, Lucus, Lukus, Ghoukas

Lucian (Latin) Surrounded by light
Luciano, Lucianus, Lucien, Lucio, Lucjan, Lukianos, Lukyan, Luce

Lucky (English) A fortunate man
Luckey, Luckee, Luckea, Lucki, Luckie

Ludlow (English) The ruler of the hill
Ludlowe

Luis (Spanish) Form of Louis, meaning "a famous warrior"
Luiz

Luke (Greek) A man from Lucania
Luc, Luken

Luthando (Latin) One who is dearly loved

Luther (German) A soldier of the people
Louther, Luter, Luthero, Lutero, Louthero, Luthus, Luthas, Luthos

Lux (Latin) A man of the light
Luxe, Luxi, Luxie, Luxee, Luxea, Luxy, Luxey

Ly (Vietnamese) A reasonable man

Lynn (English) A man of the lake
Linn, Lyn, Lynne, Linne

M

Maahes (Egyptian) Resembling a lion

Mac (Gaelic) The son of Mac (Macarthur, Mackinley, etc.)
Mack, Mak, Macky, Macki, Mackie, Mackee, Mackea

Macadam (Gaelic) The son of Adam
Macadhamh, MacAdam, McAdam, MacAdhamh

Macallister (Gaelic) The son of Alistair
MacAlister, McAlister, McAllister, Macalister

Macartan (Gaelic) The son of Artan
MacArtan, McArtan, Macarten, MacArten, McArten

Macarthur (Gaelic) The son of Arthur
MacArthur, McArthur, Macarther, MacArther, McArther

Macauslan (Gaelic) The son of Absalon
MacAuslan, McAuslan, Macauslen, MacAuslen, McAuslen

Maccoll (Gaelic) The son of Coll
McColl, Maccoll, MacColl

Maccrea (Gaelic) The son of grace
McCrea, Macrae, MacCrae, MacCray, MacCrea

Macedonio (Greek) A man from Macedonia
Macedoneo, Macedoniyo, Macedoneyo

Macgowan (Gaelic) The son of a blacksmith
MacGowan, Magowan, McGowan, McGowen, McGown, MacCowan, MacCowen

Machau (Hebrew) A gift from God

Machenry (Gaelic) The son of Henry
MacHenry, McHenry

Machk (Native American) Resembling a bear

Macintosh (Gaelic) The son of the thane
MacIntosh, McIntosh, Macintoshe, MacIntoshe, McIntoshe, Mackintosh, MacKintosh

Mackay (Gaelic) The son of fire
MacKay, McKay, Mackaye, MacKaye, McKaye

Mackinley (Gaelic) The son of the white warrior
MacKinley, McKinley, MacKinlay, McKinlay, Mackinlay, Mackinlie, MacKinlie

Macklin (Gaelic) The son of Flann
Macklinn, Macklyn, Macklynn, Macklen, Macklenn

Maclaine (Gaelic) The son of John's servant
MacLaine, Maclain, MacLain, Maclayn, McLaine, McLain, Maclane, MacLane

Macleod (Gaelic) The son of the ugly one
MacLeod, McLeod, McCloud, MacCloud

Macmurray (Gaelic) The son of Murray
MacMurray, McMurray, Macmurra, MacMurra

Macnab (Gaelic) The son of the abbot
MacNab, McNab

Macon (English / French) To make / from the city in France
Macun, Makon, Makun, Maken, Mackon, Mackun

Macrae (Gaelic) The son of Ray
MacRae, McRae, Macray, MacRay, McRay, Macraye, MacRaye, McRaye

Madden (Pakistani) One who is organized; a planner
Maddon, Maddan, Maddin, Maddyn, Maddun, Maden, Madon, Madun

Maddox (Welsh) The son of the benefactor
Madox, Madocks, Maddocks, Maddux

Madhur (Indian) A sweet man

Magee (Gaelic) The son of Hugh
MacGee, McGee, MacGhee, Maghee

Maguire (Gaelic) The son of the beige one
Magwire, MacGuire, McGuire, MacGwire, McGwire

Magus (Latin) A sorcerer
Magis, Magys, Magos, Magas, Mages

Mahant (Indian) Having a great soul
Mahante

Mahatma (Hindi) Of great spiritual development

Mahfouz (Arabic) One who is protected
Mafouz, Mahfooz, Mafooz, Mahfuz, Mafuz

Mahkah (Native American) Of the earth
Mahka, Makah, Maka

Mahmud (Arabic) One who is praiseworthy
Mahmood, Mahmoud, Mehmood, Mehmud, Mehmoud

Mailhairer (French) An ill-fated man

Maimon (Arabic) One who is dependable; having good fortune
Maymon, Maemon, Maimun, Maymun, Maemun, Mamon, Mamun

Majdy (Arabic) A glorious man
Majdey, Majdi, Majdie, Majdee, Majdea

Makaio (Hawaiian) A gift from God

Makena (Hawaiian) Man of abundance
Makenah

Makin (Arabic) Having great strength
Makeen, Makean, Makein, Makien, Makyn

Makis (Hebrew) A gift from God
Madys, Makiss, Makyss, Makisse, Madysse

Malachi (Hebrew) A messenger of God
Malachie, Malachy, Malaki, Malakia, Malakie, Malaquias, Malechy, Maleki

Malawa (African) A flourishing man

Malcolm (Gaelic) Follower of St. Columbus
Malcom, Malcolum, Malkolm, Malkom, Malkolum

Mali (Indian) A ruler; the firstborn son
Malie, Maly, Maley, Malee, Malea

Mamoru (Japanese) Of the
earth
*Mamorou, Mamorue,
Mamorew, Mamoroo*

Manchester (English) From
the city in England
*Manchestar, Manchestor,
Manchestir, Manchestyr,
Manchestur*

Mandan (Native American) A
tribal name
*Manden, Mandon, Mandun,
Mandin, Mandyn*

Mandhatri (Indian) A prince;
born to royalty
*Mandhatrie, Mandhatry,
Mandhatrey, Mandhatree,
Mandhatrea*

Mani (African) From the
mountain
*Manie, Many, Maney, Manee,
Manea*

Manjit (Indian) A conqueror
of the mind; having great
knowledge
*Manjeet, Manjeat, Manjeit,
Manjiet, Manjyt*

Manley (English) From the
man's meadow; from the
hero's meadow
*Manly, Manli, Manlie, Manlea,
Manleah, Manlee, Manleigh*

Manmohan (Indian) A hand-
some and pleasing man
*Manmohen, Manmohin,
Manmohyn*

Mannheim (German) From
the hamlet in the swamp
Manheim

Mano (Hawaiian) Resembling
a shark
Manoe, Manow, Manowe

Manohar (Indian) A delightful
and captivating man
Manoharr, Manohare

Mansel (English) From the
clergyman's house
*Mansle, Mansell, Mansele,
Manselle, Manshel, Manshele,
Manshell, Manshelle*

Mansfield (English) From the
field near the small river
Mansfeld, Maunfield, Maunfeld

Manton (English) From the
man's town; from the hero's
town
*Mantun, Manten, Mannton,
Manntun, Mannten*

Manu (African) The second-
born child
Manue, Manou, Manoo

Manuel (Spanish) Form of Emmanuel, meaning "God is with us"
Manuelo, Manuello, Manolito, Manolo, Manollo, Manny, Manni

Manya (Indian) A respected man
Manyah

Manzo (Japanese) The third son with ten-thousand-fold strength

Mar (Spanish) Of the sea
Marr, Mare, Marre

Marcel (French) The little warrior
Marceau, Marcelin, Marcellin, Marcellino, Marcell, Marcello, Marcellus, Marcelo

Marcus (Latin) Form of Mark, meaning "dedicated to Mars, the god of war"
Markus, Marcas, Marco, Markos

Mariatu (African) One who is pure; chaste
Mariatue, Mariatou, Mariatoo

Marid (Arabic) A rebellious man
Maryd

Mario (Latin) A manly man
Marius, Marios, Mariano, Marion, Mariun, Mareon

Mark (Latin) Dedicated to Mars, the god of war
Marc, Markey, Marky, Marki, Markie, Markee, Markea, Markov

Marmion (French) Our little one
Marmyon, Marmeon

Marshall (French / English) A caretaker of horses / a steward
Marchall, Marischal, Marischall, Marschal, Marshal, Marshell, Marshel, Marschall

Marston (English) From the town near the marsh
Marstun, Marsten, Marstin, Marstyn, Marstan

Martin (Latin) Dedicated to Mars, the god of war
Martyn, Mart, Martel, Martell, Marten, Martenn, Marti, Martie

Marvin (Welsh) A friend of the sea
Marvinn, Marvinne, Marven, Marvenn, Marvenne, Marvyn, Marvynn, Marvynne, Mervin

Maryland (English) Honoring Queen Mary; from the state of Maryland
Mariland, Maralynd, Marylind, Marilind

Masanao (Japanese) A good man

Masao (Japanese) A righteous man

Mason (English) One who works with stone
Masun, Masen, Masan, Masin, Masyn, Masson, Massun, Massen, Maison

Masselin (French) A young Thomas
Masselyn, Masselen, Masselan, Masselon, Masselun, Maselin, Maselyn, Maselon

Masura (Japanese) A good destiny
Masoura

Mataniah (Hebrew) A gift from God
Matania, Matanya, Matanyahu, Mattania, Mattaniah, Matanyah

Matin (Arabic) Having great strength
Maten, Matan, Matyn, Maton, Matun

Matisse (French) One who is gifted
Matiss, Matysse, Matyss, Matise, Matyse

Matlock (American) A rancher
Matlok, Matloc

Matteo (Italian) Form of Matthew, meaning "a gift from God"
Mateo

Matthew (Hebrew) A gift from God
Matt, Mathew, Matvey, Mateas, Mattix, Madteos, Matthias, Mat, Mateo, Matteo, Mateus

Matunde (African) One who is fruitful
Matundi, Matundie

Matvey (Russian) Form of Matthew, meaning "a gift from God"
Matvy, Matvee, Matvea, Matvi, Matvie, Motka, Matviyko

Maurice (Latin) A dark-skinned man; Moorish
Maurell, Maureo, Mauricio, Maurids, Maurie, Maurin, Maurio, Maurise, Baurice

Maverick (English) An independent man; a non-conformist
Maveric, Maverik, Mavrick, Mavric, Mavrik

Max (English) Form of Maxwell, meaning from Mack's spring

Maximilian (Latin) The
greatest
*Max, Macks, Maxi, Maxie,
Maxy, Maxey, Maxee, Maxea,
Maximiliano*

Maxfield (English) From
Mack's field
Mackfield, Maxfeld, Macksfeld

Maxwell (English) From
Mack's spring
*Maxwelle, Mackswell, Maxwel,
Mackswel, Mackwelle, Maxwill,
Maxwille, Mackswill*

Mayer (Latin / German /
Hebrew) A large man / a
farmer / one who is shining
bright
*Maier, Mayar, Mayor, Mayir,
Mayur, Meyer, Meir, Myer*

Mayfield (English) From the
strong one's field
*Mayfeld, Maifield, Maifeld,
Maefield, Maefeld*

Mayo (Gaelic) From the yew
tree plain
*Mayoe, Maiyo, Maeyo, Maiyoe,
Maeyoe, Mayoh, Maioh*

Mccoy (Gaelic) The son of Coy
McCoy

McKenna (Gaelic) The son of
Kenna; to ascend
*McKennon, McKennun,
McKennen, McKennan*

Mckile (Gaelic) The son of Kyle
*McKile, Mckyle, McKyle,
Mackile, Mackyle, MacKile,
MacKyle*

Medwin (German) A strong
friend
*Medwine, Medwinn, Medwinne,
Medwen, Medwenn, Medwenne,
Medwyn, Medwynn*

Meged (Hebrew) One who has
been blessed with goodness

Mehdi (Arabian) One who is
guided
*Mehdie, Mehdy, Mehdey,
Mehdee, Mehdea*

Mehetabel (Hebrew) One who
is favored by God
*Mehetabell, Mehitabel,
Mehitabell, Mehytabel,
Mehytabell*

Meilyr (Welsh) A regal ruler

Meinrad (German) A strong
counselor
*Meinred, Meinrod, Meinrud,
Meinrid, Meinryd*

Meka (Hawaiian) Of the eyes
Mekah

Melancton (Greek)
Resembling a black flower
*Melankton, Melanctun,
Melanktun, Melancten,
Melankten, Melanchton,
Melanchten, Melanchthon*

Mele (Hawaiian) One who is happy

Melesio (Spanish) An attentive man; one who is careful
Melacio, Melasio, Melecio, Melicio, Meliseo, Milesio

Meletius (Greek) A cautious man
Meletios, Meletious, Meletus, Meletos

Meli (Native American) One who is bitter
Melie, Mely, Meley, Melee, Melea, Meleigh

Melker (Swedish) A king
Melkar, Melkor, Melkur, Melkir, Melkyr

Melton (English) From the mill town
Meltun, Meltin, Meltyn, Melten, Meltan

Melville (English) From the mill town
Melvill, Melvil, Melvile, Melvylle, Melvyll, Melvyl, Melvyle

Melvin (English) A friend who offers counsel
Melvinn, Melvinne, Melven, Melvenn, Melvenne, Melvyn, Melvynn, Melvynne, Belvin

Memphis (American) From the city in Tennessee
Memfis, Memphys, Memfys, Memphus, Memfus

Menassah (Hebrew) A forgetful man
Menassa, Menass, Menas, Menasse, Menasseh

Menefer (Egyptian) Of the beautiful city
Menefar, Menefir, Menefyr, Menefor, Menefur

Menelik (African) The son of a wise man
Menelick, Menelic, Menelyk, Menelyck, Menelyc

Merlin (Welsh) Of the sea fortress; in Arthurian legend, the wizard and mentor of King Arthur
Merlyn, Merlan, Merlon, Merlun, Merlen, Merlinn, Merlynn, Merlonn

Merrill (English) Of the shining sea
Meril, Merill, Merrel, Merrell, Merril, Meryl, Merryll, Meryll

Merton (English) From the town near the lake
Mertun, Mertan, Merten, Mertin, Mertyn, Murton, Murtun, Murten

Mervin (Welsh) Form of Marvin, meaning "a friend of the sea"
Mervinn, Mervinne, Mervyn, Mervynn, Mervynne, Merven, Mervenn, Mervenne

Meshach (Hebrew) An enduring man
Meshack, Meshac, Meshak, Meeshach, Meeshack, Meeshak, Meeshac

Mhina (African) One who is delightful
Mhinah, Mheena, Mheenah, Mheina, Mheinah, Mhienah, Mhienah, Mhyna

Micah (Hebrew) Form of Michael, meaning "who is like God?"
Mica, Mycah

Michael (Hebrew) Who is like God?
Makai, Micael, Mical, Micha, Michaelangelo, Michail, Michal, Micheal, Miguel, Mick

Mick (English) Form of Michael, meaning "who is like God?"
Micke, Mickey, Micky, Micki, Mickie, Mickee, Mickea, Mickel

Mieko (Japanese) A bright man

Miguel (Portuguese / Spanish) Form of Michael, meaning "who is like God?"
Migel, Myguel

Milan (Latin) An eager and hardworking man
Mylan

Miles (German / Latin) One who is merciful / a soldier
Myles, Miley, Mily, Mili, Milie, Milee

Milford (English) From the mill's ford
Millford, Milfurd, Millfurd, Milferd, Millferd, Milforde, Millforde, Milfurde

Miller (English) One who works at the mill
Millar, Millor, Millur, Millir, Millyr, Myller, Millen, Millan

Milo (German) Form of Miles, meaning "one who is merciful"
Mylo

Milson (English) The son of Miles
Milsun, Milsen, Milsin, Milsyn, Milsan

Mimir (Norse) In mythology, a giant who guarded the well of wisdom
Mymir, Mimeer, Mimyr, Mymeer, Mymyr, Meemir, Meemeer, Meemyr

Miner (Latin / English) One who works in the mines / a youth
Minor, Minar, Minur, Minir, Minyr

Mingan (Native American) Resembling a gray wolf
Mingen, Mingin, Mingon, Mingun, Mingyn

Minh (Vietnamese) A clever man

Minster (English) Of the church
Mynster, Minstar, Mynstar, Minstor, Mynstor, Minstur, Mynstur, Minstir

Miracle (American) An act of God's hand
Mirakle, Mirakel, Myracle, Myrakle

Mirage (French) An illusion
Myrage

Mirumbi (African) Born during a period of rain
Mirumbie, Mirumby, Mirumbey, Mirumbee, Mirumbea

Mitchell (English) Form of Michael, meaning "who is like God?"
Mitch, Mitchel, Mytch, Mitchum, Mytchill, Mitcham

Mitsu (Japanese) Of the light
Mytsu, Mitsue, Mytsue

Mochni (Native American) Resembling a talking bird
Mochnie, Mochny, Mochney, Mochnee, Mochnea

Modesty (Latin) One who is without conceit
Modesti, Modestie, Modestee, Modestus, Modestey, Modesto, Modestio, Modestine

Mohajit (Indian) A charming man
Mohajeet, Mohajeat, Mohajeit, Mohajiet, Mohajyt

Mohammed (Arabic) One who is greatly praised; the name of the prophet and founder of Islam
Mahomet, Mohamad, Mohamed, Mohamet, Mohammad, Muhammad, Muhammed, Mehmet

Mohave (Native American) A tribal name
Mohav, Mojave

Mojag (Native American) One who is never quiet

Molan (Irish) The servant of the storm
Molen

Momo (American) A warring man

Mona (African) A jealous man
Monah

Mongo (African) A well-known man
Mongoe, Mongow, Mongowe

Mongwau (Native American) Resembling an owl

Monroe (Gaelic) From the mouth of the river Roe
Monro, Monrow, Monrowe, Munro, Munroe, Munrow, Munrowe

Montenegro (Spanish) From the black mountain

Montgomery (French) From Gomeric's mountain
Monty, Montgomerey, Montgomeri, Montgomerie, Montgomeree, Montgomerea

Monty (English) Form of Montgomery, meaning "from Gomeric's mountain"
Montey, Monti, Montie, Montee, Montea, Montes, Montez

Moon (American) Born beneath the moon; a dreamer

Mooney (Irish) A wealthy man
Moony, Mooni, Moonie, Maonaigh, Moonee, Moonea, Moone

Moose (American) Resembling the animal; a big, strong man
Moos, Mooze, Mooz

Moran (Irish) A great man
Morane, Morain, Moraine, Morayn, Morayne, Moraen, Moraene

Morathi (African) A wise man
Morathie, Morathy, Morathey, Morathee, Morathea

Moreland (English) From the moors
Moorland, Morland

Morley (English) From the meadow on the moor
Morly, Morleigh, Morlee, Morlea, Morleah, Morli, Morlie, Moorley

Morpheus (Greek) In mythology, the god of dreams
Morfeus, Morphius, Mofius

Mortimer (French) Of the still water; of the dead sea
Mortymer, Morty, Mortey, Morti, Mortie, Mortee, Mortea, Mort, Morte

Moses (Hebrew) A savior; in the Bible, the leader of the

Israelites; drawn from the water
Mioshe, Mioshye, Mohsen, Moke, Moise, Moises, Mose, Moshe

Mostyn (Welsh) From the mossy settlement
Mostin, Mosten, Moston, Mostun, Mostan

Moswen (African) A light-skinned man
Moswenn, Moswenne, Moswin, Moswinn, Moswinne, Moswyn, Moswynn, Moswynne

Moubarak (Arabian) One who is blessed
Mubarak, Moobarak

Mounafes (Arabic) A rival

Muhannad (Arabic) One who wields a sword
Muhanned, Muhanad, Muhaned, Muhunnad, Muhunad, Muhanned, Muhaned

Mukhtar (Arabic) The chosen one
Muktar

Mukisa (Ugandan) Having good fortune
Mukysa

Mulcahy (Irish) A war chief
Mulcahey, Mulcahi, Mulcahie, Mulcahee, Mulcahea

Mundhir (Arabic) One who cautions others
Mundheer, Mundhear, Mundheir, Mundhier, Mundhyr

Murdock (Scottish) From the sea
Murdok, Murdoc, Murdo, Murdoch, Murtagh, Murtaugh, Murtogh, Murtough

Muriel (Gaelic) Of the shining sea
Muryel, Muriell, Muryell, Murial, Muriall, Muryal, Muryall, Murell

Murphy (Gaelic) A warrior of the sea
Murphey, Murphee, Murphea, Murphi, Murphie, Murfey, Murfy, Murfee

Murray (Gaelic) The lord of the sea
Murrey, Murry, Murri, Murrie, Murree, Murrea, Murry

Murron (Celtic) A bitter man
Murrun, Murren, Murran, Murrin, Murryn

Murtadi (Arabic) One who is content
Murtadie, Murtady, Murtadey, Murtadee, Murtadea

Musad (Arabic) One who is lucky
Musaad, Mus'ad

Mushin (Arabic) A charitable man
Musheen, Mushean, Mushein, Mushien, Mushyn

Muskan (Arabic) One who smiles often
Musken, Muskon, Muskun, Muskin, Muskyn

Muslim (Arabic) An adherent of Islam
Muslym, Muslem, Moslem, Moslim, Moslym

Mustapha (Arabic) The chosen one
Mustafa, Mostapha, Mostafa, Moustapha, Moustafa

Muti (Arabic) One who is obedient
Mutie, Muty, Mutey, Mutee, Mutea, Muta

Myron (Greek) Refers to myrrh, a fragrant oil
Myrun, Myran, Myren, Myrin, Myryn, Miron, Mirun, Miran

Mystique (French) A man with an air of mystery
Mystic, Mistique, Mysteek, Misteek, Mystiek, Mistiek, Mysteeque, Misteeque

N

Nabendu (Indian) Born beneath the new moon
Nabendue, Nabendoo, Nabendou

Nabhi (Indian) The best
Nabhie, Nabhy, Nabhey, Nabhee, Nabhea

Nabil (Arabic) A highborn man
Nabeel, Nabeal, Nabeil, Nabiel, Nabyl

Nabu (Babylonian) In mythology, the god of writing and wisdom
Nabue, Naboo, Nabo, Nebo, Nebu, Nebue, Neboo

Nachshon (Hebrew) An adventurous man; one who is daring
Nachson

Nadav (Hebrew) A generous man
Nadaav

Nadif (African) One who is born between seasons
Nadeef, Nadief, Nadeif, Nadyf, Nadeaf

Nadim (Arabic) A beloved friend
Nadeem, Nadeam, Nadiem, Nadeim, Nadym

Naftali (Hebrew) A struggling man; in the Bible, one of Jacob's sons
Naphtali, Naphthali, Neftali, Nefthali, Nephtali, Nephthali, Naftalie, Naphtalie

Nagel (German) One who makes nails
Nagle, Nagler, Naegel, Nageler, Nagelle, Nagele, Nagell

Nahir (Hebrew) A clear-headed and bright man
Naheer, Nahear, Naheir, Nahier, Nahyr, Naher

Nahum (Hebrew) A compassionate man
Nahom, Nahoum, Nahoom, Nahuem

Naji (Arabic) One who is safe
Najea, Naje, Najee, Najie, Najy, Najey, Nanji, Nanjie

Najib (Arabic) Of noble descent; a highborn man
Najeeb, Najeab, Najeib, Najieb, Najyb, Nageeb, Nageab, Nagyb

Nally (Irish) A poor man
Nalley, Nalli, Nallie, Nallee, Nallea, Nalleigh

Namir (Israeli) Resembling a leopard
Nameer, Namear, Namier, Nameir, Namyr

Nandan (Indian) One who is pleasing
Nanden, Nandin, Nandyn, Nandon, Nandun

Naotau (Indian) Our new son
Naotou

Napier (French / English) A mover / one who takes care of the royal linens
Neper

Napoleon (Italian / German) A man from Naples / son of the mists
Napolean, Napolion, Napoleone, Napoleane, Napolione

Narcissus (Greek) Resembling a daffodil; self-love; in mythology, a youth who fell in love with his reflection
Narciso, Narcisse, Narkissos, Narses, Narcisus, Narcis, Narciss

Naresh (Indian) A king
Nareshe, Natesh, Nateshe

Nasih (Arabic) One who advises others
Nasyh

Natal (Spanish) Born at Christmastime
Natale, Natalino, Natalio, Natall, Natalle, Nataleo, Natica

Nathan (Hebrew) Form of Nathaniel, meaning "a gift from God"
Nat, Natan, Nate, Nathen, Nathon, Nathin, Nathyn, Nathun, Lathan

Nathaniel (Hebrew) A gift from God
Nathan, Natanael, Nataniel, Nathanael, Nathaneal, Nathanial, Nathanyal, Nathanyel, Nethanel

Navarro (Spanish) From the plains
Navaro, Navarrio, Navario, Navarre, Navare, Nabaro, Nabarro

Naveed (Persian) Our best wishes
Navead, Navid, Navied, Naveid, Navyd

Nazim (Arabian) Of a soft breeze
Nazeem, Nazeam, Naziem, Nazeim, Nazym

Nebraska (Native American) From the flat water land; from the state of Nebraska

Neckarios (Greek) Of the nectar; one who is immortal
Nectaire, Nectarios, Nectarius, Nektario, Nektarius, Nektarios, Nektaire

Neelotpal (Indian) Resembling the blue lotus
Nealotpal, Nielotpal, Neilotpal, Nilothpal, Neelothpal

Negm (Arabian) Resembling a star

Nehal (Indian) Born during a period of rain
Nehall, Nehale, Nehalle

Nehemiah (Hebrew) God provides comfort
Nehemia, Nechemia, Nechemiah, Nehemya, Nehemyah, Nechemya, Nechemyah

Neil (Gaelic) The champion
Neal, Neale, Neall, Nealle, Nealon, Neel, Neilan, Neile

Neirin (Irish) Surrounded by light
Neiryn, Neiren, Neerin, Neeryn, Neeren

Nelek (Polish) Resembling a horn
Nelec, Neleck

Nelson (English) The son of Neil; the son of a champion
Nealson, Neilson, Neillson, Nelsen, Nilson, Nilsson, Nelli, Nellie

Neptune (Latin) In mythology, god of the sea
Neptun, Neptoon, Neptoone, Neptoun, Neptoune

Neroli (Italian) Resembling an orange blossom
Nerolie, Neroly, Neroley, Neroleigh, Nerolea, Nerolee

Nevan (Irish) The little saint
Naomhan

Neville (French) From the new village
Nev, Nevil, Nevile, Nevill, Nevylle, Nevyl, Nevyle, Nevyll

Newcomb (English) From the new valley
Newcom, Newcome, Newcombe, Neucomb, Neucombe, Neucom, Neucome

Newlin (Welsh) From the new pond
Newlinn, Newlyn, Newlynn, Neulin, Neulinn, Neulyn, Neulynn

Newman (English) A newcomer
Newmann, Neuman, Neumann

Niaz (Persian) A gift
Nyaz

Nibaw (Native American) One who stands tall
Nybaw, Nibau, Nybau

Nicholas (Greek) Of the victorious people
Nick, Nicanor, Niccolo, Nichol, Nicholai, Nicholaus, Nikolai, Nicholl, Nichols, Colin, Nicolas, Nico

Nick (English) Form of Nicholas, meaning "of the victorious people"
Nik, Nicki, Nickie, Nickey, Nicky, Nickee, Nickea, Niki

Nicomedes (Greek) One who thinks of victory
Nikomedes, Nicomedo, Nikomedo

Nihal (Indian) One who is content
Neehal, Neihal, Niehal, Neahal, Neyhal, Nyhal

Nihar (Indian) Covered with the morning's dew
Neehar, Niehar, Neihar, Neahar, Nyhar

Nikan (Persian) One who brings good things
Niken, Nikin, Nikyn, Nikon, Nikun

Nikshep (Indian) One who is
treasured
Nykshep

Nikunja (Indian) From the
grove of trees

Nino (Italian / Spanish) God is
gracious / a young boy
Ninoshka

Nirad (Indian) Of the clouds
Nyrad

Niran (Thai) The eternal one
*Nyran, Niren, Nirin, Niryn,
Niron, Nirun, Nyren, Nyrin*

Nirav (Indian) One who is quiet
Nyrav

Nirbheet (Indian) A fearless
man
*Nirbhit, Nirbhyt, Nirbhay,
Nirbhaye, Nirbhai, Nirbhae*

Niremaan (Arabic) One who
shines as brightly as fire
Nyremaan, Nireman, Nyreman

Nishan (Armenian) A sign or
symbol

Nishok (Indian) Filled with
happiness
Nyshok, Nishock, Nyshock

Nissan (Hebrew) A miracle
child
Nisan

Niyol (Native American) Of
the wind

Njord (Scandinavian) A man
from the north
Njorde, Njorth, Njorthe

Noah (Hebrew) A peaceful
wanderer
Noa

Nodin (Native American) Of
the wind
*Nodyn, Noden, Nodan, Nodon,
Nodun*

Nolan (Gaelic) A famous
and noble man; a champion
of the people
*Nolen, Nolin, Nolon, Nolun,
Nolyn, Noland, Nolande*

North (English) A man from
the north
Northe

Northcliff (English) From the
northern cliff
*Northcliffe, Northclyf,
Northclyff, Northclyffe*

Norval (Scottish) From the
northern valley
*Norvall, Norvale, Norvail,
Norvaile, Norvayl, Norvayle,
Norvael, Norvaele*

Norward (English) A guardian
of the north
*Norwarde, Norwerd, Norwerde,
Norwurd, Norwurde*

Noshi (Native American) A fatherly man
Noshie, Noshy, Noshey, Noshee, Noshea, Nosh, Noshe

Notaku (Native American) Resembling a growling bear
Notakou, Notakue, Notakoo

Nuhad (Arabic) A brave young man
Nuehad, Nouhad, Neuhad

Nuncio (Spanish) A messenger
Nunzio

Nuriel (Hebrew) God's light
Nuriell, Nuriele, Nurielle, Nuryel, Nuryell, Nuryele, Nuryelle, Nooriel

Nuru (African) My light
Nurue, Nuroo, Nurou, Nourou, Nooroo

Nyack (African) One who is persistent
Niack, Nyak, Niak, Nyac, Niac

Nye (English) One who lives on the island
Nyle, Nie, Nile

O

Obedience (American) A well-behaved man
Obediance, Obedyence, Obedeynce

Oberon (German) A royal bear; having the heart of a bear
Oberron

Obert (German) A wealthy and bright man
Oberte, Oberth, Oberthe, Odbart, Odbarte, Odbarth, Odbarthe, Odhert

Ochi (African) Filled with laughter
Ochie, Ochee, Ochea, Ochy, Ochey

Odam (English) A son-in-law
Odom, Odem, Odum

Ode (Egyptian / Greek) Traveler of the road / a lyric poem

Oded (Hebrew) One who is supportive and encouraging

Oder (English) From the river
Odar, Odir, Odyr, Odur

Odin (Norse) In mythology, the supreme deity
Odyn, Odon, Oden, Odun

Odinan (Hungarian) One who is wealthy and powerful
Odynan, Odinann, Odynann

Odion (African) The first-born of twins
Odiyon, Odiun, Odiyun

Odissan (African) A wanderer; traveler
Odyssan, Odisan, Odysan, Odissann, Odyssann, Odisann, Odysann

Ofir (Hebrew) The golden son
Ofeer, Ofear, Ofyr, Ofier, Ofeir, Ofer

Oghe (Irish) One who rides horses
Oghi, Oghie, Oghee, Oghea, Oghy, Oghey

Oguz (Hungarian) An arrow
Oguze, Oguzz, Oguzze

Ohanko (Native American) A reckless man
Ohankio, Ohankiyo

Ojaswit (Indian) A powerful and radiant man
Ojaswyt, Ojaswin, Ojaswen, Ojaswyn, Ojas

Okal (African) To cross
Okall

Okan (Turkish) Resembling a horse
Oken, Okin, Okyn

Okapi (African) Resembling an animal with a long neck
Okapie, Okapy, Okapey, Okapee, Okapea, Okape

Okechuku (African) Blessed by God

Oki (Japanese) From the center of the ocean
Okie, Oky, Okey, Okee, Okea

Olaf (Scandinavian) The remaining of the ancestors
Olay, Ole, Olef, Olev, Oluf, Uolevi

Olafemi (African) A lucky young man
Olafemie, Olafemy, Olafemey, Olafemee, Olafemea

Oleg (Russian) One who is holy
Olezka

Oliver (Latin) From the olive tree
Oliviero, Olivero, Olivier, Oliviero, Olivio, Ollie

Olney (English) From the loner's field
Olny, Olnee, Olnea, Olni, Olnie, Ollaneg, Olaneg

Olumide (African) God has arrived
Olumidi, Olumidie, Olumidy, Olumidey, Olumidee, Olumidea, Olumyde, Olumydi

Omar (Arabic) A flourishing man; one who is well-spoken
Omarr, Omer

Omeet (Hebrew) My light
Omeete, Omeit, Omeite, Omeyt, Omeyte, Omit, Omeat, Omeate

Omega (Greek) The last great one; the last letter of the Greek alphabet
Omegah

Onaona (Hawaiian) Having a pleasant scent

Ond (Hungarian) The tenth-born child
Onde

Ondrej (Czech) A manly man
Ondrejek, Ondrejec, Ondrousek, Ondravsek

Onkar (Indian) The purest one
Onckar, Oncar, Onkarr, Onckarr, Oncarr

Onofrio (Italian) A defender of peace
Onofre, Onofrius, Onophrio, Onophre, Onfrio, Onfroi

Onslow (Arabic) From the hill of the enthusiast
Onslowe, Ounslow, Ounslowe

Onyebuchi (African) God is in everything
Onyebuchie, Onyebuchy, Onyebuchey, Onyebuchee, Onyebuchea

Oqwapi (Native American) Resembling a red cloud
Oqwapie, Oqwapy, Oqwapey, Oqwapee, Oqwapea

Oram (English) From the enclosure near the riverbank
Oramm, Oraham, Orahamm, Orham, Orhamm

Ordell (Latin) Of the beginning
Ordel, Ordele, Ordelle, Orde

Ordway (Anglo-Saxon) A fighter armed with a spear
Ordwaye, Ordwai, Ordwae

Oren (Hebrew / Gaelic) From the pine tree / a pale-skinned man
Orenthiel, Orenthiell, Orenthiele, Orenthielle, Orenthiem, Orenthium, Orin

Orion (Greek) A great hunter

Orleans (Latin) The golden child
Orlean, Orleane, Orleens, Orleen, Orleene, Orlins, Olryns, Orlin

Orly (Hebrew) Surrounded by light
Orley, Orli, Orlie, Orlee, Orleigh, Orlea

Ormod (Anglo-Saxon) A sorrowful man

Ormond (English) One who defends with a spear / from the mountain of bears
Ormonde, Ormund, Ormunde, Ormemund, Ormemond, Ordmund, Ordmunde, Ordmond

Ornice (Irish / Hebrew) A pale-skinned man / from the cedar tree
Ornyce, Ornise, Orynse, Orneice, Orneise, Orniece, Orniese, Orneece

Orris (Latin) One who is inventive
Orriss, Orrisse, Orrys, Orryss, Orrysse

Orson (Latin) Resembling a bear; raised by a bear
Orsen, Orsin, Orsini, Orsino, Orsis, Orsonio, Orsinie, Orsiny

Orth (English) An honest man
Orthe

Orton (English) From the settlement by the shore
Ortun, Oraton, Oratun

Orville (French) From the gold town
Orvell, Orvelle, Orvil, Orvill, Orvele, Orvyll, Orvylle, Orvyl

Orwel (Welsh) Of the horizon
Orwell, Orwele, Orwelle

Os (English) The divine

Osborn (Norse) A bear of God
Osborne, Osbourn, Osbourne, Osburn, Osburne

Oscar (English / Gaelic) A spear of the gods / a friend of deer
Oskar, Osker, Oscer, Osckar, Oscker, Oszkar, Oszcar

Osher (Hebrew) A man of good fortune

Osias (Greek) Salvation
Osyas

Oswald (English) The power of God
Oswalde, Osvald, Osvaldo, Oswaldo, Oswell, Osvalde, Oswallt, Osweald

Oswin (English) A friend of God
Oswinn, Oswinne, Oswen, Oswenn, Oswenne, Oswyn, Oswynn, Oswynne

Othniel (Hebrew) God's lion
Othniell, Othnielle, Othniele,
Othnyel, Othnyell, Othnyele,
Othnyelle

Otmar (Teutonic) A famous
warrior
Otmarr, Othmar, Othmarr,
Otomar, Ottomar

Ottokar (German) A spirited
warrior
Otokar, Otokarr, Ottokarr,
Ottokars, Otokars, Ottocar,
Otocar, Ottocars

Ouray (Native American) The
arrow
Ouraye, Ourae, Ourai

Ourson (French) Resembling
a little bear
Oursun, Oursoun, Oursen,
Oursan, Oursin, Oursyn

Ovid (Latin) A shepherd; an
egg
Ovyd, Ovidio, Ovido, Ovydio,
Ovydo, Ovidiu, Ovydiu, Ofydd

Owen (Welsh / Gaelic) Form
of Eugene, meaning "a well-
born man" / a youthful man
Owenn, Owenne, Owin,
Owinn, Owinne, Owyn,
Owynn, Owynne

Oxton (English) From the
oxen town
Oxtun, Oxtown, Oxnaton,
Oxnatun, Oxnatown

Oz (Hebrew) Having great
strength
Ozz, Ozzi, Ozzie, Ozzy,
Ozzey, Ozzee, Ozzea, Ozi

Ozni (Hebrew) One who
knows God
Oznie, Ozny, Ozney, Oznee,
Oznea

Ozuru (Japanese) Resembling
a stork
Ozurou, Ozourou, Ozuroo,
Ozooroo

P

Paavo (Finnish) Form of Paul,
meaning "a small or humble
man"
Paaveli

Pace (Hebrew / English)
Refers to Passover / a peace-
ful man
Paice, Payce, Paece, Pacey,
Pacy, Pacee, Paci, Pacie

Pacho (Spanish) An
independent man; one
who is free

Pachu'a (Native American)
Resembling a water snake

Paco (Spanish) A man from France
Pacorro, Pacoro, Paquito

Padgett (French) One who strives to better himself
Padget, Padgette, Padgete, Padgeta, Padgetta, Padge, Paget, Pagett

Padman (Indian) Resembling the lotus
Padmann

Padruig (Scottish) Of the royal family

Paine (Latin) Man from the country; a peasant
Pain, Payn, Payne, Paen, Paene, Pane, Paien

Paley (English) Form of Paul, meaning "a small or humble man"
Paly, Pali, Palie, Palee, Palea

Palladin (Greek) Filled with wisdom
Palladyn, Palladen, Palladan, Paladin, Paladyn, Paladen, Paladan

Palmer (English) A pilgrim bearing a palm branch
Pallmer, Palmar, Pallmar, Palmerston, Palmiro, Palmeero, Palmeer, Palmire

Pan (Greek) In mythology, god of the shepherds
Pann

Panama (Spanish) From the canal

Pancho (Spanish) A man from France

Pankaj (Indian) Resembling the lotus flower

Panya (African) Resembling a mouse
Panyah

Panyin (African) The first-born of twins
Panyen

Paras (Hindi) A touchstone
Parasmani, Parasmanie, Parasmany, Parasmaney, Parasmanee

Parker (English) The keeper of the park
Parkar, Parkes, Parkman, Park

Parley (Scottish) A reluctant man
Parly, Parli, Parlie, Parlee, Parlea, Parle

Parmenio (Spanish) A studious man; one who is intelligent
Parmenios, Parmenius

Parrish (Latin) Man of the church
Parish, Parrishe, Parishe, Parrysh, Parysh, Paryshe, Parryshe, Parisch

Parry (Welsh) The son of Harry
Parrey, Parri, Parrie, Parree, Parrea

Parthenios (Greek) One who is pure; chaste
Parthenius

Parthik (Greek) One who is pure; chaste
Parthyk, Parthick, Parthyck, Parthic, Parthyc

Pascal (Latin) Born during Easter
Pascale, Pascalle, Paschal, Paschalis, Pascoe, Pascual, Pascuale, Pasqual

Patamon (Native American) Resembling a tempest
Patamun, Patamen, Pataman, Patamyn, Patamin

Patch (American) Form of Peter, meaning "as solid and strong as a rock"
Pach, Patche, Patchi, Patchie, Patchy, Patchey, Patchee

Patrick (Latin) A nobleman; patrician
Packey, Padric, Pat, Patrece, Patric, Patrice, Patreece, Patricio

Patton (English) From the town of warriors
Paten, Patin, Paton, Patten, Pattin, Paddon, Padden, Paddin

Patwin (Native American) A manly man
Patwinn, Patwinne, Patwyn, Patwynne, Patwynn, Patwen, Patwenn, Patwenne

Paul (Latin) A small or humble man
Pauley, Paulie, Pauly, Paley, Paavo

Paurush (Indian) A courageous man
Paurushe, Paurushi, Paurushie, Paurushy, Paurushey, Paurushee

Pavanjit (Indian) Resembling the wind
Pavanjyt, Pavanjeet, Pavanjeat, Pavanjete

Paxton (English) From the peaceful town
Packston, Paxon, Paxten, Paxtun, Packstun, Packsten

Pazel (Hebrew) God's gold;
treasured by God
Pazell, Pazele, Pazelle

Pedro (Spanish) Form of
Peter, meaning "as solid and
strong as a rock"
*Pedrio, Pepe, Petrolino, Piero,
Pietro*

Pelham (English) From the
house of furs; from Peola's
home
Pellham, Pelam, Pellam

Pell (English) A clerk or one
who works with skins
Pelle, Pall, Palle

Pelon (Spanish) Filled with joy
Pellon

Pelton (English) From the
town by the lake
*Pellton, Peltun, Pelltun, Peltan,
Pelltan, Pelten, Pellten, Peltin*

Penda (African) One who is
dearly loved
Pendah, Penha, Penhah

Penley (English) From the
enclosed meadow
*Penly, Penleigh, Penli, Penlie,
Penlee, Penlea, Penleah, Pennly*

Pentele (Hungarian) A
merciful man
Pentelle, Pentel, Pentell

Penuel (Hebrew) The face of
God
Penuell, Penuele, Penuelle

Percival (French) One who can
pierce the vale"
*Purcival, Percy, Percey, Perci,
Percie, Percee, Percea, Persy,
Persey, Persi*

Peregrine (Latin) One who
travels; a wanderer
*Perry, Perree, Perrea, Perri,
Perrie, Perregrino*

Perez (Hebrew) To break
through
Peretz

Pericles (Greek) One who is in
excess of glory
*Perricles, Perycles, Perrycles,
Periclees, Perriclees, Peryclees,
Perryclees, Periclez*

Perkinson (English) The son of
Perkin; the son of Peter
Perkynson

Perseus (Greek) In mythology,
son of Zeus who slew Medusa
Persius, Persyus, Persies, Persyes

Perth (Celtic) From the thorny
thicket
Perthe, Pert, Perte

Perye (English) From the pear tree

Peter (Greek) As solid and strong as a rock
Peder, Pekka, Per, Petar, Pete, Peterson, Petr, Petre, Pierce, Patch, Pedro

Petuel (Hindi) The Lord's vision
Petuell, Petuele, Petuelle

Peyton (English) From the village of warriors
Payton, Peytun, Paytun, Peyten, Payten, Paiton, Paitun, Paiten

Pharis (Irish) A heroic man
Pharys, Pharris, Pharrys

Phex (American) A kind man
Phexx

Philemon (Hebrew) A loving man
Phylemon, Philimon, Phylimon, Philomon, Phylomon, Philamon, Phylamon

Philetus (Greek) A collector
Phyletus, Philetos, Phyletos

Phillip (Greek) One who loves horses
Phil, Philip, Felipe, Filipp, Phillie, Philly

Philo (Greek) One who loves and is loved

Phoebus (Greek) A radiant man
Phoibos

Phomello (African) A successful man
Phomelo

Phong (Vietnamese) Of the wind

Picardus (Hispanic) An adventurous man
Pycardus, Picardos, Pycardos, Picardas, Pycardas, Picardis, Pycardis, Picardys

Pierce (English) Form of Peter, meaning "as solid and strong as a rock"
Pearce, Pears, Pearson, Pearsson, Peerce, Peirce, Pierson, Piersson

Pin (Vietnamese) Filled with joy
Pyn

Pio (Latin) A pious man
Pyo, Pios, Pius, Pyos, Pyus

Pirro (Greek) A red-haired man
Pyrro

Pitney (English) From the island of the stubborn man
Pitny, Pitni, Pitnie, Pitnee, Pitnea, Pytney, Pytny, Pytni

Pittman (English) A laborer
Pyttman, Pitman, Pytman

Plantagenet (French)
Resembling the broom flower

Poetry (American) A romantic
man
*Poetrey, Poetri, Poetrie, Poetree,
Poetrea, Poet, Poete*

Pollux (Greek) One who is
crowned
*Pollock, Pollok, Polloc, Pollack,
Polloch*

Polo (African) Resembling an
alligator
Poloe, Poloh

Ponce (Spanish) The fifth-born
child
Ponse

Pongor (Hungarian) A mighty
man
Pongorr, Pongoro, Pongorro

Poni (African) The
second-born son
*Ponni, Ponie, Ponnie, Pony,
Ponny, Poney, Ponney, Ponee*

Pons (Latin) From the bridge
Pontius, Ponthos, Ponthus

Poornamruth (Indian) Full of
sweetness
Pournamruth

Porat (Hebrew) A productive
man

Porfirio (Greek) Refers to a
purple coloring
*Porphirios, Prophyrios, Porfiro,
Porphyrios*

Powhatan (Native American)
From the chief's hill

Prabhakar (Hindu) Of the sun

Prabhat (Indian) Born during
the morning

Pragun (Indian) One who is
straightforward; honest

Pramod (Indian) A delightful
young man

Pranit (Indian) One who is
humble; modest
Pranyt, Praneet, Praneat

Prasad (Indian) A gift from
God

Prashant (Indian) One who is
peaceful; calm
*Prashante, Prashanth,
Prashanthe*

Pratap (Hindi) A majestic man

Pravat (Thai) History

Prem (Indian) An affectionate
man

Prentice (English) A student;
an apprentice
*Prentyce, Prentise, Prentyse,
Prentiss, Prentis*

Prescott (English) From the priest's cottage
Prescot, Prestcot, Prestcott, Preostcot

Preston (English) From the priest's town
Prestin, Prestyn, Prestan, Prestun, Presten, Pfeostun

Prewitt (French) A brave young one
Prewet, Prewett, Prewit, Pruitt, Pruit, Pruet, Pruett

Prine (English) One who surpasses others
Pryne

Prometheus (Greek) In mythology, he stole fire from the heavens and gave it to man
Promitheus, Promethius, Promithius

Prosper (Latin) A fortunate man
Prospero, Prosperus

Pryderi (Celtic) Son of the sea
Pryderie, Prydery, Pryderey, Pryderee, Pryderea

Prydwen (Welsh) A handsome man
Prydwenn, Prydwenne, Prydwin, Prydwinne, Prydwinn, Prydwyn, Prydwynn, Prydwynne

Pyralis (Greek) Born of fire
Pyraliss, Pyralisse, Pyralys, Pyralyss, Pyralysse, Pyre

Qabil (Arabic) An able-bodied man
Qabyl, Qabeel, Qabeal, Qabeil, Qabiel

Qadim (Arabic) From an ancient family
Qadeem, Qadiem, Qadeim, Qadym, Qadeam

Qaiser (Arabic) A king; a ruler
Qeyser

Qamar (Arabic) Born beneath the moon
Qamarr, Quamar, Quamarr

Qimat (Hindi) A highly valued man
Qymat

Qing (Chinese) Of the deep water
Qyng

Quaddus (American) A bright man
Quadus, Quaddos, Quados

Quade (Latin) The fourth-born child
Quadrees, Quadres, Quadrys, Quadries, Quadreis, Quadreys, Quadreas, Quadrhys

Quaid (Irish) Form of Walter, meaning "the commander of the army"
Quaide, Quayd, Quayde, Quaed, Quaede

Qued (Native American) Wearing a decorated robe

Quentin (Latin) The fifth-born child
Quent, Quenten, Quenton, Quentun, Quentan, Quentyn, Quente, Qwentin

Quick (American) One who is fast; a witty man
Quik, Quicke, Quic

Quillan (Gaelic) Resembling a cub
Quilan, Quillen, Quilen, Quillon, Quilon

Quilliam (Gaelic) Form of William, meaning "the determined protector"
Quilhelm, Quilhelmus, Quilliams, Quilliamson

Quimby (Norse) From the woman's estate
Quimbey, Quimbee, Quimbea, Quimbi, Quimbie

Quincy (English) The fifth-born child; from the fifth son's estate
Quincey, Quinci, Quincie, Quincee, Quinncy, Quinnci, Qúyncy, Quyncey

Quinlan (Gaelic) A strong and healthy man
Quindlan, Quinlen, Quindlen, Quinian, Quinlin, Quindlin, Quinlyn, Quindlyn

Quinn (Gaelic) One who provides counsel; an intelligent man
Quin, Quinne, Qwinn, Quynn, Qwin, Quiyn, Quyn, Qwinne

Quintavius (American) The fifth-born child
Quintavios, Quintavus, Quintavies

Quinto (Spanish) The fifth-born child
Quynto, Quintus, Quintos, Quinty, Quinti, Quintie

Quinton (Latin) From the queen's town or settlement
Laquinton

Quintrell (English) An elegant and dashing man
Quintrel, Quintrelle, Quyntrell, Quyntrelle, Quyntrel, Quyntrele, Quintrele

Quirinus (Latin) One who wields a spear
Quirinos, Quirynus, Quirynos, Quirinius, Quirynius

Quito (Spanish) A lively man
Quyto, Quitos, Quytos

Quoc (Vietnamese) A patriot
Quok, Quock

Qutub (Indian) One who is tall

R

Rabbaanee (African) An easy-going man

Rabbi (Hebrew) The master

Rach (African) Resembling a frog

Radames (Egyptian) A hero
Radamays, Radamayes, Radamais, Radamaise

Radford (English) From the red ford
Radforde, Radferd, Radfurd, Radferde, Radfurde

Rafael (Spanish) Form of Raphael, meaning "one who is healed by God"
Raphael, Raphaello, Rafaello

Rafe (Irish) A tough man
Raffe, Raff, Raf, Raif, Rayfe, Raife, Raef, Raefe

Rafi (Arabic) One who is exalted
Rafie, Rafy, Rafey, Rafea, Rafee, Raffi, Raffie, Raffy

Rafiki (African) A gentle friend
Rafikie, Rafikea, Rafikee, Rafiky, Rafikey

Rafiya (African) A dignified man
Rafeeya, Rafeaya, Rafeiya, Rafieya

Raghib (Arabic) One who is desired
Ragheb, Ragheeb, Ragheab, Raghyb, Ragheib, Raghieb

Ragnar (Norse) A warrior who places judgment
Ragnor, Ragner, Ragnir, Ragnyr, Ragnur, Regnar

Rahim (Arabic) A compassionate man
Rahym, Raheim, Rahiem, Raheem, Raheam

Raiden (Japanese) In mythology, the god of thunder and lightning
Raidon, Rayden, Raydon, Raeden, Raedon, Raden

Raimi (African) A
compassionate man
*Raimie, Raimy, Raimey,
Raimee, Raimea*

Rajab (African) A glorified
man

Rajan (Indian) A king
Raj, Raja, Rajah

Rajarshi (Indian) The king's
sage
*Rajarshie, Rajarshy, Rajarshey,
Rajarshee, Rajarshea*

Rajesh (Hindi) The king's rule

Rajit (Indian) One who is
decorated
*Rajeet, Rajeit, Rajiet, Rajyt,
Rajeat*

Rajiv (Hindi) To be striped
Rajyv, Rajeev, Rajeav

Ralph (English) Wolf counsel
*Ralf, Ralphe, Ralfe, Ralphi,
Ralphie, Ralphee, Ralphea,
Ralphy, Raoul*

Rami (Arabic) A loving man
*Ramee, Ramea, Ramie, Ramy,
Ramey*

Ramiro (Portuguese) A famous
counselor; a great judge
*Ramyro, Rameero, Rameyro,
Ramirez, Ramyrez, Rameerez*

Ramsey (English) From the
raven island; from the island
of wild garlic
*Ramsay, Ramsie, Ramsi,
Ramsee, Ramsy, Ramsea,
Ramzy, Ramzey*

Rand (German) One who
shields others
Rande

Randall (German) The wolf
shield
*Randy, Randal, Randale,
Randel, Randell, Randl,
Randle, Randon, Rendall*

Randolph (German) The wolf
shield
*Randy, Randolf, Ranolf,
Ranolph, Ranulfo, Randulfo,
Randwulf, Ranwulf, Randwolf*

Randy (English) Form of
Randall or Randolph,
meaning "the wolf shield"
*Randey, Randi, Randie,
Randee, Randea*

Rang (English) Resembling a
raven
Range

Ranjan (Indian) A delightful boy

Raoul (French) Form of Ralph,
meaning "wolf counsel"
*Raoule, Raul, Roul, Rowl,
Raule, Roule, Rowle*

Raqib (Arabic) A glorified man
Raqyb, Raqeeb, Raqeab, Rakib, Rakeeb, Rakeab, Rakyb

Rashaun (American) Form of Roshan, meaning "born during the daylight"
Rashae, Rashane, Rashawn, Rayshaun, Rayshawn, Raishaun, Raishawn, Raeshaun

Ratul (Indian) A sweet man
Ratule, Ratoul, Ratoule, Ratool, Ratoole

Raulo (Spanish) One who is wise
Rawlo

Ravi (Hindi) From the sun
Ravie, Ravy, Ravey, Ravee, Ravea

Ravid (Hebrew) A wanderer; one who searches
Ravyd, Raveed, Ravead, Raviyd, Ravied, Raveid

Ravindra (Indian) The strength of the sun
Ravyndra

Ravinger (English) One who lives near the ravine
Ravynger

Rawlins (French) From the renowned land
Rawlin, Rawson, Rawlinson, Rawlings, Rawling, Rawls, Rawl, Rawle

Ray (English) Form of Raymond, meaning "a wise protector"
Rae, Rai, Rayce, Rayder, Rayse, Raye, Rayford, Raylen

Rayfield (English) From the field of roe deer
Rayfeld

Rayhurn (English) From the roe deer's stream
Rayhurne, Rayhorn, Rayhorne, Rayhourn, Rayhourne

Raymond (German) A wise protector
Ray, Raemond, Raemondo, Raimond, Raimondo, Raimund, Raimundo, Rajmund, Ramon

Rebel (American) An outlaw
Rebell, Rebele, Rebelle, Rebe, Rebbe, Rebbi, Rebbie, Rebbea

Reeve (English) A bailiff
Reve, Reave, Reeford, Reeves, Reaves, Reves, Reaford

Regal (American) Born into royalty
Regall

Regan (Gaelic) Born into royalty; the little ruler
Raegan, Ragan, Raygan, Reganne, Regann, Regane, Reghan, Reagan

Reggie (Latin) Form of Reginald, meaning "the king's advisor"
Reggi, Reggy, Reggey, Reggea, Reggee, Reg

Reginald (Latin) The king's advisor
Reggie, Reynold, Raghnall, Rainault, Rainhold, Raonull, Raynald, Rayniero, Regin, Reginaldo

Regine (French) One who is artistic
Regeen, Regeene, Regean, Regeane, Regein, Regeine, Regien, Regiene

Reid (English) A red-haired man; one who lives near the reeds
Read, Reade, Reed, Reede, Reide, Raed

Reilly (Gaelic) An outgoing man
Reilley, Reilli, Reillie, Reillee, Reilleigh, Reillea

Remington (English) From the town of the raven's family
Remyngton, Remingtun, Remyngtun

Renweard (Anglo-Saxon) The guardian of the house
Renward, Renwarden, Renwerd

Renzo (Japanese) The third-born son

Reuben (Hebrew) Behold, a son!
Reuban, Reubin, Reuven, Rouvin, Rube, Ruben, Rubin, Rubino

Rex (Latin) A king
Reks, Recks, Rexs

Rexford (English) From the king's ford
Rexforde, Rexferd, Rexferde, Rexfurd, Rexfurde

Reynold (English) Form of Reginald, meaning "the king's advisor"
Reynald, Reynaldo, Reynolds, Reynalde, Reynolde

Rhett (Latin) A well-spoken man
Rett, Rhet

Rhys (Welsh) Having great enthusiasm for life

Richard (English) A powerful ruler
Rick, Rich, Ricard, Ricardo, Riccardo, Richardo, Richart, Richerd, Rickard, Rickert

Richmond (French / German)
From the wealthy hill / a
powerful protector
*Richmonde, Richmund,
Richmunde*

Rick (English) Form of
Richard, meaning "a powerful
ruler"
*Ric, Ricci, Ricco, Rickie, Ricki,
Ricky, Rico, Rik*

Riddock (Irish) From the
smooth field
*Ridock, Riddoc, Ridoc,
Ryddock, Rydock, Ryddoc,
Rydoc, Ryddok*

Ridgeway (English) One who
lives on the road near the
ridge
Rydgeway, Rigeway, Rygeway

Rigg (English) One who lives
near the ridge
*Rig, Ridge, Rygg, Ryg, Rydge,
Rige, Ryge, Riggs*

Riley (English) From the rye
clearing
*Ryly, Ryli, Rylie, Rylee,Ryleigh,
Rylea, Ryleah*

Riordain (Irish) A bright man
*Riordane, Riordayn, Riordaen,
Reardain, Reardane, Reardayn,
Reardaen*

Riordan (Gaelic) A royal poet;
a bard or minstrel
*Riorden, Rearden, Reardan,
Riordon, Reardon*

Ripley (English) From the
noisy meadow
*Riply, Ripleigh, Ripli, Riplie,
Riplea, Ripleah, Riplee, Rip*

Rishley (English) From the
untamed meadow
*Rishly, Rishli, Rishlie, Rishlee,
Rishlea, Rishleah, Rishleigh*

Rishon (Hebrew) The first-
born son
*Ryshon, Rishi, Rishie, Rishea,
Rishee, Rishy, Rishey*

Risley (English) From the
brushwood meadow
*Risly, Risli, Rislie, Risleigh,
Rislea, Risleah, Rislee*

Riston (English) From the
brushwood settlement
Ryston, Ristun, Rystun

Ritter (German) A knight
Rytter, Ritt, Rytt

River (American) From the
river
Ryver, Rivers, Ryvers

Roald (Norse) A famous ruler
Roal

Roam (American) One who wanders, searches
Roami, Roamie, Roamy, Roamey, Roamea, Roamee

Roark (Gaelic) A champion
Roarke, Rorke, Rourke, Rork, Rourk, Ruark, Ruarke

Robert (German) One who is bright with fame
Bob, Rupert, Riobard, Roban, Robers, Roberto, Robertson, Robartach

Rochester (English) From the stone fortress

Rockford (English) From the rocky ford
Rockforde, Rokford, Rokforde, Rockferd, Rokferd, Rockfurd, Rokfurd

Roderick (German) A famous ruler
Rod, Rodd, Roddi, Roddie, Roddy, Roddee, Roddea

Rodney (German / English) From the famous one's island / from the island's clearing
Rodny, Rodni, Rodnie

Rogelio (Spanish) A famous soldier
Rogelo, Rogeliyo, Rogeleo, Rogeleyo, Rojelio, Rojeleo

Roland (German) From the renowned land
Roeland, Rolando, Roldan, Roley, Rollan, Rolland, Rollie, Rollin

Roman (Latin) A citizen of Rome
Romain, Romaine, Romeo

Romeo (Italian) Traveler to Rome

Ronald (Norse) The king's advisor
Ranald, Renaldo, Ronal, Ronaldo, Rondale, Roneld, Ronell, Ronello

Ronan (Gaelic) Resembling a little seal
Ronin

Rong (Chinese) Having glory

Rook (English) Resembling a raven
Rooke, Rouk, Rouke, Ruck, Ruk

Rooney (Gaelic) A red-haired man
Roony, Rooni, Roonie, Roonea, Roonee, Roon, Roone

Roosevelt (Danish) From the field of roses
Rosevelt

Roper (English) One who makes rope
Rapere

Rory (Gaelic) A red-haired man
Rori, Rorey, Rorie, Rorea, Roree, Rorry, Rorrey, Rorri

Roshan (Hindi) Born during the daylight
Rashaun

Roslin (Gaelic) A little red-haired boy
Roslyn, Rosselin, Rosslyn, Rozlin, Rozlyn, Rosling, Rozling

Roswald (German) Of the mighty horses
Rosswald, Roswalt, Rosswalt

Roswell (English) A fascinating man
Rosswell, Rozwell, Roswel, Rozwel

Roth (German) A red-haired man
Rothe

Rousseau (French) A little red-haired boy
Roussell, Russo, Rousse, Roussel, Rousset, Rousskin

Rowdy (English) A boisterous man
Rowdey, Rowdi, Rowdie, Rowdee, Rowdea

Roy (Gaelic / French) A red-haired man / a king
Roye, Roi, Royer, Ruy

Royce (German / French) A famous man / son of the king
Roice, Royse, Roise

Ruadhan (Irish) A red-haired man; the name of a saint
Ruadan, Ruadhagan, Ruadagan

Ruarc (Irish) A famous ruler
Ruarck, Ruarcc, Ruark, Ruarkk, Ruaidhri, Ruaidri

Rubio (Spanish) Resembling a ruby

Rudeger (German) A friendly man
Rudegar, Rudger, Rudgar, Rudiger, Rudigar

Rudolph (German) A famous wolf
Rodolfo, Rodolph, Rodolphe, Rodolpho, Rudy, Rudey, Rudi, Rudie

Rudyard (English) From the red paddock

Rufus (Latin) A red-haired man
Ruffus, Rufous, Rufino

Ruiz (Spanish) A good friend

Rujul (Indian) An honest man
Rujool, Rujoole, Rujule, Rujoul, Rujoule

Rumford (English) From the broad ford
Rumforde, Rumferd, Rumferde, Rumfurd

Rupert (English) Form of Robert, meaning "one who is bright with fame"
Ruprecht

Rushford (English) From the ford with rushes
Rusheford, Rushforde, Rusheforde, Ryscford

Russell (French) A little red-haired boy
Russel, Roussell, Russ, Rusel, Rusell

Russom (African) The chief; the boss
Rusom, Russome, Rusome

Rusty (English) One who has red hair or a ruddy complexion
Rustey, Rusti, Rustie, Rustee, Rustea, Rust, Ruste, Rustice

Rutherford (English) From the cattle's ford
Rutherfurd, Rutherferd, Rutherforde, Rutherfurde

Ryan (Gaelic) The little ruler; little king
Rian, Rien, Rion, Ryen, Ryon, Ryun, Rhyan, Rhyen

Ryder (English) An accomplished horseman
Rider, Ridder, Ryden, Rydell, Rydder

Ryker (Danish) Form of Richard, meaning "a powerful ruler"
Riker

Rylan (English) Form of Ryland, meaning "from the place where rye is grown"
Ryelan, Ryle

Ryland (English) From the place where Rye is grown

S

Saarik (Hindi) Resembling a small songbird
Saarick, Saaric, Sarik, Sarick, Saric, Saariq, Sareek, Sareeq

Saber (French) Man of the sword
Sabere, Sabr, Sabre

Sabir (Arabic) One who is patient
Sabyr, Sabeer, Sabear, Sabeir, Sabier, Sabri, Sabrie, Sabree

Saddam (Arabic) A powerful ruler; the crusher
Saddum, Saddim, Saddym

Sadiq (Arabic) A beloved friend
Sadeeq, Sadyq, Sadeaq, Sadeek, Sadeak, Sadyk, Sadik

Saga (American) A storyteller
Sago

Sagar (Indian / English) A king / one who is wise
Saagar, Sagarr, Saagarr

Sagaz (Spanish) One who is clever
Sagazz

Sagiv (Hebrew) Having great strength
Sagev, Segiv, Segev

Sailor (American) Man who sails the seas
Sailer, Sailar, Saylor, Sayler, Saylar, Saelor

Saith (English) One who is well-spoken
Saithe, Sayth, Saythe, Saeth, Saethe, Sath, Sathe

Sajal (Indian) Resembling a cloud
Sajall, Sajjal, Sajjall

Sajan (Indian) One who is dearly loved
Sajann, Sajjan, Sajjann

Saki (Japanese) One who is cloaked
Sakie, Saky, Sakey, Sakee, Sakea

Salaam (African) Resembling a peach

Salehe (African) A good man
Saleh, Salih

Salim (Arabic) One who is peaceful
Saleem, Salem, Selim

Salvador (Spanish) A savior
Sal, Sally, Salvadore, Xalvador

Samanjas (Indian) One who is proper

Samarth (Indian) A powerful man; one who is efficient
Samarthe

Sameen (Indian) One who is treasured
Samine, Sameene, Samean, Sameane, Samyn, Samyne

Sami (Arabic) One who has been exalted
Samie, Samy, Samey, Samee, Samea

Sammohan (Indian) An attractive man

Samson (Hebrew) As bright as the sun; in the Bible, a man with extraordinary strength
Sampson, Sansom, Sanson, Sansone

Samuel (Hebrew) God has heard
Sam, Sammie, Sammy, Samuele, Samuello, Samwell, Samuelo, Sammey

Samuru (Japanese) The name of God

Sandburg (English) From the sandy village
Sandbergh, Sandberg, Sandburgh

Sandon (English) From the sandy hill
Sanden, Sandan, Sandun, Sandyn, Sandin

Sanford (English) From the sandy crossing
Sandford, Sanforde, Sandforde, Sanfurd, Sanfurde, Sandfurd, Sandfurde

Sang (Vietnamese) A bright man
Sange

Sanjiro (Japanese) An admirable man
Sanjyro

Sanjiv (Indian) One who lives a long life
Sanjeev, Sanjyv, Sanjeiv, Sanjiev, Sanjeav, Sanjivan

Sanorelle (American) An honest man
Sanorell, Sanorel, Sanorele

Santana (Spanish) A saintly man
Santanna, Santanah, Santannah, Santa

Santiago (Spanish) Refers to St. James

Santo (Italian) A holy man
Sante, Santino, Santos, Santee, Santi, Santie, Santea, Santy

Sapan (Indian) A dream or vision
Sapann

Sar (Anglo-Saxon) One who inflicts pain
Sarlic, Sarlik

Sarbajit (Indian) The conqueror
Sarbajeet, Sarbajyt, Sarbajeat, Sarbajet, Sarvajit, Sarvajeet, Sarvajyt, Sarvajeat

Sarojin (Hindu) Resembling a lotus
Saroj

Sarosh (Persian) One who prays
Saroshe

Satayu (Hindi) In Hinduism, the brother of Amavasu and Vivasu
Satayoo, Satayou, Satayue

Satoshi (Japanese) Born from the ashes
Satoshie, Satoshy, Satoshey, Satoshee, Satoshea

Satparayan (Indian) A good-natured man

Saturn (Latin) In mythology, the god of agriculture
Saturnin, Saturno, Saturnino

Satyankar (Indian) One who speaks the truth
Satyancar, Satyancker

Saville (French) From the willow town
Savil, Savile, Savill, Savyile, Savylle, Savyle, Sauville, Sauvile

Savir (Indian) A great leader
Savire, Saveer, Saveere, Savear, Saveare, Savyr, Savyre

Sawyer (English) One who works with wood
Sayer, Saer

Saxon (English) A swordsman
Saxen, Saxan, Saxton, Saxten, Saxtan

Sayad (Arabic) An accomplished hunter

Scand (Anglo-Saxon) One who is disgraced
Scande, Scandi, Scandie, Scandee, Scandea

Sceotend (Anglo-Saxon) An archer

Schaeffer (German) A steward
Schaffer, Shaeffer, Shaffer, Schaeffur, Schaffur, Shaeffur, Shaffur

Schelde (English) From the river
Shelde

Schneider (German) A tailor
Shneider, Sneider, Snider, Snyder

Schubert (German) One who makes shoes
Shubert, Schuberte, Shuberte, Schubirt, Shubirt, Schuburt, Shuburt

Scirocco (Italian) Of the warm wind
Sirocco, Scyrocco, Syrocco

Scott (English) A man from Scotland
Scot, Scottie, Scotto, Scotty, Scotti, Scottey, Scottee, Scottea

Seabury (English) From the village by the sea
Seaburry, Sebury, Seburry, Seaberry, Seabery, Seberry

Seaman (English) A mariner

Sean (Irish) Form of John, meaning "God is gracious"
Shaughn, Shawn, Shaun, Shon, Shohn, Shonn, Shaundre, Shawnel

Seanachan (Irish) One who is wise

Seanan (Hebrew / Irish) A gift from God / an old, wise man
Sinon, Senen, Siobhan

Sebastian (Greek) The revered one
Sabastian, Seb, Sebastiano, Sebastien, Sebestyen, Sebo, Sebastyn, Sebestyen

Sedgwick (English) From the place of sword grass
Sedgewick, Sedgewyck, Sedgwyck, Sedgewic, Sedgewik, Sedgwic, Sedgwik, Sedgewyc

Seerath (Indian) A great man
Seerathe, Searath, Searathe

Sef (Egyptian) Son of yesterday
Sefe

Seferino (Greek) Of the west wind
Seferio, Sepherino, Sepherio, Seferyno, Sepheryno

Seignour (French) Lord of the house

Selas (African) Refers to the Trinity
Selassi, Selassie, Selassy, Selassey, Selassee, Selassea

Selestino (Spanish) One who is heaven-sent
Selestyno, Selesteeno, Selesteano

Sellers (English) One who dwells in the marshland
Sellars, Sellurs, Sellirs, Sellyrs

Seminole (Native American) A tribal name
Semynole

Septimus (Latin) The seventh-born child
Septymus

Seraphim (Hebrew) The burning ones; heavenly winged angels
Sarafino, Saraph, Serafin, Serafino, Seraph, Seraphimus, Serafim

Sereno (Latin) One who is calm; tranquil

Serfati (Hebrew) A man from France
Sarfati, Serfatie, Sarfatie, Serfaty, Sarfaty, Serfatey, Sarfatey, Serfatee

Sergio (Latin) An attendant; a servant
Seargeoh, Serge, Sergei, Sergeo, Sergey, Sergi, Sergios, Sergiu

Seth (Hebrew) One who has been appointed
Sethe, Seath, Seathe, Zeth

Seung (Korean) A victorious successor

Sewati (Native American) Resembling a bear claw
Sewatie, Sewaty, Sewatey, Sewatee, Sewatea

Sexton (English) The church's custodian
Sextun, Sextan, Sextin, Sextyn

Seymour (French) From the French town of Saint Maur
Seamore, Seamor, Seamour, Seymore

Shaan (Hebrew) A peaceful man

Shade (English) A secretive man
Shaid, Shaide, Shayd, Shayde, Shaed, Shaede

Shadi (Persian / Arabic) One who brings happiness and joy / a singer
Shadie, Shady, Shadey

Shadrach (Hebrew) Under the command of the moon god Aku
Shadrack, Shadrick, Shad

Shah (Persian) The king

Shai (Hebrew) A gift from God

Shail (Indian) A mountain rock
Shaile, Shayl, Shayle, Shael, Shaele, Shale

Shaka (African) A tribal leader
Shakah

Shakir (Arabic) One who is grateful
Shakeer, Shaqueer, Shakier, Shakeir, Shakear, Shakar, Shaker, Shakyr

Shane (English) Form of John, meaning "God is gracious"
Shayn, Shayne, Shaine, Shain

Shannon (Gaelic) Having ancient wisdom
Shanan, Shanen, Shannan, Shannen, Shanon

Shardul (Indian) Resembling a tiger
Shardule, Shardull, Shardulle

Shashi (Indian) Of the moon-beam
Shashie, Shashy, Shashey, Shashee, Shashea, Shashhi

Shaw (English) From the woodland
Shawe

Shaykeen (American) A successful man
Shaykean, Shaykein, Shakeyn, Shakine

Shea (Gaelic) An admirable man / from the fairy fortress
Shae, Shai, Shay, Shaye, Shaylon, Shays

Sheen (English) A shining man
Sheene, Shean, Sheane

Sheffield (English) From the crooked field
Sheffeld

Sheldon (English) From the steep valley
Shelden, Sheldan, Sheldun, Sheldin, Sheldyn, Shel

Shelley (English) From the meadow's ledge
Shelly, Shelli, Shellie, Shellee, Shellea, Shelleigh, Shelleah

Shelton (English) From the farm on the ledge
Shellton, Sheltown, Sheltun, Shelten, Shelny, Shelney, Shelni, Shelnie

Shem (Hebrew) Having a well-known name

Shepherd (English) One who herds sheep
Shepperd, Shep, Shepard, Shephard, Shepp, Sheppard

Sheridan (Gaelic) A seeker
Sheredan, Sheridon, Sherridan, Seireadan, Sheriden, Sheridun, Sherard, Sherrard

Sherlock (English) A fair-haired man
Sherlocke, Shurlock, Shurlocke

Sherman (English) One who cuts wool cloth
Shermon, Scherman, Schermann, Shearman, Shermann, Sherm, Sherme

Sherrerd (English) From the open field
Shererd, Sherrard, Sherard

Shields (Gaelic) A faithful protector
Sheelds, Shealds

Shikha (Indian) A fiery man
Shykha

Shiloh (Hebrew) He who was sent
Shilo, Shyloh, Shylo

Shing (Chinese) A victorious man
Shyng

Shino (Japanese) A bamboo stem
Shyno

Shipton (English) From the ship town; from the sheep town

Shiro (Japanese) The fourth-born son
Shyro

Shreshta (Indian) The best; one who is superior

Shubhang (Indian) A handsome man

Shuraqui (Arabic) A man from the east

Siamak (Persian) A bringer of joy
Syamak, Siamack, Syamack, Siamac, Syamac

Sidor (Russian) One who is talented
Sydor

Sierra (Spanish) From the jagged mountain range
Siera, Syerra, Syera, Seyera, Seeara

Sigehere (English) One who is victorious
Sygehere, Sigihere, Sygihere

Sigenert (Anglo-Saxon) A king
Sygenert, Siginert, Syginert

Sigmund (German) The victorious protector
Siegmund, Sigmond, Zsigmond, Zygmunt

Sihtric (Anglo-Saxon) A king
Sihtrik, Sihtrick, Syhtric, Syhtrik, Syhtrick, Sihtryc, Sihtryk, Sihtryck

Sik'is (Native American) A friendly man

Silas (Latin) Form of Silvanus, meaning "a woodland dweller"

Silny (Czech) Having great strength
Silney, Silni, Silnie, Silnee, Silnea

Simbarashe (African) The power of God
Simbarashi, Simbarashie, Simbarashy, Simbarashey, Simbarashee

Simcha (Hebrew) Filled with joy
Symcha, Simha, Symha

Simmons (Hebrew) The son of Simon
Semmes, Simms, Syms, Simmonds, Symonds, Simpson, Symms, Simson

Simon (Hebrew) God has heard
Shimon, Si, Sim, Samien, Semyon, Simen, Simeon, Simone

Sinai (Hebrew) From the clay desert

Sinclair (English) Man from Saint Clair
Sinclaire, Sinclare, Synclair, Synclaire, Synclare

Singer (American) A vocalist
Synger

Sion (Armenian) From the fortified hill
Sionne, Syon, Syonne

Sirius (Greek) Resembling the brightest star
Syrius

Siyavash (Persian) One who owns black horses
Siyavashe

Skerry (Norse) From the rocky island
Skereye, Skerrey, Skerri, Skerrie, Skerree, Skerrea

Slade (English) Son of the valley
Slaid, Slaide, Slaed, Slaede, Slayd, Slayde

Sladkey (Slavic) A glorious man
Sladky, Sladki, Sladkie, Sladkee, Sladkea

Smith (English) A blacksmith
Smyth, Smithe, Smythe, Smedt, Smid, Smitty, Smittee, Smittea

Solange (French) An angel of the sun

Solaris (Greek) Of the sun
Solarise, Solariss, Solarisse, Solarys, Solaryss, Solarysse, Solstice, Soleil

Somer (French) Born during the summer
Somers, Sommer, Sommers, Sommar, Somar

Somerset (English) From the summer settlement
Sommerset, Sumerset, Summerset

Songaa (Native American) Having great strength
Songan

Sophocles (Greek) An ancient playwright
Sofocles

Sorley (Irish) Of the summer vikings
Sorly, Sorlee, Sorlea, Sorli, Sorlie

Soumil (Indian) A beloved friend
Soumyl, Soumille, Soumylle, Soumill, Soumyll

Southern (English) Man from the south
Sothern, Suthern

Sovann (Cambodian) The golden son
Sovan, Sovane

Spark (English / Latin) A gallant man / to scatter
Sparke, Sparki, Sparkie, Sparky, Sparkey, Sparkee, Sparkea

Spencer (English) One who dispenses provisions
Spenser

Squire (English) A knight's companion; the shield-bearer
Squier, Squiers, Squires, Squyre, Squyres

Stanford (English) From the stony ford
Standford, Standforde, Standforde, Stamford

Stanhope (English) From the stony hollow
Stanhop

Stanton (English) From the stone town
Stantown, Stanten, Staunton, Stantan, Stantun

Stark (German) Having great strength
Starke, Starck, Starcke

Stavros (Greek) One who is crowned

Steadman (English) One who lives at the farm
Stedman, Steadmann, Stedmann, Stedeman

Steed (English) Resembling a stallion
Steede, Stead, Steade

Stephen (Greek) Crowned with garland
Staffan, Steba, Steben, Stefan, Stefano, Steffan, Steffen, Steffon, Steven, Steve

Sterling (English) One who is highly valued
Sterlyng, Stirling, Sterlyn

Stian (Norse) A voyager; one who is swift
Stig, Styg, Stygge, Stieran, Steeran, Steeren, Steeryn, Stieren

Stilwell (Anglo-Saxon) From the quiet spring
Stillwell, Stilwel, Stylwell, Styllwell, Stylwel, Stillwel

Stobart (German) A harsh man
Stobarte, Stobarth, Stobarthe

Stockley (English) From the meadow of tree stumps
Stockly, Stockli, Stocklie, Stocklee, Stockleigh

Storm (American) Of the tempest; stormy weather; having an impetuous nature
Storme, Stormy, Stormi, Stormie, Stormey, Stormee, Stormea

Stratford (English) From the street near the river ford
Strafford, Stratforde, Straford, Strafforde, Straforde

Stratton (Scottish) A home-body
Straton, Stratten, Straten, Strattan, Stratan, Strattun, Stratun

Strider (English) A great warrior
Stryder

Striker (American) An aggressive man
Strike, Stryker, Stryke

Struthers (Irish) One who lives near the brook
Struther, Sruthair, Strother, Strothers

Stuart (English) A steward; the keeper of the estate
Steward, Stewart, Stewert, Stuert, Stu, Stew

Suave (American) A smooth and sophisticated man
Swave

Subhi (Arabic) Born during the early morning hours
Subhie, Subhy, Subhey, Subhee, Subhea

Suffield (English) From the southern field
Suffeld, Suthfeld, Suthfield

Sullivan (Gaelic) Having dark eyes
Sullavan, Sullevan, Sullyvan

Sully (English) From the southern meadow
Sulley, Sulli, Sullie, Sulleigh, Sullee, Sullea, Sulleah, Suthley

Sultan (African / American) A ruler / one who is bold
Sultane, Sulten, Sultun, Sulton, Sultin, Sultyn

Suman (Hindi) A wise man

Sundiata (African) Resembling a hungry lion
Sundyata, Soundiata, Soundyata, Sunjata

Su'ud (Arabic) One who has good luck
Suoud

Swahili (Arabic) Of the coastal people
Swahily, Swahiley, Swahilee, Swahiley, Swaheeli, Swaheelie, Swaheely, Swaheeley

Sylvester (Latin) Man from the forest
Silvester, Silvestre, Silvestro, Sylvestre, Sylvestro, Sly, Sevester, Seveste

Syon (Indian) One who is followed by good fortune

Szemere (Hungarian) A man of small stature
Szemir, Szemeer, Szemear, Szemyr

T

Tabari (Arabic) A famous historian
Tabarie, Tabary, Tabarey, Tabaree, Tabarea

Tabbai (Hebrew) A well-behaved boy
Tabbae, Tabbay, Tabbaye

Tabbart (German) A brilliant man
Tabbert, Tabart, Tabert, Tahbert, Tahberte

Tacari (African) As strong as a warrior
Tacarie, Tacary, Tacarey, Tacaree, Tacarea

Tadao (Japanese) One who is satisfied

Tadeusuz (Polish) One who is worthy of praise
Tadesuz

Tadi (Native American) Of the wind
Tadie, Tady, Tadey, Tadee, Tadea

Tadzi (American / Polish) Resembling the loon / one who is praised
Tadzie, Tadzy, Tadzey, Tadzee, Tadzea

Taft (French / English) From the homestead / from the marshes
Tafte

Taggart (Gaelic) Son of a priest
Taggert, Taggort, Taggirt, Taggyrt

Taghee (Native American) A chief
Taghea, Taghy, Taghey, Taghi, Taghie

Taheton (Native American) Resembling a hawk

Tahoe (Native American) From the big water
Taho

Tahoma (Native American) From the snowy mountain peak
Tehoma, Tacoma, Takoma, Tohoma, Tocoma, Tokoma, Tekoma, Tecoma

Taishi (Japanese) An ambitious man
Taishie, Taishy, Taishey, Taishee, Taishea

Taj (Indian) One who is crowned
Tahj, Tajdar

Tajo (Spanish) Born during the daytime

Taksony (Hungarian) One who is content; well-fed
Taksoney, Taksoni, Taksonie, Taksonee, Taksonea, Tas

Talasi (Native American) Resembling a cornflower
Talasie, Talasy, Talasey, Talasee, Talasea

Talford (English) From the high ford
Talforde, Tallford, Tallforde

Talmon (Hebrew) One who is oppressed
Talman, Talmin, Talmyn, Talmen

Talo (Finnish) From the homestead

Tam (Vietnamese / Hebrew) Having heart / one who is truthful

Taman (Hindi) One who is needed

Tamarius (American) A stubborn man
Tamarias, Tamarios, Tamerius, Tamerias, Tamerios

Tameron (American) Form of Cameron, meaning "having a crooked nose"
Tameren, Tameryn, Tamryn, Tamerin, Tamren, Tamrin, Bamron

Tammany (Native American) A friendly chief
Tammani, Tammanie, Tammaney, Tammanee, Tammanea

Tanafa (Polynesian) A drumbeat

Taneli (Hebrew) He will be judged by God
Tanelie, Tanely, Taneley, Tanelee, Tanelea

Tanish (Indian) An ambitious man
Tanishe, Taneesh, Taneeshe, Taneash, Taneashe, Tanysh, Tanyshe

Tanjiro (Japanese) The prized second-born son
Tanjyro

Tanner (English) One who makes leather
Tannere, Tannor, Tannar, Tannir, Tannyr, Tannur, Tannis

Tannon (German) From the fir tree
Tannan, Tannen, Tannin, Tansen, Tanson, Tannun, Tannyn

Tano (Ghanese) From the river
Tanu

Tao (Chinese) One who will have a long life

Taos (Spanish) From the city in New Mexico

Tapani (Hebrew) A victorious man
Tapanie, Tapany, Tapaney, Tapanee, Tapanea

Tapko (American) Resembling an antelope

Tappen (Welsh) From the top of the cliff
Tappan, Tappon, Tappin, Tappyn, Tappun

Taran (Gaelic) Of the thunder
Taren, Taron, Tarin, Taryn, Tarun

Taranga (Indian) Of the waves

Taregan (Native American) Resembling a crane
Taregen, Taregon, Taregin, Taregyn

Tarit (Indian) Resembling lightning
Tarite, Tareet, Tareete, Tareat, Tareate, Taryt, Taryte

Tarn (Norse) From the mountain pool

Tarquin (Latin) One who is impulsive
Tarquinn, Tarquinne, Tarquen, Tarquenn, Tarquenne, Tarquyn, Tarquynn, Tarquynne

Tarrant (American) One who upholds the law
Tarrent, Tarrint, Tarrynt, Tarront, Tarrunt

Tarun (Indian) A youthful man
Taroun, Taroon, Tarune, Taroune, Taroone

Tashi (Tibetan) One who is prosperous
Tashie, Tashy, Tashey, Tashee, Tashea

Tate (English) A cheerful man; one who brings happiness to others
Tayt, Tayte, Tait, Taite, Taet, Taete

Tausiq (Indian) One who provides strong backing
Tauseeq, Tauseaq, Tausik, Tauseek, Tauseak

Tavaris (American) Of misfortune; a hermit
Tavarius, Tavaress, Tavarious, Tavariss, Tavarous, Tevarus, Tavorian, Tavarian

Tavas (Hebrew) Resembling a peacock

Tavi (Aramaic) A good man
Tavie, Tavy, Tavey, Tavee, Tavea

Tavin (German) Form of Gustav, meaning "of the staff of the gods"
Tavyn, Taven, Tavan, Tavon, Tavun, Tava, Tave

Tawa (Native American) Born beneath the sun
Tawah

Tay (Scottish) From the river
Taye, Tae, Tai

Taylor (English) Cutter of cloth, one who alters garments

Teagan (Gaelic) A handsome man
Teegan, Teygan, Tegan, Teigan

Ted (English) Form of Theodore, meaning "a gift from God"
Tedd, Teddy, Teddi, Teddie, Teddee, Teddea, Teddey, Tedric

Teetonka (Native American) One who talks too much
Teitonka, Tietonka, Teatonka, Teytonka

Tegene (African) My protector
Tegeen, Tegeene, Tegean, Tegeane

Teiji (Japanese) One who is righteous
Teijo

Teilo (Welsh) A saintly man

Teka (African) He has replaced

Tekeshi (Japanese) A formidable and brave man
Tekeshie, Tekeshy, Tekeshey, Tekeshee, Tekeshea

Telly (Greek) The wisest man
Telley, Tellee, Tellea, Telli, Tellie

Temman (Anglo-Saxon) One who has been tamed

Temple (Latin) From the sacred place
Tempel, Templar, Templer, Templo

Teon (Anglo-Saxon) One who harms others

Teris (Irish) The son of Terence
Terys, Teriss, Teryss, Terris, Terrys, Terriss, Terryss

Terrance (Latin) From an ancient Roman clan
Tarrants, Tarrance, Tarrence, Tarrenz, Terencio, Terance, Terrence, Terrey, Terry

Terrian (American) One who is strong and ambitious
Terrien, Terriun, Terriyn

Terron (English) Form of Terence, meaning "from an ancient Roman clan"
Tarran, Tarren, Tarrin

Teshi (African) One who is full of laughter
Teshie, Teshy, Teshey, Teshee, Teshea

Tessema (African) One to whom people listen

Tet (Vietnamese) Born on New Year's

Teteny (Hungarian) A chieftain

Teva (Hebrew) A natural man
Tevah

Thabo (African) Filled with happiness

Thackary (English) Form of Zachary, meaning "the Lord remembers"
Thackery, Thakary, Thakery, Thackari, Thackarie, Thackarey, Thackaree, Thackarea

Thaddeus (Aramaic) Having heart
Tad, Tadd, Taddeo, Taddeusz, Thad, Thadd, Thaddaios, Thaddaos

Thandiwe (African) One who is dearly loved
Thandie, Thandi, Thandy, Thandey, Thandee, Thandea

Thanus (American) One who owns land

Thao (Vietnamese) One who is courteous

Thatcher (English) One who fixes roofs
Thacher, Thatch, Thatche, Thaxter, Thacker, Thaker, Thackere, Thakere

Thayer (Teutonic) Of the nation's army

Theodore (Greek) A gift from God
Ted, Teddy, Teddie, Theo, Theodor

Theron (Greek) A great hunter
Therron, Tharon, Theon, Tharron

Theseus (Greek) In mythology, hero who slew the Minotaur
Thesius, Thesyus

Thinh (Vietnamese) A prosperous man

Thomas (Aramaic) One of twins
Tam, Tamas, Tamhas, Thom, Thomason, Thomson, Thompson, Tomas

Thor (Norse) In mythology, god of thunder
Thorian, Thorin, Thorsson, Thorvald, Tor, Tore, Turo, Thorrin

Thorburn (Norse) Thor's bear
Thorburne, Thorbern, Thorberne, Thorbjorn, Thorbjorne, Torbjorn, Torborg, Torben

Thormond (Norse) Protected by Thor
Thormonde, Thormund, Thormunde, Thurmond, Thurmonde, Thurmund, Thurmunde, Thormun

Thorne (English) From the thorn bush
Thorn

Thuong (Vietnamese) One who loves tenderly

Thurston (English) From Thor's town; Thor's stone
Thorston, Thorstan, Thorstein, Thorsten, Thurstain, Thurstan, Thursten, Torsten

Thuy (Vietnamese) One who is kind

Tiassale (African) It has been forgotten

Tiberio (Italian) From the Tiber river
Tibero, Tyberio, Tybero, Tiberius, Tiberios, Tyberius, Tyberios

Tibor (Slavic) From the sacred place

Tiburon (Spanish) Resembling a shark

Tiernan (Gaelic) Lord of the manor
Tiarnan, Tiarney, Tierney, Tierny, Tiernee, Tiernea, Tierni, Tiernie

Tilian (Anglo-Saxon) One who strives to better himself
Tilien, Tiliun, Tilion

Tilon (Hebrew) A generous man
Tilen, Tilan, Tilun, Tilin, Tilyn

Tilton (English) From the fertile estate
Tillton, Tilten, Tillten, Tiltan, Tilltan, Tiltin, Tilltin, Tiltun

Timir (Indian) Born in the darkness
Timirbaran

Timothy (Greek) One who honors God
Tim, Timmo, Timmothy, Timmy, Timo, Timofei, Timofeo

Tin (Vietnamese) A great thinker

Tino (Italian) A man of small stature
Teeno, Tieno, Teino, Teano, Tyno

Tisa (African) The ninth-born child
Tisah, Tysa, Tysah

Titus (Greek / Latin) Of the giants / a great defender
Tito, Titos, Tytus, Tytos, Titan, Tytan, Tyto

Toa (Polynesian) A brave-hearted woman

Toan (Vietnamese) One who is safe
Toane

Tobias (Hebrew) The Lord is good
Toby

Todd (English) Resembling a fox
Tod

Todor (Bulgarian) A gift from God
Todos, Todros

Tohon (Native American) One who loves the water

Tokala (Native American) Resembling a fox
Tokalo

Tomer (Hebrew) A man of tall stature
Tomar, Tomur, Tomir, Tomor, Tomyr

Tomi (Japanese / African) A wealthy man / of the people
Tomie, Tomee, Tomea, Tomy, Tomey

Tonauac (Aztec) One who possesses the light

Torger (Norse) The power of Thor's spear
Thorger, Torgar, Thorgar, Terje, Therje

Torht (Anglo-Saxon) A bright man
Torhte

Torin (Celtic) One who acts as chief
Toran, Torean, Toren, Torion, Torran, Torrian, Toryn

Tormaigh (Irish) Having the spirit of Thor
Tormey, Tormay, Tormaye, Tormai, Tormae

Torr (English) From the tower
Torre

Torrence (Gaelic) From the little hills
Torence, Torrance, Torrens, Torrans, Toran, Torran, Torrin, Torn, Torry

Torry (Norse / Gaelic) Refers to Thor / form of Torrence, meaning "from the little hills"
Torrey, Torree, Torrea, Torri, Torrie, Tory, Torey, Tori

Toshiro (Japanese) One who is talented and intelligent
Toshihiro

Tostig (English) A well-known earl
Tostyg

Toviel (Hebrew) The Lord is good
Toviell, Toviele, Tovielle, Tovi, Tovie, Tovee, Tovea, Tovy

Toyo (Japanese) A man of plenty

Tracy (Gaelic) One who is warlike
Tracey, Traci, Tracie, Tracee, Tracea, Treacy, Trace, Tracen

Travis (French) To cross over
Travys, Traver, Travers, Traviss, Trevis, Trevys, Travus, Traves

Treffen (German) One who socializes
Treffan, Treffin, Treffon, Treffyn, Treffun

Tremain (Celtic) From the town built of stone
Tramain, Tramaine, Tramayne, Tremaine, Tremayne, Tremaen, Tremaene, Tramaen

Tremont (French) From the three mountains
Tremonte, Tremount, Tremounte

Trenton (English) From the town near the rushing rapids
Trent, Trynt, Trenten, Trentyn

Trevin (English) From the fair town
Trevan, Treven, Trevian, Trevion, Trevon, Trevyn, Trevonn

Trevor (Welsh) From the large village
Trefor, Trevar, Trever, Treabhar, Treveur, Trevir, Trevur

Trey (English) The third-born child
Tre, Trai, Trae, Tray, Traye, Trayton, Treyton, Trayson

Trigg (Norse) One who is truthful
Trygg

Tripp (English) A traveler
Trip, Trypp, Tryp, Tripper, Trypper

Tripsy (American) One who enjoys dancing
Tripsey, Tripsee, Tripsea, Tripsi, Tripsie

Tristan (Celtic) A sorrowful man; in Arthurian legend, a knight of the Round Table
Trystan, Tris, Tristam, Tristen, Tristian, Tristin, Triston, Tristram

Trong (Vietnamese) One who is respected

Troy (Gaelic) Son of a foot-soldier
Troye, Troi

Trumbald (English) A bold man
Trumbold, Trumbalde, Trumbolde

Trygve (Norse) One who wins with bravery

Tse (Native American) As solid as a rock

Tsidhqiyah (Hebrew) The Lord is just
Tsidqiyah, Tsidhqiya, Tsdqiya

Tucker (English) One who makes garments
Tuker, Tuckerman, Tukerman, Tuck, Tuckman, Tukman, Tuckere, Toukere

Tuketu (Native American) Resembling a running bear
Tuketue, Tuketoo, Tuketou, Telutci, Telutcie, Telutcy, Telutcey, Telutcee

Tulsi (Indian) A holy man
Tulsie, Tulsy, Tulsey, Tulsee, Tulsea

Tumaini (African) An optimist
*Tumainie, Tumainee,
Tumainy, Tumainey, Tumayni,
Tumaynie, Tumaynee,
Tumayney*

Tunde (African) One who
returns
*Tundi, Tundie, Tundee,
Tundea, Tundy, Tundey*

Tunleah (English) From the
town near the meadow
*Tunlea, Tunleigh, Tunly,
Tunley, Tunlee, Tunli, Tunlie*

Tupac (African) A messenger
warrior
Tupack, Tupoc, Tupock

Tushar (Indian) Of the snow
Tusharr, Tushare

Tusita (Chinese) One who is
heaven-sent

Txanton (Basque) Form
of Anthony, meaning "a
flourishing man; of an
ancient Roman family"
*Txantony, Txantoney,
Txantonee, Txantoni,
Txantonie, Txantonea*

Tybalt (Latin) He who sees the
truth
Tybault, Tybalte, Tybaulte

Tye (English) From the
fenced-in pasture
Tyg, Tyge, Tie, Tigh, Teyen

Tyfiell (English) Follower of
the god Tyr
Tyfiel, Tyfielle, Tyfiele

Tyler (English) A tiler of roofs
*Tilar, Tylar, Tylor, Tiler, Tilor,
Ty, Tye, Tylere*

Typhoon (Chinese) Of the
great wind
*Tiphoon, Tyfoon, Tifoon,
Typhoun, Tiphoun, Tyfoun,
Tifoun*

Tyrone (French) From Owen's
land
*Terone, Tiron, Tirone, Tyron,
Ty, Kyrone*

Tyson (French) One who is
high-spirited; fiery
*Thyssen, Tiesen, Tyce, Tycen,
Tyeson, Tyssen, Tysen, Tysan*

U

Uaithne (Gaelic) One who is
innocent; green
*Uaithn, Uaythne, Uaythn,
Uathne, Uathn, Uaethne,
Uaethn*

Ualan (Scottish) Form of Valentine, meaning "one who is strong and healthy"
Ualane, Ualayn, Ualayne, Ualen, Ualon

Uba (African) One who is wealthy; lord of the house
Ubah, Ubba, Ubbah

Uberto (Italian) Form of Hubert, meaning "having a shining intellect"
Ulberto, Umberto

Udath (Indian) One who is noble
Udathe

Uddhar (Indian) One who is free; an independent man
Uddharr, Udhar, Udharr

Udell (English) From the valley of yew trees
Udale, Udel, Udall, Udayle, Udayl, Udail, Udaile, Udele

Udi (Hebrew) One who carries a torch
Udie, Udy, Udey, Udee, Udea

Udup (Indian) Born beneath the moon's light
Udupp, Uddup, Uddupp

Udyan (Indian) Of the garden
Uddyan, Udyann, Uddyann

Ugo (Italian) A great thinker

Uland (English) From the noble country
Ulande, Ulland, Ullande, Ulandus, Ullandus

Ulhas (Indian) Filled with happiness
Ulhass, Ullhas, Ullhass

Ulmer (German) Having the fame of the wolf
Ullmer, Ullmar, Ulmarr, Ullmarr, Ulfmer, Ulfmar, Ulfmaer

Ultman (Indian) A godly man
Ultmann, Ultmane

Umrao (Indian) One who is noble

Unai (Basque) A shepherd
Unay, Unaye, Unae

Unathi (African) God is with us
Unathie, Unathy, Unathey, Unathee, Unathea

Uncas (Native American) Resembling a fox
Unkas, Unckas

Ungus (Irish) A vigorous man
Unguss

Unique (American) Unlike others; the only one
Unikue, Unik, Uniqui, Uniqi, Uniqe, Unikque, Unike, Unicke

Uolevi (Finnish) Form of Olaf, meaning "the remaining of the ancestors"
Uolevie, Uolevee, Uolevy, Uolevey, Uolevea

Uri (Hebrew) Form of Uriah, meaning "the Lord is my light"
Urie, Ury, Urey, Uree, Urea

Uriah (Hebrew) The Lord is my light
Uri, Uria, Urias, Urija, Urijah, Uriyah, Urjasz, Uriya

Urjavaha (Hindu) Of the Nimi dynasty

Urtzi (Basque) From the sky
Urtzie, Urtzy, Urtzey, Urtzee, Urtzea

Usher (Latin) From the mouth of the river
Ushar, Ushir, Ussher, Usshar, Usshir

Ushi (Chinese) As strong as an ox
Ushie, Ushy, Ushey, Ushee, Ushea

Utsav (Indian) Born during a celebration
Utsavi, Utsave, Utsava, Utsavie, Utsavy, Utsavey, Utsavee, Utsavea

Utt (Arabic) One who is kind and wise
Utte

Uzi (Hebrew) Having great power
Uzie, Uzy, Uzey, Uzee, Uzea, Uzzi, Uzzie, Uzzy

Uzima (African) One who is full of life
Uzimah, Uzimma, Uzimmah, Uzyma

Uzziah (Hebrew) The Lord is my strength
Uzzia, Uziah, Uzia, Uzzya, Uzzyah, Uzyah, Uzya, Uzziel

Vachel (French) Resembling a small cow
Vachele, Vachell

Vachlan (English) One who lives near water

Vadar (Dutch) A fatherly man
Vader, Vadyr

Vadhir (Spanish) Resembling a rose
Vadhyr, Vadheer

Vadim (Russian) A good-
looking man
*Vadime, Vadym, Vadyme,
Vadeem, Vadeeme*

Vaijnath (Hindi) Refers to
Lord Shiva
Vaejnath, Vaijnathe, Vaejnathe

Valdemar (German) A well-
known ruler
*Valdemarr, Valdemare, Valto,
Valdmar, Valdmarr, Valdimar,
Valdimarr*

Valentine (Latin) One who is
strong and healthy
*Val, Valentin, Valentino,
Valentyne, Ualan*

Valerian (Latin) One who is
strong and healthy
*Valerien, Valerio, Valerius,
Valery, Valeryan, Valere, Valeri,
Valerii*

Valin (Hindi) The monkey
king

Valle (French) From the glen
Vallejo

Valri (French) One who is
strong
Valrie, Valry, Valrey, Valree

Vance (English) From the
marshland
Vanse

Vandy (Dutch) One who
travels; a wanderer
Vandey, Vandi, Vandie, Vandee

Vandyke (Danish) From the
dike
Vandike

Vanir (Norse) Of the ancient
gods

Varante (Arabic) From the
river

Varg (Norse) Resembling a
wolf

Varick (German) A protective
ruler
Varrick, Warick, Warrick

Varius (Latin) A versatile man
Varian, Varinius

Variya (Hindi) The excellent
one

Vasava (Hindi) Refers to Indra

Vashon (American) The Lord
is gracious
*Vashan, Vashawn, Vashaun,
Vashone, Vashane, Vashayn,
Vashayne*

Vasin (Indian) A great ruler
*Vasine, Vaseen, Vaseene, Vasyn,
Vasyne*

Vasuki (Hindi) In Hinduism, a serpent king
Vasukie, Vasuky, Vasukey, Vasukee, Vasukea

Vasuman (Indian) Son born of fire

Vasyl (Slavic) A king
Vasil, Vassil, Wasyl

Vatsa (Indian) Our beloved son
Vathsa

Vatsal (Indian) One who is affectionate

Velyo (Bulgarian) A great man
Velcho, Veliko, Velin, Velko

Vere (French) From the alder tree

Verge (Anglo-Saxon) One who owns four acres

Vernon (French) From the alder-tree grove
Vern, Vernal, Vernard, Verne, Vernee, Vernen, Verney, Vernin

Verrill (French) One who is faithful
Verill, Verrall, Verrell, Verroll, Veryl, Veryll, Verol, Verall

Vibol (Cambodian) A man of plenty
Viboll, Vibole, Vybol, Vyboll, Vybole

Victor (Latin) One who is victorious; the champion
Vic, Vick, Victoriano

Vidal (Spanish) A giver of life
Videl, Videlio, Videlo, Vidalo, Vidalio, Vidas

Vidar (Norse) Warrior of the forest; in mythology, a son of Odin
Vidarr

Vien (Vietnamese) One who is complete; satisfied

Vincent (Latin) One who prevails; the conqueror
Vicente, Vicenzio, Vicenzo, Vin, Vince, Vincens, Vincente, Vincentius

Viorel (Romanian) Resembling the bluebell
Viorell, Vyorel, Vyorell

Vipin (Indian) From the forest
Vippin, Vypin, Vypyn, Vyppin, Vyppyn, Vipyn, Vippyn

Virgil (Latin) The staff-bearer
Verge, Vergil, Vergilio, Virgilio, Vergilo, Virgilo, Virgilijus

Vitéz (Hungarian) A courageous warrior

Vito (Latin) One who gives life
Vital, Vitale, Vitalis, Vitaly, Vitas, Vitus, Vitali, Vitaliy, Vid

Vitus (Latin) Giver of life
Wit

Vladimir (Slavic) A famous prince
Vladamir, Vladimeer, Vladimyr, Vladimyre, Vladamyr, Vladamyre, Vladameer, Vladimer

Vladislav (Slavic) One who rules with glory

Volodymyr (Slavic) To rule with peace
Wolodymyr

Vulcan (Latin) In mythology, the god of fire
Vulkan, Vulckan

Vyacheslav (Russian) Form of Wenceslas, meaning "one who receives more glory"

W

Wade (English) To cross the river ford
Wayde, Waid, Waide, Waddell, Wadell, Waydell, Waidell, Waed

Wadley (English) From the meadow near the ford
Wadly, Wadlee, Wadli, Wadlie, Wadleigh

Wadsworth (English) From the estate near the ford
Waddsworth, Wadsworthe, Waddsworthe

Wafi (Arabic) One who is trustworthy
Wafie, Wafy, Wafey, Wafee, Wafiy, Wafiyy

Wahab (Indian) A big-hearted man

Wainwright (English) One who builds wagons
Wainright, Wainewright, Wayneright, Waynewright, Waynwright

Wakil (Arabic) A lawyer; a trustee
Wakill, Wakyl, Wakyle, Wakeel, Wakeele

Wakiza (Native American) A desperate fighter
Wakyza, Wakeza, Wakieza, Wakeiza

Walbridge (English) From the Welshman's bridge
Wallbridge, Walbrydge, Wallbrydge

Walker (English) One who trods the cloth
Walkar, Walkir, Walkor

Wallace (Scottish) A Welshman, a man from the South
Wallach, Wallas, Wallie, Wallis, Wally, Wlash, Welch

Walter (German) The commander of the army
Walther, Walt, Walte, Walder, Wat, Wouter, Wolter, Woulter, Galtero, Quaid

Wanikiy (Native American) A savior
Wanikiya, Wanikie, Wanikey, Waniki, Wanikee

Wanjala (African) Born during a famine
Wanjalla, Wanjal, Wanjall

Warford (English) From the ford near the weir
Warforde, Weirford, Weirforde, Weiford, Weiforde

Warley (English) From the meadow near the weir
Warly, Warleigh, Warlee, Warlea, Warleah, Warli, Warlie, Weirley

Warner (German) Of the defending army
Werner, Wernher, Warnher, Worner, Wornher

Warra (Aboriginal) Man of the water
Warrah, Wara, Warah

Warren (English / German) From the fortress

Warrick (English) Form of Varick, meaning "a protective ruler"
Warrik, Warric, Warick, Warik, Waric, Warryck, Warryk, Warryc

Warrigal (Aboriginal) One who is wild
Warrigall, Warigall, Warigal, Warygal, Warygall

Warwick (English) From the farm near the weir
Warwik, Warwyck, Warwyk

Wasswa (African) The first-born of twins
Waswa, Wasswah, Waswah

Wasyl (Ukrainian) Form of Vasyl, meaning "a king"
Wasyle, Wasil, Wasile

Watson (English) The son of Walter
Watsin, Watsen, Watsan, Watkins, Watckins, Watkin, Watckin, Wattekinson

Waylon (English) From the roadside land

Wayne (English) One who builds wagons
Wain, Wanye, Wayn, Waynell, Waynne, Guwayne

Webster (English) A weaver
Weeb, Web, Webb, Webber, Weber, Webbestre, Webestre, Webbe

Wei (Chinese) A brilliant man; having great strength

Wenceslas (Polish) One who receives more glory
Wenceslaus, Wenzel, Vyacheslav

Wendell (German) One who travels; a wanderer
Wendel, Wendale, Wendall, Wendele, Wendal, Windell, Windel, Windal

Wesley (English) From the western meadow
Wes, Wesly, Wessley, Westleigh, Westley, Wesli, Weslie, Wesleigh

Westby (English) From the western farm
Westbey, Wesby, Wesbey, Westbi, Wesbi, Westbie, Wesbie, Westbee

Weston (English) From the western town

Whit (English) A white-skinned man
White, Whitey, Whitt, Whitte, Whyt, Whytt, Whytte, Whytey

Whitby (English) From the white farm
Whitbey, Whitbi, Whitbie, Whitbee, Whytbey, Whytby, Whytbi, Whytbie

Whitfield (English) From the white field
Whitfeld, Whytfield, Whytfeld, Witfield, Witfeld, Wytfield, Wytfeld

Whitley (English) From the white meadow
Whitly, Whitli, Whitlie, Whitlee, Whitleigh, Whytley, Whytly, Whytli

Whitman (English) A white-haired man
Whitmann, Witman, Witmann, Whitmane, Witmane, Whytman, Whytmane, Wytman

Wildon (English) From the wooded hill
Willdon, Wilden, Willden

Wiley (English) One who is crafty; from the meadow by the water
Wily, Wileigh, Wili, Wilie, Wilee, Wylie, Wyly, Wyley

Wilford (English) From the willow ford
Willford, Wilferd, Willferd, Wilf, Wielford, Weilford, Wilingford, Wylingford

William (German) The determined protector
Wilek, Wileck, Wilhelm, Wilhelmus, Wilkes, Wilkie, Wilkinson, Will, Guillaume, Quilliam

Willow (English) Of the willow tree
Willowe, Willo, Willoe

Wilmer (German) A strong-willed and well-known man
Wilmar, Wilmore, Willmar, Willmer, Wylmer, Wylmar, Wyllmer, Wyllmar

Winston (English) Of the joy stone; from the friendly town
Win, Winn, Winsten, Winstonn, Wynstan, Wynsten, Wynston, Winstan

Winthrop (English) From the friendly village
Winthrope, Wynthrop, Wynthrope, Winthorp, Wynthorp

Winton (English) From the enclosed pastureland
Wintan, Wintin, Winten, Wynton, Wyntan, Wyntin, Wynten

Wirt (Anglo-Saxon) One who is worthy
Wirte, Wyrt, Wyrte, Wurt, Wurte

Wit (Polish) Form of Vitus, meaning "giver of life"
Witt

Wlodzimierz (Polish) To rule with peace
Wlodzimir, Wlodzimerz

Wolfric (German) A wolf ruler
Wolfrick, Wolfrik, Wulfric, Wulfrick, Wulfrik, Wolfryk, Wolfryck, Wolfryc

Woorak (Aboriginal) From the plains
Woorack, Woorac

Wyatt (English) Having the strength of a warrior
Wyat, Wyatte, Wyate, Wiatt, Wiatte, Wiat, Wiate, Wyeth

Wyndham (English) From the windy village
Windham

Xakery (American) Form of Zachery, meaning "the Lord remembers"
Xaccary, Xaccery, Xach, Xacharie, Xachery, Xack, Xackarey, Xackary

Xalvador (Spanish) Form of Salvador, meaning "a savior"
Xalvadore, Xalvadoro, Xalvadorio, Xalbador, Xalbadore, Xalbadorio, Xalbadoro, Xabat

Xannon (American) From an ancient family
Xanon, Xannen, Xanen, Xannun, Xanun

Xanthus (Greek) A blond-haired man
Xanthos, Xanthe, Xanth

Xavier (Basque / Arabic) Owner of a new house / one who is bright
Xaver, Xever, Xabier, Xaviere, Xabiere, Xaviar, Xaviare, Xavior

Xenocrates (Greek) A foreign ruler

Xesus (Galician) Form of Jesus, meaning "God is my salvation"

Xoan (Galician) Form of John, meaning "God is gracious"
Xoane, Xohn, Xon

Xue (Chinese) A studious young man

Y

Yael (Israeli) Strength of God
Yaele

Yagil (Hebrew) One who rejoices, celebrates
Yagill, Yagyl, Yagylle

Yahto (Native American) Having blue eyes; refers to the color blue
Yahtoe, Yahtow, Yahtowe

Yahweh (Hebrew) Refers to God
Yahveh, Yaweh, Yaveh, Yehowah, Yehweh, Yehoveh

Yakiv (Ukrainian) Form of Jacob, meaning "he who supplants"
Yakive, Yakeev, Yakeeve, Yackiv, Yackeev, Yakieve, Yakiev, Yakeive

Yakout (Arabian) As precious as a ruby

Yale (Welsh) From the fertile upland
Yayle, Yayl, Yail, Yaile

Yanai (Aramaic) God will answer
Yanae, Yana, Yani

Yankel (Hebrew) Form of Jacob, meaning "he who supplants"
Yankell, Yanckel, Yanckell, Yankle, Yanckle

Yaotl (Aztec) A great warrior
Yaotyl, Yaotle, Yaotel, Yaotyle

Yaphet (Hebrew) A handsome man
Yaphett, Yapheth, Yaphethe

Yaqub (Arabic) Form of Jacob, meaning "he who supplants"
Ya'qub, Yaqob, Yaqoub

Yardley (English) From the fenced-in meadow
Yardly, Yardleigh, Yardli, Yardlie, Yardlee, Yardlea, Yarley, Yarly

Yaromir (Russian) Form of Jaromir, meaning "from the famous spring"
Yaromire, Yaromeer, Yaromeere, Yaromyr, Yaromyre

Yas (Native American) Child of the snow

Yasahiro (Japanese) One who is peaceful and calm

Yasin (Arabic) A wealthy man
Yasine, Yaseen, Yaseene, Yasyn, Yasyne, Yasien, Yasiene, Yasein

Yasir (Arabic) One who is well-off financially
Yassir, Yasser, Yaseer, Yasr, Yasyr, Yassyr, Yasar, Yassar

Yegor (Russian) Form of George, meaning "one who works the earth; a farmer"
Yegore, Yegorr, Yegeor, Yeorges, Yeorge, Yeorgis

Yenge (African) A hard-working man
Yengi, Yengie, Yengy, Yengey, Yengee

Yeoman (English) A man-servant
Youman, Yoman

Yestin (Welsh) One who is just and fair
Yestine, Yestyn, Yestyne

Yigil (Hebrew) He shall be redeemed
Yigile, Yigyl, Yigyle, Yigol, Yigole, Yigit, Yigat

Yishachar (Hebrew) He will be rewarded
Yishacharr, Yishachare, Yissachar, Yissachare, Yisachar, Yisachare

Yiska (Native American) The night has gone

Yngve (Scandinavian) Refers to the god Ing

Yoav (Hebrew) Form of Joab, meaning "the Lord is my father"
Yoave, Yoavo, Yoavio

Yochanan (Hebrew) Form of John, meaning "God is gracious"
Yochan, Yohannan, Yohanan, Yochannan

Yohan (German) Form of John, meaning "God is gracious"
Yohanan, Yohann, Yohannes, Yohon, Yohonn, Yohonan

Yonatan (Hebrew) Form of Jonathan, meaning "a gift of God"
Yonaton, Yohnatan, Yohnaton, Yonathan, Yonathon, Yoni, Yonie, Yony

Yong (Korean) One who is courageous

York (English) From the yew settlement
Yorck, Yorc, Yorke

Yovanny (English) Form of Giovanni, meaning "God is gracious"
Yovanni, Yovannie, Yovannee, Yovany, Yovani, Yovanie, Yovanee

Yukon (English) From the settlement of gold
Youkon, Yucon, Youcon, Yuckon, Youckon

Yuliy (Russian) Form of Julius, meaning "one who is youthful"
Yuli, Yulie, Yulee, Yuleigh, Yuly, Yuley, Yulika, Yulian

Yuudai (Japanese) A great hero
Yudai, Yuudae, Yudae, Yuuday, Yuday

Yves (French) A young archer
Yve, Yvo, Yvon, Yvan, Yvet, Yvete

Zabian (Arabic) One who worships celestial bodies
Zabion, Zabien, Zaabian

Zabulon (Hebrew) One who is exalted
Zabulun, Zabulen

Zacchaeus (Hebrew) Form of Zachariah, meaning "The Lord remembers"
Zachaeus, Zachaios, Zaccheus, Zackaeus, Zacheus, Zackaios, Zaccheo

Zachariah (Hebrew) The Lord remembers
Zacaria, Zacarias, Zaccaria, Zaccariah, Zachaios, Zacharia, Zacharias, Zacherish

Zachary (Hebrew) Form of Zachariah, meaning "the Lord remembers"
Zaccary, Zaccery, Zach, Zacharie, Zachery, Zack, Zackarey, Zackary, Thackary, Xakery

Zaci (African) In mythology, the god of fatherhood

Zaden (Dutch) A sower of seeds
Zadin, Zadan, Zadon, Zadun, Zede, Zeden, Zedan

Zadok (Hebrew) One who is righteous; just
Zadoc, Zaydok, Zadock, Zaydock, Zaydoc, Zaidok, Zaidock, Zaidoc

Zador (Hungarian) An ill-tempered man
Zador, Zadoro, Zadorio

Zafar (Arabic) The conquerer; a victorious man
Zafarr, Zaffar, Zhafar, Zhaffar, Zafer, Zaffer

Zahid (Arabic) A pious man
Zahide, Zahyd, Zahyde, Zaheed, Zaheede, Zaheide, Zahiede, Zaheid

Zahir (Arabic) A radiant and flourishing man
Zahire, Zahireh, Zahyr, Zahyre, Zaheer, Zaheere, Zaheir, Zahier

Zahur (Arabic) Resembling a flower
Zahure, Zahureh, Zhahur, Zaahur

Zale (Greek) Having the strength of the sea
Zail, Zaile, Zayl, Zayle, Zael, Zaele

Zamir (Hebrew) Resembling a songbird
Zamire, Zameer, Zameere, Zamyr, Zamyre, Zameir, Zameire, Zamier

Zander (Slavic) Form of Alexander, meaning "a helper and defender of mankind"
Zandros, Zandro, Zandar, Zandur, Zandre

Zane (English) form of John, meaning "God is gracious"
Zayne, Zayn, Zain, Zaine

Zareb (African) The protector; guardian
Zarebb, Zaareb, Zarebe, Zarreb, Zareh, Zaareh

Zared (Hebrew) One who has been trapped
Zarede, Zarad, Zarade, Zaared, Zaarad

Zasha (Russian) A defender of the people
Zashah, Zosha, Zoshah, Zashiya, Zoshiya

Zayden (Arabic) Form of Zayd, meaning "To become greater, to grow"
Zaiden

Zeke (English) Form of Ezekiel, meaning "strengthened by God"
Zekiel, Zeek, Zeeke, Zeeq

Zene (African) A handsome man
Zeene, Zeen, Zein, Zeine

Zereen (Arabic) The golden one
Zereene, Zeryn, Zeryne, Zerein, Zereine, Zerrin, Zerren, Zerran

Zeroun (Armenian) One who is respected for his wisdom
Zeroune, Zeroon, Zeroone

Zion (Hebrew) From the citadel
Zionn, Zione, Zionne

Ziv (Hebrew) A radiant man
Zive, Ziiv, Zivi, Zivie, Zivee, Zivy, Zivey

Ziyad (Arabic) One who betters himself; growth
Ziad

Zlatan (Croatian) The golden son
Zlattan, Zlatane, Zlatann, Zlatain, Zlatayn, Zlaten, Zlaton, Zlatin

Zorion (Basque) Filled with happiness
Zorian, Zorien

Zoticus (Greek) Full of life
Zoticos, Zoticas

Zubair (Arabic) One who is pure
Zubaire, Zubayr, Zubayre, Zubar, Zubarr, Zubare, Zubaer

Zuberi (African) Having great strength
Zuberie, Zubery, Zuberey, Zuberee, Zubari, Zubarie, Zubary, Zubarey

Zubin (English) One with a toothy grin
Zubine, Zuben, Zuban, Zubun, Zubbin

Zuzen (Basque) One who is just and fair
Zuzenn, Zuzan, Zuzin

Zvonimir (Croatian) The sound of peace
Zvonimirr, Zvonimeer

My Favorite Names

My Favorite Names

My Favorite Names

My Favorite Names